The Maudsley Reader in Phenomenological Psychiatry

The Maudsley Reader in Phenomenological Psychiatry

Edited by

Matthew R. Broome
Associate Clinical Professor of Psychiatry, Division of Mental Health and Wellbeing,
Warwick Medical School, University of Warwick, Coventry; Honorary Consultant Psychiatrist in
Early Intervention, Coventry and Warwickshire Partnership Trust; and
Honorary Senior Lecturer, Department of Psychosis Studies, Institute of Psychiatry,
King's College London, UK

Robert Harland
Consultant in General Adult Psychiatry, Psychosis Clinical Academic Group, Maudsley Hospital,
South London and Maudsley NHS Foundation Trust, London, UK

Gareth S. Owen
Wellcome Trust Clinical Research Fellow, Institute of Psychiatry, King's College London, and
Honorary Consultant Psychiatrist, South London and Maudsley NHS Foundation Trust, London, UK

Argyris Stringaris
Senior Lecturer and Wellcome Trust Clinical Research Fellow, Institute of Psychiatry, King's College
London; and Honorary Consultant Child and Adolescent Psychiatrist, Mood Disorder Clinic,
Maudsley Hospital, South London and Maudsley NHS Foundation Trust, London, UK

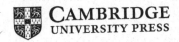
CAMBRIDGE
UNIVERSITY PRESS

CAMBRIDGE
UNIVERSITY PRESS

University Printing House, Cambridge CB2 8BS, United Kingdom

Cambridge University Press is part of the University of Cambridge.

It furthers the University's mission by disseminating knowledge in the pursuit of education, learning and research at the highest international levels of excellence.

www.cambridge.org
Information on this title: www.cambridge.org/9780521709279

© Matthew R. Broome, Robert Harland, Gareth S. Owen and Argyris Stringaris 2012

First published 2012
Reprinted 2014

A catalogue record for this publication is available from the British Library

Library of Congress Cataloguing in Publication data

The Maudsley reader in phenomenological psychiatry / edited by Matthew Broome . . . [et al.].
    p.   cm.
  Includes bibliographical references and index.
  ISBN 978-0-521-88275-0 (Hardback) – ISBN 978-0-521-70927-9 (Paperback)
    1. Phenomenological psychology.   2. Phenomenology.
3. Psychiatry.   I. Broome, Matthew R.
  BF204.5.M23 2012
  150.19′52–dc23

                                                          2012008944

ISBN 978-0-521-88275-0 Hardback
ISBN 978-0-521-70927-9 Paperback

Contents

v

Prologue

This book contains texts from the past. Interpreting the themes and using them to concern ourselves intelligently with the future is present, unfinished, business. We have assembled a range of texts which we read as young psychiatrists, training at the Maudsley Hospital over the last ten years. We had been attracted to the Maudsley, in part, because of the intellectual history of the institution: its blend of empirical inquiry and conceptual scholarship. When we arrived, we were confronted with patients: their unusual states of mind and their suffering, but also a space to think about them and interact as peers. We took to reading widely and meeting to discuss in an informal reading group. This group developed and over time became the Maudsley Philosophy Group which is now a registered charity, and of whose work this book is part. Inevitably, the writings we were drawn to concerned mental states and their structures. Quite quickly the arena of phenomenology and phenomenological psychiatry opened up and we spent a number of years grappling with the dispersed and difficult material that makes up that field.

Preparing this *Reader* was a complex undertaking in finding (in some cases translating), selecting and editing these texts. Equally challenging was understanding them, setting them in relation to one another and getting to the point where we could think critically about them. We think this project was worthwhile and is by no means complete or definitive; particularly in terms of providing a robust critique. Progress, we believe, will be aided by psychiatrists and other researchers not having to search around for the writings of the various authors as we had to. Therefore, this book seeks to provide the anthology we wished had been available to us when we started out as clinicians.

Approaching phenomenology

A lot has been written about what phenomenology is or what relationship it had (or didn't have) with psychiatry (Berrios 1993; Wiggins and Schwartz 1997). We deal more fully with what phenomenology is, philosophically, in the introduction to Part I and with the phenomenological approaches to psychiatry in the introduction to Part II. Insisting upon definitional precision is sometimes better avoided. Words may, instead, refer to family resemblances. We think the definition of phenomenology is an instance of this. One of the interesting outcomes for us in producing this book is that we have come to think that the differences in the approaches taken by the phenomenologists are as instructive as the similarities. Likewise, we have found tensions and differences within the phenomenological approaches to psychiatry which we think are as enlightening as any single mission statement the approach may have settled upon.

Jaspers' two-way divide

In the history of psychiatry, Karl Jaspers famously allowed psychopathology to be open to two methods: that which could be understood and that which could be explained. Understanding was to be achieved through empathy and explanation through the scientific study of causation. Both approaches are supported and exhaustively elucidated in sections of his *General Psychopathology* (Jaspers 1963). It is less well known that Jaspers also added a domain of *Existenz* – becoming in his later years an existential philosopher – recognizing that any modelling of the human being on understanding and explanation alone was limited. In his psychiatric writings *Existenz* remains largely empty of content and therefore of interest to a psychiatrist only in somewhat indirect terms. You might say that Jaspers' two-way divide has endured *because* of its limited phenomenological or existential ambitions. Alternatively, you might say he remains the quintessential phenomenological psychiatrist because he is both philosophical and anti-philosophical. He draws close to philosophy, only to pull back worried and exercised about the overextension of philosophy into a medical speciality.

The experience of becoming a psychiatrist

Today, the young psychiatrist coming into the field is often anxious, and shares this existential feeling with Jaspers. Leaving behind the objective certainties of medical pathology, for the models of psychiatry, renders much of the mechanical knowledge acquired in medical school less obviously applicable. He may bring a useful working knowledge of internal medicine and neurology, but he soon becomes aware that the neuroscientific hypotheses – that underpin psychiatry as part of medicine – lack predictive and discriminatory power. On this less stable footing, he is trained to elicit symptoms, acknowledge syndromes and formulate cases; drawing on and enriched by both explanation and understanding. While a formulation may lead to a professional consensus, the psychopathology most often cannot be confirmed, or disproved, on the basis of further investigations.

In this context, acute psychosis comes as a huge relief. The force of meeting a person suffering their first episode cannot be overstated. Hearing a textbook list of bizarre symptoms described spontaneously and unprompted by the unschooled patient convinces many of the medical reality of psychotic illness and ushers in the prospect of a biomedical basis for the whole subject; the belief that psychosis is a biomedical entity is a common consensus amongst many trainees (Harland et al. 2009).

However, the burgeoning experience of the young psychiatrist brings him into contact with distortions of human character and experience that undermine, or at least complicate, this picture. Trainees tend to develop their own model of psychopathology and find patient groups and forms of research or clinical practice that accord to it. Dementia, psychosis and the pervasive developmental disorders (such as autism) paradigmatically submit to a biomedical model, while mood, anxiety and personality disorders less so. In reality of course the field is more contentious with advocates for a variety of approaches existing in all areas.

But while there are divisions and professional debate, the broad conceptual distinctions that frame them often remain close to those found in Jaspers. Explanation – including (among others) heredity, the findings of cognitive neuroscience and environmental

risk – and understanding in terms of empathically mediated meaningful connections; both are still given more or less prominence in formulating diverse clinical material, allowing a pragmatic Jasperian truce to continue.[1]

Back to Jaspers: a three-way divide or the human being as a whole

But, as Jaspers could not help but admit, psychiatry must also be about the category of existence. A Heideggerian would surely draw our attention to the existential encounter in psychiatry between one human being, existing within a world, in relation to others and facing their own mortality, who is meeting a physician and asking for, or being forced to accept, their help. A good training in psychiatry accepts this fact, in that it is as much about developing resilience of emotional and intellectual character, as it is about applying a simple rubric to elicit symptoms and formulate a case. Put another way, the human being *as a whole* is confronted in psychiatry: whether it is with a 'biopsychosocial' (Engel 1977) formulation of a person, in honest deliberations about the nature of psychiatric diagnoses, or in the ethics of involuntary treatment. Here, given his under-theorized third category (of existence), Jaspers is less helpful, or at least is only one writer among a number who provide importantly different answers. If psychiatric confidence and expertise is found in a sound response to questions located in this area, then there is a need for trainees to be aware of the philosophers and psychiatrists who have tried to address them.

---

[1] Recent work by Bolton and Hill (2004) has suggested that cognitive clinical psychology overcomes the causality/meaning distinction. It is argued that cognitive algorithms carry meaning within a causal pathway that can be studied empirically. This approach draws on the philosophy of language found in the later Wittgenstein. It is controversial, but does not in substance undermine the established Jasperian consensus of admitting, in practice, both meanings and causes alongside one another. It might be cautioned that removing the historical opposition means the tensions between them are less likely to be scrutinised. Bolton expresses the view that unhelpful philosophical distinctions (derived from language use) are overcome, leaving *the science* to decide the value of a variety of previously distinctive fields (psychology and neuroscience for example) now seen as existing alongside one another. [Editors' note]

Psychiatry cannot flourish in an historical or cultural vacuum

This book focuses on one response: the phenomenological movement. Phenomenology is of particular interest to psychiatry because it is, in part, a philosophy of human experience. With different emphases the philosophers in this tradition wanted to distinguish a form of knowledge that could be considered primary – a 'return to the things in themselves'. Described differently as an analysis of the structures of subjectivity or the life-world (Husserl), an analysis of that being for whom being was itself a question (Heidegger) or a honing of a kind of asymbolic intuition (Scheler) it found unity in its suspicion of the claims of an unexamined scientific reduction, including forms of knowing that were not grounded primarily in human experience. That philosophy of this kind can be applied to psychiatry – a subject defined by characteristic pathological distortions of human experience – was apparent to many influential psychiatrists who lived contemporaneously with, and in many cases personally knew, these philosophers. Binswanger and Schneider, among many others, used philosophical phenomenology.

In psychiatry today, the descriptive phenomenology found in taxonomies such as ICD-10 (World Health Organization 1992) aims to be a-theoretical: here through the description of symptoms clustered into syndrome categories. There is, as in Jaspers, a clinical pragmatism and scientific value in this project. But every a-theoretical syndrome and symptom category contains within it, however hidden, a conceptual history. Although biological psychiatry, descriptive psychology, psychoanalysis and medical sociology lay important claims to that history, an equally important one is made by the phenomenological psychiatry introduced in this book. Furthermore a familiarity with this tradition, we maintain, enriches conceptual thinking and therefore (as above) strengthens professional resilience.

> *Our patient's whole relation to the outside world is affected in the most comprehensive way. The knowledge of all these disturbances is a fruitful field for the investigation of mental life, not only revealing many of its universal laws, but also giving a deep insight into the development of the human mind, both in the individual and in the [human] race. It also provides us with the proper scale for comprehending the numerous intellectual, moral, religious, and artistic currents and phenomena of our social life. But it is not these variously branching scientific relations to so many of the most important questions of human existence which make a knowledge of psychical disturbances indispensable to the physician; it is rather their extraordinary practical importance. [Psychiatric illness], even its mildest forms, involves the greatest suffering that physicians have to meet.*

This is not a 'phenomenological psychiatrist' speaking. It is Kraepelin (1913, p. 2). He believed passionately that psychiatry was a branch of medicine, and he was also alive to the specialness of that branch. Here the doctor meets, more directly than in the rest of medicine, disturbances in the human being as a whole and it is not appropriate for him to negotiate these disturbances in a cultural vacuum ill-equipped with cultural knowledge and without a capacity for critique.

How to read this book

We hope that the *Reader* will be of interest to clinicians primarily, but also to those in academia whether in neuroscience research, in social science research or in philosophy. As mentioned above, one of our goals in assembling the texts in a book was to allow the reader to access classical writings in phenomenological psychopathology.

We hope the book can serve as a teaching resource. The editors are all part of institutions that offer postgraduate courses in philosophy and psychiatry, and typically these courses do include sessions on phenomenology. Thus, this book can provide readings ready to hand for both tutors and students. We have used the material for teaching with very positive feedback.

We would also suggest that this book may serve as a helpful companion or guide when approaching much of the contemporary work done in phenomenology and psychiatry.[1] We think being able to refer to Minkowski, Heidegger or Schneider easily, for example, when reading the recent literature would help the contemporary work become more accessible and its study yield greater benefits.

The book is not meant to be comprehensive and we are aware that arguments can be fielded for the inclusion of a certain text or the exclusion of one we have included. Our selection can only have been partial and based on what we ourselves have found useful and what resonates with recently published work in phenomenological psychiatry. As such, the book does not offer a central narrative and although we have imposed a structure, there is no clear progression through the texts. We would suggest that it is read in the order of greatest interest, to be picked up and reviewed when a clinical or conceptual issue arises. It is a compendium of ideas and reflections relevant to psychiatry, not a treatise or a practical handbook.

Our hope is that this book will help clinicians realize the depth and scope of human experience and bear it in mind when they interview and try to understand others.

---

[1] There has been a burgeoning of interest and research in phenomenology and psychiatry and medicine: contemporary writers include Havi Carel, John Cutting, Thomas Fuchs, Shaun Gallagher, Nassir Ghaemi, Gerrit Glas, Eric Matthews, Iain McGilchrist, Aaron Mishara,

Paul Mullen, Katherine Morris, Louis Sass, Michael Schwartz, Matthew Ratcliffe, Josef Parnas, Giovanni Stanghellini, Phil Thomas, Osborne Wiggins and Dan Zahavi.

Acknowledgements

This project has been made possible by donors to the Maudsley Philosophy Group Trust. We thank them for supporting a philosophical psychiatry. We thank our editors at Cambridge University Press for their patience on a project that has taken five years and has been carried out in the spare moments of four psychiatrists working across clinical and research jobs.

Many people have been of assistance in the preparation of this book. In particular, we would like to thank the psychiatrist John Cutting for his inspiration and generosity and the library at the Institute of Psychiatry, London for holding on to such a rich variety of texts in phenomenological psychiatry from the interwar and postwar years. For help with philosophical questions we would like to thank Matthew Ratcliffe, Keith Ansell-Pearson and Wayne Martin. The editors would like to thank the Heidegger family for their kindness in allowing us to extract from Martin Heidegger's lectures. For help with translations we would like to thank Nikola Kern and Aaron Mishara. For bibliographic assistance we would like to thank Adam Thomas and Martin Guha. Alex Linklater gave us some useful editorial feedback for which we are grateful. Professor Sir Robin Murray has supported the Maudsley Philosophy Group since its inception and that helped this project find the light of day.

The editors would like to thank their families for their love and support during the preparation of the book.

Endorsements

The Maudsley Reader in Phenomenological Psychiatry is a unique, and most welcome, addition to the resources available to students of philosophy and psychiatry alike. The editors have done a judicious job in identifying and excerpting key writings pertaining to the intellectual background of phenomenology, the development of essential phenomenological themes and concepts, and canonical applications of those concepts to the fields of psychology and psychiatry. Clear, critical chapter introductions and brief editorial commentaries on texts dealing with psychiatric disorders reliably orient the reader without overwhelming the writings themselves. Since the material gathered here stems from widely dispersed and often not readily available sources, *The Maudsley Reader* should become the standard reference work in this area. It is certainly a splendid basis from which to set out in exploring the powerful insights that a phenomenological perspective can contribute to psychiatry today.

Steven Crowell, Joseph and Joanna Nazro Mullen
Professor of Philosophy, Rice University

In its origins modern psychiatry was closely connected to phenomenology – the school of philosophy which begins from the study of consciousness, and which distinguishes human understanding from scientific explanation. Some of the most subtle accounts of psychological phenomena have been given by members of this school – Max Scheler's essays on sympathy, shame and resentment, for example, or the accounts of self-consciousness in Jaspers and Heidegger. Here, gathered together in one volume, are texts from the phenomenological tradition that are essential reading for students and practitioners of psychiatry. From these essays the reader will learn of methods and forms of understanding that should have a place in the thinking of all practitioners, and also of anyone who wants to know how self-consciousness really works.

Roger Scruton
Visiting Professor, University of Oxford and
University of St Andrews

This remarkable book covers a wide range of authors and topics in philosophical phenomenology and phenomenological psychiatry, from Brentano to Merleau-Ponty, from Jaspers to Blankenburg, from obsessions to schizophrenia.

Indispensable for young clinicians who, coming into the field, want to leave behind the presumed objective certainties of the biomedical model and are interested in the life-worlds real patients live in.

Giovanni Stanghellini
Professor of Dynamic Psychology and Psychopathology,
G. d'Annunzio University, Chieti, Italy

Careful observation of individual human beings, in all their complex diversity and in all the complex diversity of the illnesses that afflict them, is the heart and soul of medicine and of psychiatry. This fine book tethers modern psychiatry to its intellectual and philosophical roots, providing access to texts from the 19th and 20th centuries that have previously been difficult to access, especially in a single volume. Great credit goes to the Maudsley group for making these readings available to 21st century readers. I wish every psychiatrist would buy it, read it, and (most importantly) apply its teachings in contemporary practice.

Nancy Andreasen, Andrew H. Woods
Chair of Psychiatry and Director of the
Neuroimaging Research Center and the Mental
Health Clinical Research Center,
The University of Iowa Carver College of Medicine

The Maudsley Hospital is much to be admired for its blend of clinical and conceptual research out of which this reader arose. It is likely to be uniquely useful to those interested in the interface between philosophy and psychiatry. It brings together texts from both philosophers and clinicians which are otherwise difficult to access; many are newly translated. The editors have done excellent work in selecting, explaining and abbreviating the basic philosophical texts, including those of Jaspers and Heidegger, who are notoriously long-winded and intentially obscure authors. I found it absorbing and illuminating.

Baroness Mary Warnock House of Lords

People get sad, angry, euphoric, delusional – and sometimes they are sick. How can we tell whether someone has a disease or not? How can these experiences be understood as part of psychiatric diagnoses? When are they simply human experiences? These important questions – which are the basis of phenomenology – are infrequently asked in a psychiatry of checklists and drugs for symptoms. *The Maudsley Reader* provides classic historical sources that can begin the process of asking these questions again, and beginning to answer them.

Nassir Ghaemi
Mood Disorders Program, Department of Psychiatry, Tufts Medical Center, United States and Tufts University School of Medicine, Boston, MA, USA

This reader is a delight. The collective who produced the book have gone beyond compiling texts to produce a challenge to contemporary psychiatry and psychology. For many clinicians, the best place to begin reading may be with Chapter 16 on schizophrenia then move to the theoretical basis. It is traditional in a book boost to recommend all one's fellow professionals to buy it and read it. In this instance it is my heartfelt prayer. If only...

Paul E. Mullen
Department of Psychological Medicine, Monash University and Victorian Institute of Forensic Mental Health, Victoria, Australia

Introduction

This chapter gives a selection of purely philosophical texts which influenced the phenomenological approach to psychiatry. They make up a tradition which has been called the 'phenomenological movement' in European thought (Spiegelberg 1969; Spiegelberg 1972). Before presenting these individual philosophers we offer a brief account of their unifying features. This is treacherous territory because the question 'What is phenomenology?' has been highly resistant to one answer. Furthermore, it is a question for philosophers and historians of ideas and we write here as psychiatrists. With these two important cautions in mind some points can be made. Firstly, phenomenology is not synonymous with the notion of subjectivity ordinarily understood. It is not simply the detailed description of mental events (Ratcliffe 2009). Secondly, phenomenology is not a doctrine nor primarily is it a school. Indeed, rather like the conceptual analysis of Moore and Russell, it is a method of inquiry first and foremost, despite real disagreements existing within the phenomenological movement as to the precise nature of that method (Spiegelberg 1969). As such, it can be applied to different areas of concern and is by no means limited to mental phenomena. 'Phenomenon' for Husserl and others is simply 'that which appears'. Hence, a phenomenological psychiatry is by no means confined to studying abnormal mental phenomena, but can include the phenomenon of the clinical consultation, of inpatient services, the science of psychiatry, how mental illness manifests to wider society in the media, amongst other themes. Many of these themes have yet to be addressed systematically by phenomenological psychiatry.

Simon Glendinning (Glendinning 2007) offers some ideas about phenomenology's relationship to philosophy and about the nature of phenomenological inquiry itself. He tries to identify some shared features of philosophers typically recognized as 'phenomenologists'.

- Phenomenology is a way of doing philosophy, and in particular, has a role to play in developing a critique of the default natural scientific outlook, the 'natural attitude'.
- Phenomenology eschews any constructive theoretical work: phenomenology does not seek to advances theses or defend positions.
- Phenomenology emphasizes description or elucidation rather than explanation or analysis. Phenomenology is an effort to make explicit that which was implicit, to become reflectively aware of that which was already evident.
- Phenomenology works to avoid 'blinkers' and prejudice: perhaps the strongest appeal to empirically minded psychiatrists lies in this idea of avoiding theoretical assumptions and distortions. Phenomenology urges us to return to what is given as given, as phenomena.
- Phenomenology eschews a 'narrow argument' style of persuasion but rather seeks that the reader or listener comes reflectively to terms with something pre-reflectively before his or her eyes. Rather than taking the reader through a series of argumentative steps, phenomenology seeks to show the world in a clear and explicit way: hence, being 'convinced' is more akin to 'seeing' things in a certain way and hence obviously true, rather than being persuaded of the truths of certain propositions.

We now offer some very brief introductions to individual philosophers, either phenomenologists themselves or others who influenced the movement, together with sample texts.

Chapter

2

Franz Brentano (1838–1917)

Editors' introduction

Brentano was an important impetus to both Husserl and Jaspers. Further, his work continues to be of crucial importance to philosophy of mind and cognitive science through his notion of intentionality as a defining feature of the mental (Smith 1994). The other crucial notion from Brentano of importance for phenomenological psychiatry is that of descriptive psychology. We will discuss both these concepts briefly; selections from his writings where he presents these notions follow.

For Brentano, psychology is an immature science. He believes that psychology waits on advances from physiology to mature. Hence, Brentano makes a distinction between 'genetic' or 'explanatory' psychology and 'descriptive' psychology. The explanatory psychology is based on physics and physiology and answers causal questions whereas descriptive psychology is relatively freer from this dependence on basic science. Rather, for Brentano, descriptive psychology is akin to philosophy of mind and philosophical psychology (Mulligan 2004). However, he still thinks that in some sense descriptive psychology is empirical, and refers to it as such, due to a belief that it is based on 'inner' perception. Mulligan helpfully describes Brentano's conception of descriptive psychology thus:

> ... conceptual truths about and analyses of psychological phenomena in which classifications, the identification of the fundamental types of psychological phenomena, and claims about relations of necessary co-existence are prominent (p. 67)
>
> (Mulligan 2004).

Descriptive psychology is prior to explanatory psychology: one needs to have a clear account of the nature of the mental phenomenon to be investigated prior to causal and explanatory claims being made. Whereas descriptive psychology yields exact and exceptionless truths, explanatory psychology will reveal contingent causal mechanism that could logically be different from mental phenomenon yet still underpin them.

The notion of intentionality has widely been taken up as a mark of the mental, the defining characteristic of mental states. For something to be intentional is to say that it intends or is about something. Thus intentionality is the aboutness of thought (Jacquette 2004). Further, there are no mental acts without a presentation, without an intended object. Intentionality allows Brentano to adopt a dualism based upon this idea of content: physical phenomena lack intentionality, whereas intentionality is the defining characteristic of mental phenomena. It is worth stressing, however, that this notion of 'aboutness' and intentionality doesn't necessarily imply the idea of the mind somehow stretching out of the body toward the world, but rather suggests the mind taking on properties of the intended object. Part of the reason for this is Brentano's indebtedness to Aristotle. For Aristotle, the soul takes in sensory and intelligible forms and thus, 'Sensing and thinking, for a Brentanian Aristotelian is, to repeat, a form of taking in' (Smith 1994, p. 41), a taking in of the form, but not the matter. So intentionality is not so much about the mind being directed to external objects, but rather, such aboutness is towards objects that are immanently within the mind, having been taken up by the senses.

Brentano, F. (1888–9), 'The concept of descriptive psychology'

From (1983/1995) *Descriptive Psychology*. Edited and translated by Benito Müller. London: Routledge: 137–8. Originally a lecture given in 1888–9.

1. By this I understand the analysing description of our phenomena.
2. By phenomena, however, [I understand] that which is perceived by us, in fact, what is perceived by us in the strict sense of the word.
3. This, for example, is not the case for the external world.

4. To be a phenomenon, something must exist in itself [*in sich sein*]. It is wrong to set phenomena in opposition to what exists in itself [*an sich Seiendes*].

5. Something can be a phenomenon, however, without being a thing in itself, such as, for example, what is presented as such [*das Vorgestellte als solches*], or what is desired as such.

6. One is telling the truth if one says the phenomena are objects of inner perception, even though the term 'inner' is actually superfluous. All phenomena are to be called inner because they all belong to one reality, be it as constituents or as correlates.

7. By calling the description of phenomena descriptive psychology one particularly emphasizes the contemplation of psychical realities. Genetic psychology is then added to it as the second part of psychology.

8. Physiology has to intervene forcefully in the latter, whereas descriptive psychology is relatively independent of it.

9. Descriptive psychology is the prior part (of psychology). The relationship between it and genetic psychology is similar to the one between anatomy and physiology.

10. *The value of descriptive psychology.*

   (a) It is the foundation of genetic psychology.
   (b) It has a value in itself because of the dignity of the psychical domain.

Brentano, F. (1874), 'The distinction between mental and physical phenomena'

From (1995) *Psychology from an Empirical Standpoint*. Edited by Oscar Kraus and Linda L. McAlister, translated by Antos C. Rancurello, D. B. Terrell and Linda L. McAlister. London, Routledge: 77–100. Originally published in 1874.

All the data of our consciousness are divided into two great classes – the class of physical and the class of mental phenomena ...

Our aim is to clarify the meaning of the two terms "*physical phenomenon*" and "*mental phenomenon*," removing all misunderstanding and confusion concerning them. And it does not matter to us what means we use, as long as they really serve to clarify these terms.

Every idea or presentation which we acquire either through sense perceptions or imagination is an example of a mental phenomenon. By presentation I do not mean that which is presented, but rather the act of presentation. Thus, hearing a sound, seeing a colored object, feeling warmth or cold, as well as similar states of imagination are examples of what I mean by this term. I also mean by it the thinking of a general concept, provided such a thing actually does occur. Furthermore, every judgement, every recollection, every expectation, every inference, every conviction or opinion, every doubt, is a mental phenomenon. Also to be included under this term is every emotion: joy, sorrow, fear, hope, courage, despair, anger, love, hate, desire, act of will, intention, astonishment, admiration, contempt, etc.

*****

Every mental phenomenon is characterized by what the Scholastics of the Middle Ages called the intentional (or mental) inexistence of an object, and what we might call, though not wholly unambiguously, reference to a content, direction toward an object (which is not to be understood here as meaning a thing), or immanent objectivity. Every mental phenomenon includes something as object within itself, although they do not all do so in the same way. In presentation something is presented, in judgement something is affirmed or denied, in love loved, in hate hated, in desire desired and so on.

This intentional in-existence is characteristic exclusively of mental phenomena. No physical phenomenon exhibits anything like it. We can, therefore, define mental phenomena by saying that they are those phenomena which contain an object intentionally within themselves.

*****

Another characteristic which all mental phenomena have in common is the fact that they are only perceived in inner consciousness, while in the case of physical phenomena only external perception is possible. ... However, besides the fact that it has a special object, inner perception possesses another distinguishing characteristic: its immediate, infallible self-evidence. Of all the types of knowledge of the objects of experience, inner perception alone possesses this characteristic. Consequently, when we say that mental phenomena are those which are apprehended by means of inner perception, we say that their perception is immediately evident.

*****

Let us, in conclusion, summarize the results of the discussion about the difference between mental and physical phenomena. First of all, we illustrated the specific nature of the two classes by means of *examples*. We then defined mental phenomena as *presentations* or as phenomena which are based *upon presentations*; all the other phenomena being physical phenomena. Next we spoke of *extension*, which psychologists have asserted to be the specific characteristic of all physical phenomena, while all mental phenomena are supposed to be unextended. This assertion, however, ran into contradictions which can only be clarified by later investigations. All that can be determined now is that all mental phenomena really appear to be unextended. Further we found that the *intentional in-existence*, the reference to something as an object, is a distinguishing characteristic of all mental phenomena. No physical phenomena are the exclusive *object of inner perception*; they alone, therefore, are perceived with immediate evidence. Indeed, in the strict sense of the word, they alone are perceived. On this basis we proceeded to define them as the only phenomena which possess *actual existence* in addition to intentional existence. Finally, we emphasized as a distinguishing characteristic the fact that the mental phenomena which we perceive, in spite of all their multiplicity, *always* appear to us *as a unity*, while physical phenomena, which we perceive at the same time, do not all appear in the same way as parts of one single phenomenon.

That feature which best characterizes mental phenomena is undoubtedly their intentional in-existence. By means of this and the other characteristics listed above, we may now consider mental phenomena to have been clearly differentiated from physical phenomena.

Our explanations of mental and physical phenomena cannot fail to place our earlier definitions of psychology and natural science in a clearer light. . . .

We must consider only mental phenomena in the sense of real states as the proper object of psychology. And it is in reference only to these phenomena that we say that psychology is the science of mental phenomena.

Chapter 3

Wilhelm Dilthey (1833–1911)

Editors' introduction

Dilthey's influence on phenomenological psychiatry is crucial and is most clearly illustrated by Jaspers' adoption of *Verstehen* or 'interpretative understanding' (Outhwaite 1986; Rickman 1987). Although understanding another is clearly a complex activity, for the German hermeneutic tradition there is nothing particularly mystical or technical about the concept of *Verstehen*: it is simply the everyday understanding of another, whether a real individual or a fictional or historical figure, which we all engage in. In contemporary philosophical terminology this is often termed folk psychology.

Dilthey's hermeneutic project was similar to that of the neo-Kantians (Broome 2008). He was interested in the 'historical sciences' and his Kantian question was the reflection on the possibility of sciences that took the human mind as their object of study (Outhwaite 1986). Dilthey's work on *verstehende Psychologie* is a crucial part of this wider concern. 'Understanding', as Outhwaite puts it (p. 27) is on this conception, experiencing another person's 'thoughts and emotions from the inside by "putting oneself in their shoes" (*sich hineinversetzten*) and reliving their experiences (*nacherleben*)' (Outhwaite 1986). For Dilthey, such an approach should work in parallel with causal understanding. Further, *Verstehen* should never be complete, incapable of error, and explicitly relies on imagination. Its goal is to attempt to understand the individual and works by analogy (Makkreel 1998).

Dilthey, W. (1894), 'Ideas about a descriptive and analytical psychology'

From (1976) *Dilthey: Selected Writings*. Edited by H. P. Rickman. Cambridge University Press: 88–97. Originally published in 1894.

The task of laying a psychological foundation for the human studies

Explanatory psychology, which at present absorbs such a large measure of work and interest, establishes a causal nexus which claims to explain all mental phenomena. It tries to explain the constitution of the mental world according to its constituents, forces and laws, in the same way as physics and chemistry explain the physical world.... The difference between explanatory and descriptive science assumed here, corresponds to ordinary usage. By an explanatory science we understand the subsumption of a range of phenomena under a causal nexus by means of a limited number of unambiguously defined elements (i.e. constituents of the nexus). This concept describes an ideal science which has been shaped particularly by the development of atomic physics. So explanatory psychology tries to subsume mental phenomena under a causal nexus by means of a limited number of unambiguously defined elements. This is an extraordinarily bold idea containing the possibility of an immeasurable development of the human studies into a strict system of causal knowledge corresponding to that of the physical sciences. Every psychology wants to make the causal relationships of mental life conscious but the distinguishing mark of explanatory psychology is that it is convinced that it can produce a complete and transparent knowledge of mental phenomena from a limited number of unambiguously defined elements. It would be even more precisely characterized by the name constructive psychology.

*****

[T]he human studies must work towards more definite procedures and principles within their own sphere by trying them out on their own subject-matter, just as the physical sciences have done. We do not show ourselves genuine disciples of the great scientific thinkers simply by transferring their methods to our sphere; we must adjust our knowledge to the nature of our subject-matter and thus treat it as the scientists treated theirs. We conquer nature by submitting to it. The human studies differ from the sciences because the latter deal with facts which present themselves to consciousness as external and separate phenomena, while the former deal with the living connections of reality experienced in the mind. It follows that the sciences arrive at connections within nature through inferences by means of a combination of hypotheses while the human sciences are based on directly given mental connections. We explain nature but we understand mental life. Inner experience grasps the processes by which we accomplish something as well as the combination of individual functions of mental life into a whole. The experience of the whole context comes first; only later do we distinguish its individual parts. This means that the methods of studying mental life, history and society differ greatly from those used to acquire knowledge of nature.

Descriptive and analytical psychology

If we try to gain knowledge of the comprehensive and uniform pattern of mental life we shall see if a descriptive psychology can be developed. Psychological analysis has certainly established many individual connections in our mental life. We can follow the processes which lead from an outer impression to the development of a perceptual image; we can pursue its transformation into a memory; we can describe the formation of fantasies and concepts. We can also describe motive, choice and purposive action. But all these particular patterns must be co-ordinated into a general pattern of mental life. The question is can we pave the way for this?

The decisive fact for the study of mental structure is that *the transitions from one state to another, the effect of one on another are part of inner experience. We experience this structure.* We understand human life, history and all the hidden depths of the human mind because we experience these transitions and effects and so become aware of this structure which embraces all passions, sufferings and human destinies. Who has not experienced how images thrusting themselves on the imagination suddenly arouse strong desire which, confronted with great difficulties, urges us towards an act of will? In these and other concrete connections we become aware of particular transitions and effects; these inner experiences recur and one connection or another is repeated until the whole structure becomes secure, empirical, knowledge in our inner consciousness. It is not only the major parts of this structure which have an inner connection in our experience, we can become aware of such relationships within the parts themselves. The process of mental life in all its forms, from the lowest to the highest, is from the beginning a unified whole. Mental life does not arise from parts growing together; it is not compounded of elementary units; it does not result from interacting particles of sensation or feeling; it is always an encompassing unity. Mental functions have been differentiated in it but they remain tied to their context. This has reached its highest form of development in the unity of consciousness and the unity of the person and completely distinguishes mental life from the whole physical world. Knowledge of this context of life makes the new theory that mental processes are single, unconnected representations of a pattern of physical events, completely unacceptable.

Max Weber (1864–1920)

Editors' introduction

Jaspers acknowledges a great debt to the sociologist Max Weber, both as a friend but also as the means by which he was introduced to Husserl and Heidegger (Jaspers 1981). Intellectually, Weber's conception of 'ideal types' has had a profound influence in phenomenological psychiatry (Schwartz and Wiggins 1987; Ghaemi 2009), both in it being used to try to clarify what is thought of as a 'typical' presentation or symptom, but perhaps more strongly, used as an equivalent term as 'essence' when talking about the defining features of a given psychopathology (Broome 2006). However, although psychiatrists may think in terms of prototypical features, it would be mistaken to conflate this with Husserl's concept of essence, as discussed below.

On most readings, Weber's concept of ideal type is a construct one uses to interrogate the social world (i.e. phenomena involving meaning and value) ('The construction of abstract ideal-types recommends itself not as an end but as a means' (p. 90) (Weber 1904/ 2004)). Husserlian essences, however, are the result of performing the eidetic reduction (see below, pp. 15–16, 24–35). Thus, one measures empirical reality using the ideal type and compares the ideal type to empirical reality but this is done interpretatively rather than statistically. Husserlian essences, however, are obtained by bracketing away empirical reality. In other ways too, Weber's notion of ideal types differs from Husserl's notion of essence: in particular, Weber suggested that ideal types are variable for any question, depending upon the researcher's question (Weber 1904/2004, p. 91; Parkin 2002), whereas essence is necessary and a priori. Further, ideal types do not exist in reality ('In its conceptual purity, this mental construct (*Gedankenbild*) cannot be found anywhere in reality. It is a utopia.' (Weber 1904/2004, p. 90)). As such, we should not, for Weber, expect anything we encounter to match the ideal type perfectly.

Burger offers a useful definition of Weber's notoriously hard to pin down idea (Burger 1976, p. 134):

> Ideal types are statements of general form asserting the existence of certain constellations of elements which are empirically only approximated by the instances of the class of phenomena to which each type refers.

Thus, ideal types vary, their structure is determined by the investigators' concerns and the problems studied, and are never fully instantiated in empirical reality. Hence, the ideal type may serve as an extreme end of continuum that actual existent cases only approximate towards (the clearest, most distinct example of delusion we use to recognize other delusions but never expect to meet in reality, for example). The subject matter of psychiatry, given its proximity to the phenomena of meaning, intentions, values and interpretations, and given its pragmatic nature, may find the notion of 'ideal types' more germane than that of essences as developed by Husserl initially in the fields of mathematics, logic, grammar and geometry.

Weber, M. (1904), '"Objectivity" in social science and social policy'

From (2004) *The Methodology of the Social Sciences.* Translated by Edward A. Shils and Henry A. Finch. Jaipur, India: ABD Publishers: 49–112. Originally published by Free Press in 1949.

We have in abstract economic theory an illustration of those synthetic constructs which have been designated as "*ideas*" of historical phenomena. It offers us an ideal picture of events on the commodity-market under conditions of a society organized on the principles of an exchange economy, free competition and rigorously rational conduct. This conceptual pattern brings together certain relationships and events of historical life into a complex, which is conceived as an internally consistent system. Substantively, this construct in itself is like a *utopia* which has been arrived at by the analytical accentuation of certain elements of reality. Its relationship to the empirical data consists solely in the fact that where market-conditioned relationships of the type referred to by the abstract construct are discovered or suspected to exist in reality to some extent, we can make the *characteristic* features of this relationship pragmatically *clear* and *understandable* by reference to an *ideal-type*. This procedure can be indispensable for heuristic as well as expository purposes. The ideal typical concept will help to develop our skill in imputation in *research*: it is no "hypothesis" but it offers guidance to the construction of hypotheses. It is not a *description* of reality but it aims to give unambiguous means of expression to such a description. It is thus the "idea" of the *historically* given modern society, based on an exchange economy, which is developed for us by quite the same logical principles as are used in constructing the idea of the medieval "city economy" as a "genetic" concept. When we do this, we construct the concept "city economy" not as an average of the economic structures actually existing in all the cities observed but as an *ideal-type*. An ideal type is formed by the one-sided *accentuation* of one or more points of view and by the synthesis of a great many diffuse, discrete, more or less present and occasionally absent *concrete individual* phenomena, which are arranged according to those one-sidedly emphasized viewpoints into a unified *analytical* construct [*Gedankenbild*]. In its conceptual purity, this mental construct [*Gedankenbild*] cannot be found empirically anywhere in reality. It is a *utopia*.

*****

When a genetic definition of the content of the concept is sought, there remains only the ideal-type in the sense explained above. It is a conceptual construct [*Gedankenbild*] which is neither historical reality nor even the "true" reality. It is even less fitted to serve as a schema under which a real situation or action is to be subsumed as one *instance*. It has the significance of a purely ideal *limiting* concept with which the real situation or action is *compared* and surveyed for the explication of certain of its significant components. Such concepts are constructs in terms of which we formulate relationships by the application of the category of objective possibility. By means of this category, the adequacy of our imagination, oriented and disciplined by reality, is *judged*.

In this function especially, the ideal-type is an attempt to analyze historically unique configurations or their individual components by means of genetic concepts. Let us take for instance the concepts "church" and "sect." They may be broken down purely classificatorily into complexes of characteristics whereby not only the distinction between them but also the content of the concept must constantly remain fluid. If however I wish to formulate the concept of "sect" genetically, e.g., with reference to certain important cultural significances which the "sectarian spirit" has had for modern culture, certain characteristics of both become *essential* because they stand in an adequate causal relationship to those influences. However, the concepts thereupon become ideal-typical in the sense that they appear in full conceptual *integrity* either not at all or only in individual instances. Here as elsewhere every concept which is not purely classificatory diverges from reality. But the discursive nature of our knowledge, i.e., the fact that we comprehend reality only through a chain of intellectual modifications postulates such a conceptual short-hand. Our imagination can often dispense with explicit conceptual formulations as a means of *investigation*. But as regards exposition, formulations in the sphere of cultural analysis is in many cases absolutely necessary. Whoever disregards it entirely must confine himself to the formal aspect of cultural phenomena, e.g., to legal history. The universe of legal norms is naturally clearly definable and is valid (in the *legal* sense!) for historical reality. But social science in our sense is concerned with practical *significance*. This significance however can very often be brought unambiguously to mind only by relating the empirical data to an ideal limiting case.

Henri Bergson (1859–1941)

Editors' introduction

Bergson is not commonly acknowledged as an influence on phenomenological psychiatry, and perhaps this state of affairs is similar to his rather under-acknowledged and diffuse influence on philosophy more generally (Matthews 1996; Gutting 2001; Mullarkey 2010). For our purposes, Bergson's work was a direct influence upon both Scheler and the French psychiatrist Minkowski. In particular, it was Bergson's early work, translated as *Time and Free Will*, that impacted upon psychopathology. Here, Bergson offers a sustained critique of how mental life is viewed, and specifically how the tools and ways of thinking about the physical, external, world have been imported into the discourse of how we think about our mental life. For Bergson, using the language of mechanism in the domain of the living is, as it were, a category mistake (Guerlac 2006). Newtonian physics presents a world of quantity, of measurement and mathematization, and importantly for Bergson, the idea of reversibility. Equations can be reformulated in the opposite direction, reversed, yet, we are unable to draw this parallel with mental life and specifically for Bergson, time, and thinking in time, is irreversible (Guerlac 2006). The quantitative differences in the physical world, captured in measurement, are, Bergson argues, not present in mental life where the differences that occur are those of quality. The dominant psychology of Bergson's day led to the danger of thinking of these distinct qualities as quantitative differences in intensity and hence, trying to measure them (Guerlac 2006), viewing them as differences in degree rather than kind. From these concerns about the science of psychology Bergson's important work uses these insights to discuss the living, the nature of consciousness and, importantly, time and free will. Bergson situates his own work as a response to Kant: praising Kant for his Newtonianism and demonstrating the importance of external apperception in the experience of space, but argues against Kant and Kantians employing these insights in thinking about inner life, and also in their seeming conflation of space with the radical alterity that is time. Unlike space, time is not a homogenous mileu (Guerlac 2006).

Bergson, H. (1910), Selections from *Time and Free Will: An Essay on the Immediate Data of Consciousness*

From (2008) *Time and Free Will: An Essay on the Immediate Data of Consciousness.* Translated by S. L. Pogson. New York: Cosimo: 10–155. Originally published in 1910.

Neither inner joy nor passion is an isolated inner state which at first occupies the corner of the soul and gradually spreads. At its lowest level it is very like a turning of our states of consciousness towards the future. Then, as if their weight were diminished by this attraction, our ideas and sensations succeed one another with greater rapidity; our movements no longer cost us the same effort. Finally, in cases of extreme joy, our perceptions and memories become tinged with an indefinable quality, as with a kind of heat or light, so novel that now and then, as we stare at our own self, we wonder how it can really exist. Thus there are several characteristic forms of purely inward joy, all of which are successive stages corresponding to qualitative alterations in the whole of our psychic states. But the number of states which are concerned with each of these alterations is more or less considerable, and, without explicitly counting them, we know very well whether, for example, our joy pervades all the impressions which we receive in the course of the day or whether any escape from its influence. We thus set up points of division in the interval which separate two successive forms of joy, and this gradual transition from one to the other makes them appear in their turn as different intensities of one and the same feeling, which is thus supposed to change in magnitude.

*****

If, in order to count states of consciousness, we have to represent them symbolically in space, is it not likely that this symbolic representation will alter the normal conditions of inner perception? Let us recall what we said a short time ago about the intensity of certain psychic states. Representative sensation, looked at in itself, is pure quality; but, seen through the medium of extensity, this quality becomes in a certain sense quantity, and is called intensity. In the same way, our projection of our psychic states into space in order to form a discrete multiplicity is likely to influence these states themselves and to give them in a reflective consciousness a new form, which immediate perception did not attribute to them. Now, let us notice that when we speak of *time*, we generally think of a homogeneous medium in which our conscious states are ranged alongside one another as in space, so as to form a discrete multiplicity. Would not time, thus understood, be to the multiplicity of our psychic states what intensity is to certain of them, – a sign, a symbol, absolutely distinct from true duration? Let us ask consciousness to isolate itself from the external world, and, by a vigorous effort of abstraction, to become itself again. We shall then put this question to it: does the multiplicity of our conscious states bear the slightest resemblance to the multiplicity of the units of a number? Has true duration anything to do with space?

*****

In truth, it is not a wish to meet the requirements of positive science, but rather a psychological mistake which has caused this abstract principle of mechanics to be set up as a universal law. As we are not accustomed to observe ourselves directly, but perceive ourselves through forms borrowed from an external world, we are led to believe that real duration, the duration lived by consciousness, is the same as the duration which glides over the inert atoms without penetrating and altering them. Hence it is that we do not see any absurdity in putting things back in their place after a lapse of time, in supposing the same motives acting afresh on the same persons, and in concluding that these causes would again produce the same effect. ... For the present let us simply show that, if once we enter upon this path, we are of course led to set up the principle of the conservation of energy as a universal law. For we have thereby got rid of just that difference between the outer and the inner world which a close examination shows to be the main one: we have identified true duration with apparent duration. ... Thus, while we ought only to say (if we kept aloof from all presuppositions concerning free will) that the law of the conservation of energy governs physical phenomena and *may*, one day, be extended to all phenomena if psychological facts also prove favourable to it, we go far beyond this, and, under the influence of a metaphysical prepossession, we lay down the principle of the conservation of energy as a law which *should* govern all phenomena whatever, or must be supposed to do so until psychological facts have actually spoken against it. Science, properly so called, has therefore nothing to do with all this. We are simply confronted with a confusion between concrete duration and abstract time, two very different things.

Edmund Husserl (1859–1938)

6

Editors' introduction

Commentators differ on viewing Husserl as being a systematic, coherent, philosopher building on work from 1900 until his death to being a philosopher with distinct 'phases' in his philosophy. For example, Smith (Smith 2007) refers to Husserl as a 'holographic writer', where each piece of writing focuses on a specific theme, yet refers to his wider philosophical project, largely set out in his *Logical Investigations* of 1901. Conversely, Moran, using Husserl's own assistant's, Fink's, categorization suggests three phases: psychologism (1887–1901), descriptive phenomenology (1901–1913) and transcendental phenomenology (1913–1938) with a shift in the latter two phases from a more Humean/Brentanian view of the self and ego to one more informed by Cartesian and Kantian concepts (Moran 2000). The final phase is also increasingly concerned with issues such as embodiment and being with others.

As discussed when offering a preliminary definition of phenomenology, Husserl sees his method as a descriptive enterprise rather than one that offers theory construction (Crowell 2009). As such, its goal is clarification rather than explanation. Further, it is described as 'eidetic': that is, it is not an enquiry into finding out all the facts about a particular entity, but rather, it focuses on its essence and as such what properties make it a thing of this certain kind rather than another (Crowell 2009). Lastly, Crowell suggests that Husserlian phenomenology is marked by being 'reflective': unlike the natural sciences, it is not concerned directly with entities but rather our experience of entities. Hence, we should not abstract from our experience when attempting to clarify the essential conditions of *X*, but rather, concern ourselves as to how *X* is given in experience.

Naturalism and the natural attitude

Naturalism as a target for Husserl, argues that psychology and mental life can be understood wholly by reference to rigid laws. For Husserl the normativity of mental life, of intentional states, cannot be explained by causal laws alone and reason is required to allow experiences, beliefs, and judgements to interrelate with one another in a rational manner (Crowell 2009). As Crowell puts it:

> Phenomenology thus becomes the study of how the meaningful world of our experience is constituted. . . . And because natural science is itself a tissue of meaning, its own theses (and so those of philosophical naturalism) are founded by the meaningful relations uncovered by phenomenology'
>
> (Crowell 2009, p. 17).

Hence, phenomenology is prior to natural science and will seek to make explicit the assumptions, and how they relate to one another, that science takes for granted. A further distinction useful for understanding Husserl is that between immanent and transcendent. Immanence is the part of the object that is contained within the mental act; the transcendent is that which is outside of the act and the mind. As such, the intentional object is immanent and is the goal of phenomenological enquiry. This discussion of naturalism and immanence/transcendence lead to Husserl's important concepts of the 'natural attitude' and the 'reductions', the latter being used to uncover and reveal the assumptions and default position that make up the 'natural attitude'.

The natural attitude is nothing terribly obscure ultimately: it is simply the default common-sense view of the world we all share. We believe, for example, that things we encounter in our day-to-day world are as they present themselves, are real, will interact in our common-sense, physical conception of the world. The world of the natural attitude is there for all of us, not just me (Russell 2006). Even with errors in this world, such as hallucination and illusions, they can occur only against a background, or horizon, of the world that remains constant and firm (Crowell 2009). You can doubt within the world and the natural attitude, but it itself cannot be doubted. This thesis bares some striking resemblance to the arguments regarding doubt and belief advanced by Wittgenstein in *On Certainty* (Wittgenstein 1969).

For Husserl, the natural attitude is thus positing the world as the horizon of being; as Russell puts it:

> essential to the natural attitude is the positing of the world itself (not just individual entities) as independent of my experience of it, as extending beyond my field of spatial experience, as extending beyond my temporal experience, and so forth. This 'positing' of the world, which sets up the 'universal horizon', is what Husserl calls 'the general positing which characterises the natural attitude'
>
> (Russell 2006, pp. 60–1).

Hence, as with Kant, objects do not simply give us the categories of time, space, causality, etc., we place them in such a world. We assume in advance entities exist independently of us, interact by physical laws, are three-dimensional, and are thus predisposed to discover such objects. Further, this leads us to experience spatiality, temporality and causality as basic features of the world and as constitutive of experience. Natural science builds itself upon the natural attitude and the assumptions of the attitude are what drives and governs the methodology and paradigm of science. Thus, Husserl suggests a division of labour where science studies the world as we experience it in the natural attitude; philosophy must free itself from those assumptions to investigate experience.

One of Husserl's crucial contributions to the method of phenomenology is the idea of the 'reduction'. There are two main 'reductions' Husserl discusses, the eidetic reduction used for the analysis of essences, and the transcendental phenomenological reduction used to free ourselves of the natural attitude and to determine the meaning of entities as given to us in consciousness. This latter reduction is given various names throughout Husserl's work by combining the terms phenomenological or transcendental with either reduction or epoché (ἐποχή). Following Crowell (2009) and Russell (2006) we will refer to this reduction as having two stages: the psychological stage or epoché, and the latter stage the transcendental phenomenological reduction.

The epoché (ἐποχή) or psychological reduction.

The epoché is the first step to peel back the natural attitude. It is not so much an attempt at extreme doubt and scepticism, for example as in Descartes, but rather, as the first step in the phenomenological reduction. The epoché takes the existence of objects we encounter no longer for granted: it 'brackets' world belief and sets aside the real being of what presents itself to us. The purpose of the epoché is to put belief in the world-horizon to one side and hence, importantly, all the explanatory theories that come with it (such as the theories of natural science and of psychology). Thus, the epoché allows the intentional mental state to be viewed apart from the reality of what it is intending, free of belief as to its causal structure, and freeing it from being merely another entity in the world to be examined naturalistically. 'The phenomenological epoché entails abstaining from all judgements that rely upon the general positing of the world' (Russell 2006, p. 66). The epoché, if you will, is a 'brake', something to be applied to stop our default ontological and causal assumption from running free. It brackets out all aspects of being 'outside' leaving only immanent mental acts as the subject matter for phenomenology. Consciousness becomes everything and the world drops away.

It is worth noting, before addressing the reduction further, that other phenomenologists, in particular Heidegger and Merleau-Ponty, felt that the epoché was either unnecessary or impossible, and that phenomenology need not aspire to such ontological neutrality. For Scheler, by contrast, the reduction did not go far enough and missed out on revealing more interesting facets to our experience.

The transcendental phenomenological reduction

The epoché strips away the default meaning we have in the natural attitude, the transcendental phenomenological reduction focuses on the meaning of the object as it is given to us. This reduction allows us to examine how objects are intentionally constituted, what their sense or meaning is in consciousness. Further, it shows us that there is a radical separability of psychical acts from the world, due to the immanence of mental events.

As Crowell puts it:

> The basic idea is relatively simple. The same entity can be experienced in a variety of ways: this rock, which I kick out of the way as an impediment, is subsequently picked up by my geologist neighbour as a fine specimen of Texas granite. The same rock is given each time with

a different meaning. According to Husserl, we must attribute these differences not solely to the thing itself (though they belong to it) but to the consciousness that experiences them in these ways, because only the conscious act explains why at this moment just these aspects of the object are experienced, why my experience has this content'

(Crowell 2009, p. 21).

The transcendental reduction leaves us with a realm to investigate independent of the world, and in doing so, makes conspicuous facts of the world that had previously been hidden from us. Phenomenology sees consciousness as primal and primary, the object that grants all others their status, whereas psychology, as part of the natural attitude, sees consciousness as an object to be studied alongside others (Russell 2006).

Russell sums up where the reductions leave us:

phenomenology is about staying with the conscious experience of the world itself, tarrying awhile, observing it in all its variety and in all of its dimensions, and then describing it according to its structures'

(Russell 2006, p. 73).

The eidetic reduction

For Husserl one of the key features of phenomenology is that it can serve as an a-priori science of essences.

For Husserl, the elucidation of essence is in fact not linked to concrete empirical data. Phenomenology, as the study of essences, suggests each empirical science will rest upon this a-priori science. Phenomenology examines the most general essences in what Husserl terms 'formal ontology', and the specific essences relevant to each subject domain in 'material or regional ontology'.

As Zahavi writes:

The work of formal ontology is consequently to be found in the elucidation of such categories as quality, property, relation, identity, whole, part and so on. In contrast, the material (or regional) ontology examines the essential structures belonging to a given region or kind of object and seeks to determine that which holds true with necessity for any member of the region in question.

(Zahavi 2003, p. 38).

Reading Husserl (Husserl 1973/1999, p. 293) we find a definition of essence and advice on how to carry out the 'eidetic reduction':

The essence proves to be that without which an object of a particular kind cannot be thought, i.e., without which the object cannot be intuitively imagined as such. This general essence is the eidos, the idea in the Platonic sense, but apprehended in its purity and free from all metaphysical interpretations, therefore taken exactly as it is given to us immediately and intuitively in the vision of the idea which arises in this way.

Similar to the notion of ideal types, however, the elucidation of essences is not dependent upon empirical perception but rather the use of the investigator's imagination (Husserl 1973/1999, p. 294; Held 2003, pp. 16–17). The method to discover such essences is that of 'free variation' whereby an experience or object is imagined in a variety of determinations until our variations lead it to becoming something else, losing its identity. This process allows recognition of the conceptual limits of the item under investigation. The data used for such an eidetic reduction need not actually be empirical. Husserl is emphatic about this point:

For a pure eidos, the factual actuality of the particular cases by means of which we progress in the variation is completely irrelevant. And this must be taken literally. The actualities must be treated as possibilities among other possibilities, in fact as arbitrary possibilities of the imagination. This treatment is achieved only when every connection to pregiven actuality is most carefully excluded

(Husserl, 1973/1999, p. 298).

If this is correct, then empirical data have no place in the determination of phenomenological essence. To relate this back to psychiatry, if we assume that there is a regional or material ontology, using Husserlian terminology that consists of the entities of psychiatry or psychopathology, then, firstly, it seems that an eidetic analysis can take place without any empirical data. We do not need to interview any patients to reach the essence of, for example, schizophrenia. Secondly, when we perform the eidetic variation in fantasy we will discover the essence of schizophrenia when we hit the boundary of the disorder. That is to say, when any further variation leads to the loss of identity: 'The variation consequently allows us to distinguish between the accidental properties, i.e. the properties that could have been different, and the essential properties, i.e. the invariant structures that make the phenomenon be of the type it is' (Parnas and Zahavi 2002, p. 157). However, and this is perhaps where Husserl means that phenomenology is an eidetic science, to do this we must already know, a priori, pre-empirically, if only implicitly, the boundary conditions of all the entities of the regional ontology we are investigating. Rather like Socratic dialectic reminding us of our knowledge of the Eternal Forms, Husserlian eidetic reduction makes explicit the boundary conditions of concepts we use routinely. However, with reference to psychiatric entities, there is controversy as to whether crisp and discrete boundaries, with invariant and essential properties, are to be found. We merely possess empirical constructs, it can be argued, and these must stand or fall in relation to how well they enable us to predict, control, manipulate, etc. Yet the question 'What is schizophrenia?', for example, remains and here the notion of essence returns. Purely empirical work also has difficulties resolving disputes that to some extent are conceptual and definitional, e.g. whether the property of 'personality or intellectual decline' is essential to schizophrenia.

The selections below focus firstly on Husserl's understanding of the natural attitude and of the epoché (*Ideas 1*). Here, Husserl uses the Greek ἐποχή consistently to refer to the epoché. The second reading details his characterization of the eidetic reduction (*Experience and Judgment*).

Husserl, E. (1919), Selections from *Ideas 1*

From (1998) *Ideas 1*. Dordrecht: Kluwer Academic Publishers: 51–73. Originally published as (1919) *Ideen zu einer reinen Phänomenologie und phänomenologischen Philosophie. Erstes Buch: Allgemeine Einführung in die reine Phänomenologie [Ideas: General Introduction to Pure Phenomenology]*. Halle: Max Niemeyer Verlag. Original footnotes have been removed in this extract.

The Positing which Belongs to the Natural Attitude and its Eclusion

§27.   The World of the Natural Attitude: I and My Surrounding World

We begin our consideration as human beings who are living naturally, objectivating, judging, feeling, willing "in the natural attitude." What that signifies we shall make clear in simple meditations which can best be carried out in the first person singular.

I am conscious of a world endlessly spread out in space, endlessly becoming and having, endlessly become in time. I am conscious of it: that signifies, above all, that intuitively I find it immediately, that I experience it. By my seeing, touching, hearing, and so forth, and in the different modes of sensuous perception, corporeal physical things with some spatial distribution or other are *simply there for me, "on hand"* in the literal or the figurative sense, whether or not I am particularly heedful of them and busied with them in my considering, thinking, feeling, or willing. Animate beings too, human beings, let us say – are immediately there for me: I look up; I see them; I hear their approach; I grasp their hands; talking with them I understand immediately what they objectivate and think, what feelings stir within them, what they wish or will. They are also present as actualities in my field of intuition even when I do not heed them. But it is not necessary that they, and likewise that other objects, be found directly in my *field of perception*. Along with the ones now perceived, other actual objects are there for me as determinate, as more or less well known, without being themselves perceived or, indeed, present in any other mode of intuition. I can let my attention wander away from the writing table which was just now seen and noticed, out through the unseen parts of the room which are behind my back, to the verandah, into the garden, to the children in the arbor, etc., to all the Objects I directly "know of" as being there and here in the surroundings of which there is also consciousness – a "knowing of them" which involves no conceptual thinking and which changes into a clear intuiting only with the advertence of attention, and even then only partially and for the most part very imperfectly.

But not even with the domain of this intuitionally clear or obscure, distinct or indistinct, *co present* which makes up a constant halo around the field of actual perception – is the world exhausted which is "on hand" for me in the manner peculiar to consciousness at every waking moment. On the contrary, in the fixed order of its being, it reaches into the unlimited. What is now perceived and what is more or less clearly co-present and determinate (or at least somewhat determinate), are penetrated and surrounded by an *obscurely intended to horizon of indeterminate actuality*. I can send rays of the illuminative regard of attention into this horizon with varying results. Determining presentations, obscure at first and then becoming alive, haul something out for me; a chain of such quasi-memories is linked together; the sphere of determinateness becomes wider and wider, perhaps so wide that connection is made with the field of actual perception as my *central* surroundings. But generally the result is different: an empty mist of obscure indeterminateness is populated with intuited possibilities or likelihoods; and only the "form" of the world, precisely as "the world," is predelineated. Moreover, my indeterminate surroundings are infinite, the misty and never fully determinable horizon is necessarily there.

What is the case with the world as existing in the order of the spatial present, which I have just been tracing, is also the case with respect to its *order in the sequence of time*. This world, on hand for me now and manifestly in every waking Now, has its two-sidedly infinite temporal horizon, its known and unknown, immediately living and lifeless past and future. In the free activity of experiencing which makes what is present intuited, I can trace these interrelations of the actuality immediately surrounding me.

I can change my standpoint in space and time, turn my regard in this or that direction, forwards or backwards in time; I can always obtain new perceptions and presentations, more or less clear and more or less rich in content, or else more or less clear images in which I illustrate to myself intuitionally what is possible or likely within the fixed forms of a spatial and temporal world.

In my waking consciousness I find myself in this manner at all times, and without ever being able to alter the fact, in relation to the world which remains one and the same, though changing with respect to the composition of its contents. It is continually "on hand" for me and I myself am a member of it. Moreover, this world is there for me not only as a world of mere things, but also with the same immediacy as a *world of objects with values, a world of goods, a practical world*. I simply find the physical things in front of me furnished not only with merely material determinations but also with value-characteristics, as beautiful and ugly, pleasant and unpleasant, agreeable and disagreeable, and the like. Immediately, physical things stand there as Objects of use, the "table" with its "books," the "drinking glass," the "vase," the "piano," etc. These value-characteristics and practical characteristics also belong *constitutively to the Objects "on hand" as Objects*, regardless of whether or not I turn to such characteristics and the Objects. Naturally this applies not only in the case of the "mere physical things," but also in the case of humans and brute animals belonging

to my surroundings. They are my "friends" or "enemies," my "servants" or "superiors," "strangers" or "relatives," etc.

§28. The Cogito. My Natural Surrounding World and the Ideal Surrounding Worlds

The complexes of my manifoldly changing *spontaneities* of consciousness then relate to this world, *the world in which I find myself and which is, at the same time, my surrounding world* – complexes of investigative inspecting, of explicating and conceptualizing in descriptions, of comparing and distinguishing, of collecting and counting, of presupposing and inferring: in short, of theorizing consciousness in its different forms and at its different levels. Likewise the multiform acts and states of emotion and of willing: liking and disliking, being glad and being sorry, desiring and shunning, hoping and fearing, deciding and acting. All of them – including the simple Ego-acts in which I, in spontaneous advertence and seizing, am conscious of the world as *immediately* present – are embraced by the one Cartesian expression, *cogito*. Living along naturally, I live continually in *this fundamental form of* "active" ["*aktuellen*"] *living* whether, while so living, I state the cogito, whether I am directed "reflectively" to the Ego and the cogitare. If I am directed to them, a new cogito is alive, one that, for its part, is not reflected on and thus is not objective for me. I always find myself as someone who is perceiving, objectivating in memory or in phantasy, thinking, feeling, desiring etc.; and I find myself actively related in these activities *for the most part* to the actuality continually surrounding me. For I am not always so related; not every cogito in which I live has as its cogitatum physical things, human beings, objects or affair-complexes of some kind or other that belong to my surrounding world. I busy myself, let us say, with pure numbers and their laws: Nothing like that is present in the surrounding world, this world of "real actuality." The world of numbers is likewise there for me precisely as the Object-field of arithmetical busiedness; during such busiedness single numbers of numerical formations will be at the focus of my regard, surrounded by a partly determinate, partly indeterminate arithmetical horizon; but obviously this factual being-there-for-me, like the factually existent itself, is of a different sort. *The arithmetical world is there for me only if, and as long as, I am in the arithmetical attitude*. The *natural* world, however, the world in the usual sense of the word is, and has been, *there for me continuously* as long as I go on living naturally. As long as this is the case, I am *"in the natural attitude,"* indeed both signify precisely the same thing. That need not be altered in any respect whatever if, at the same time, I appropriate to myself the arithmetical world and other similar "worlds" by effecting the suitable attitudes. In that case the natural world *remains "on hand:"* afterwards, as well as before, I am in the natural attitude, *undisturbed* in it *by the new attitudes.* If my cogito is moving *only* in the worlds pertaining to these new attitudes, the natural world remains outside consideration; it is a background for my act-consciousness, but it is *not a horizon within which an arithmetical world finds a place.* The two worlds simultaneously present are *not connected,* disregarding their Ego-relation by virtue of which I can freely direct my regard and my acts into the one or the other.

§29. The "Other" Ego-subjects 'and the Intersubjective Natural Surrounding World

All that which holds for me myself holds, as I know, for all other human beings whom I find present in my surrounding world. Experiencing them as human beings, I understand and accept each of them as an Ego-subject just as I myself am one, and as related to his natural surrounding world. But I do this in such a way that I take their surrounding world and mine Objectively as one and the same world of which we all are conscious, only in different modes. Each has his place from which he sees the physical things present; and, accordingly, each has different physical-thing appearances. Also, for each the fields of actual perception, actual memory, etc., are different, leaving aside the fact that intersubjectively common objects of consciousness in those fields are intended to as having different modes, different manners of apprehension, different degrees of clarity and so forth. For all that, we come to an understanding with our fellow human beings and in common with them posit an Objective spatiotemporal actuality as *our factually existent surrounding world to which we ourselves nonetheless belong.*

§30. The General Positing which Characterizes the Natural Attitude

What we presented as a characterization of the givenness belonging to the natural attitude, and therefore

as a characterization of that attitude itself, was a piece of pure description *prior to any "theory."* In these investigations, we keep theories – here the word designates preconceived opinions of every sort – strictly at a distance. Only as facts of our surrounding world, not as actual or supposed unities of validity, do theories belong in our sphere. But we do not set for ourselves now the task of continuing the pure description and raising it to the status of a systematically comprehensive characterization, exhausting the breadths and depths of what can be found as data accepted in the natural attitude (to say nothing of the attitudes which can be harmoniously combined with it). Such a task can and must be fixed – as a scientific task; and it is an extraordinarily important one, even though barely seen up to now. It is not our task here. For us, who are striving toward the entrance-gate of phenomenology, everything needed along that line has already been done; we need only a few quite universal characteristics of the natural attitude which have already come to the fore with a sufficiently *full clarity* in our descriptions. Just this full clarity was of particular consequence to us.

Once more, in the following propositions we single out something most important: As what confronts me, I continually find the one spatiotemporal actuality to which I belong like all other human beings who are to be found in it and who are related to it as I am. I find the "actuality," the word already says it, as a *factually existent actuality and also accept it as it presents itself to me as factually existing.* No doubt about or rejection of data belonging to the natural world alters in any respect the *general positing which characterizes the natural attitude.* "The" world is always there as an actuality; here and there it is at most "otherwise" than I supposed; this or that is, so to speak, to be struck *out of it* and given such titles as "illusion" and "hallucination," and the like; <it is to be struck out of "the" world> which – according to the general positing – is always factually existent. To cognize "the" world more comprehensively, more reliably, more perfectly in every respect than naive experiential cognizance can, to solve all the problems of scientific cognition which offer themselves within the realm of the world, that is the aim of the *sciences belonging to the natural attitude.*

§31. Radical Alteration of the Natural Positing. "Excluding," "Parenthesizing"

Instead of remaining in this attitude, we propose to alter it radically. What we now must do is to convince ourselves of the essential possibility of the alteration in question.

The general positing, by virtue of which there is not just any continual apprehensional consciousness of the real surrounding world, but a consciousness of it as a *factually existing* "actuality," naturally does *not consist of a particular act,* perchance an articulated judgment *about* existence. It is, after all, something that lasts continuously throughout the whole duration of the attitude, i.e., throughout natural waking life. That which at any time is perceived, is clearly or obscurely presentiated – in short, everything which is, before any thinking, an object of experiential consciousness issuing, from the natural world – bears, in its total unity and with respect to all articulated saliencies in it, the characteristic "there," "on hand;" and it is essentially possible to base on this characteristic: an explicit (predicative) judgment of existence agreeing with it. If we state such a judgment, we nevertheless know that in it we have only made thematic and conceived as a predicate what already was somehow inherent, as unthematic, unthought, unpredicated, in the original experiencing or, correlatively, in the experienced, as the characteristic of something "on hand."

We can now proceed with the potential and inexplicit positing precisely as we can with the explicit judgment-positing. One procedure, possible at any time, is the *attempt to doubt universally* which *Descartes* carried out for an entirely different purpose with a view toward bringing out a sphere of absolutely indubitable being. We start from here, but at the same time emphasize that the attempt to doubt universally shall serve us only as a *methodic expedient* for picking out certain points which, as included in its essence, can be brought to light and made evident by means of it.

The attempt to doubt universally belongs to the realm of our *perfect freedom:* we can *attempt to doubt* anything whatever, no matter how firmly convinced of it, even assured of it in an adequate evidence, we may be.

Let us reflect on what lies in the essence of such an act. Someone who attempts to doubt some "being" or other, or predicatively explicated, a "that exists," a "that is how it is," or the like. The sort of being does not matter. For example, someone who doubts whether an object, the being of which he does not doubt, in qualified thus and so, doubts precisely the *being-qualified-thus-and-so.* Obviously this is carried over from doubting to *attempting* to doubt. Furthermore, it is clear that we cannot doubt a being and, in the same consciousness (with the form of unity belonging to the simultaneous) posit the substrate of this being, thus being conscious of the substrate it as having the characteristic, "on hand." Equivalently the same material of being cannot be simultaneously doubted and held to be certain. In like manner, it is clear that the *attempt* to doubt anything intended to as something *on hand* necessarily *effects a certain annulment of positing* and precisely this interests us. The annulment in question is not a transmutation of positing into counter positing, of position into negation; it is also not a transmutation into uncertain presumption, deeming possible, undecidedness, into a doubt (in any sense whatever of the word): nor indeed is anything like that within the sphere of our free choice. *Rather it is something wholly peculiar. We do not give up the positing we effected, we do not in any respect alter our conviction* which remains in itself as it is as long as we do not introduce new judgment-motives: precisely this is what we do not do. Nevertheless the positing undergoes a modification while it in itself remains what it is, we, so to speak, "put it out of action," we "exclude it," we "parenthesize it." It is still there, like the parenthesized in the parentheses, like the excluded outside the context of inclusion [*wie das Ausgeschaltete außerhalb des Zusammenhanges der Schaltung*]. We can also say: The positing is a mental process, *but we make "no use" of it,* and this is not understood, naturally, as implying that we are deprived of it (as it would if we said of someone who was not conscious, that he made no use of a positing); rather, in the case of this expression and all parallel expressions it is a matter of indicative designations of a definite, *specifically peculiar mode of consciousness* which is added to the original positing simpliciter (whether this is or not an actional [*aktuelle*] and even a predicative *positing* of existence) and, likewise in a specifically peculiar manner, changes its value. *This changing of value is a matter in which we are perfectly free, and it stands over against all cogitative position-takings coordinate* with the positing and incompatible with the positing in the unity of the "simultaneous," as well as over against all position-takings in the proper sense of the term.

In the attempt to doubt which accompanies a positing which, as we presuppose, is certain and continued, the "excluding" is brought about in and with a modification of the counter positing, namely the "*supposition*" *of non-being* which is, therefore, part of the substratum of the attempt to doubt. In Descartes this part is so predominant that we can say that his attempt to doubt universally is properly an attempt to negate universally. Here we disregard this part; we are not interested in every analytically distinguishable component of the attempt to doubt, and consequently we are not interested in the exact and fully sufficient analysis of it. *We single out only the phenomenon of "parenthesizing" or "excluding"* which, while obviously not restricted to the phenomenon of attempting to doubt, is particularly easy to analyze out and which can, on the contrary, make its appearance *also in other combinations* and, equally well, *alone.* With regard to *any* positing we can quite freely exercise this peculiar ἐποχή, *a certain refraining from judgment which is compatible with the unshaken conviction of truth, even with the unshakable conviction o/ evident truth.* The positing is "put out of action," parenthesized, converted into the modification, "parenthesized positing"; the judgment simpliciter is converted into the *"parenthesized judgment."*

Naturally one must not identify this consciousness with the consciousness called "mere phantasying," let us say, that nymphs are performing a round dance. In the latter consciousness, after all, *no excluding* of a living conviction, which remains alive, takes place. The consciousness of which we are speaking is even further from being a matter of just thinking of something in the sense *of "assuming" or presupposing,* which, in ordinary equivocal language, can also be expressed by "It seems to me (I make the assumption) that such and such is the case."

It should also be said that nothing prevents *speaking correlatively of parenthesizing* with respect to a *positable objectivity* belonging to no matter what region and category. When speaking thus, we mean that *every positing related to this objectivity is to be excluded* and converted into its parenthetical modification. Furthermore, when the metaphor of parenthesizing is closely examined it is seen to be, from the very beginning, more suitable to the object-sphere; just as the locution of "putting out of action" is better suited to the act- or consciousness-sphere.

§32. The Phenomenological ἐποχή

We could now let the universal ἐποχή, in our sharply determinate and novel sense of the term, take the place of the Cartesian attempt to doubt universally. But with good reason we *limit* the universality of that.

Since we are completely free to modify every positing and every judging [*Urteil*] and to parenthesize every objectivity which can be judged about if it were as comprehensive as possible, then no province would be left for unmodified judgments, to say nothing of a province for science. But our purpose is to discover a new scientific domain, one that is to be gained *by the method of parenthesizing* which, therefore, must be a definitely restricted one.

The restriction can be designated in a word.

We put out of action the general positing which belongs to the essence, of the natural attitude; we parenthesize everything which that positing encompasses with respect to being: *thus the whole natural world* which is continually "there for us," "on hand," and which will always remain there according to consciousness as an "actuality" even if we choose to parenthesize it.

If I do that, as I can with complete freedom, then I am *not negating* this "world" as though I were a sophist; I am *not doubting its factual being* as though 1 were a skeptic; rather I am exercising the "phenomenological" ἐποχή which also *completely shuts me off from any judgment about spatiotemporal factual being.*

Thus I exclude all sciences relating to this natural world no matter how firmly they stand there for me, no matter how much I admire them, no matter how little I think of making even the least objection to them; I make *absolutely no use of the things posited in them* [*von ihren Geltungen*]. *Nor do I make my own a single one of the propositions belonging to <those sciences>, even though it be perfectly evident; none is accepted by me; none gives me a foundation* – let this be well noted: as long as it is understood as it is presented in one of those sciences as a truth *about actualities* of this world. I *must not accept such a proposition until after I have put parenthesis around it.* That signifies that I may accept such a proposition only in the modified consciousness, the consciousness of judgment-excluding, and therefore *not as it is in science, a proposition which claims validity and the validity of which I accept and use.*

The ἐποχή in question here is not to be mistaken for the one which positivism requires, but which indeed, as we had to persuade ourselves, is itself violated by such positivism. It is not now a matter of excluding all prejudices that cloud the pure objectivity of research, not a matter of constituting a science "free of theories," "free of metaphysics," by groundings all of which go back to the immediate findings, nor a matter of means for attaining such ends, about the value of which there is, indeed, no question. What *we* demand lies in another direction. The whole pre-discovered world posited in the natural attitude, actually found in experience and taken with perfect "freedom from theories" as it is actually experienced, as it clearly shows itself in the concatenations of experience, is now without validity for us; without being tested and also without being contested, it shall be parenthesized. In like manner all theories and sciences which relate to this world, no matter how well they may be grounded positivistically or otherwise, shall meet the same fate.

Consciousness and Natural Actuality

§33. Preliminary Indication of "Pure" or "Transcendental" Consciousness As the Phenomenological Residuum

We have learned to understand the sense of the phenomenological ἐποχή but not by any means its possible effect. Above all, it is not clear to what extent the previous delimitation of the total sphere of the ἐποχή actually involves a restriction of its universality. *What can remain, if the whole world, including ourselves with all our cogitare, is excluded?*

Since the reader already knows that the interest governing these meditations concerns a new eidetics, he will at first expect that, more particularly, the world as matter of fact is excluded but not the *world as Eidos,* not any other sphere of essences. Indeed, the exclusion of the world actually does not signify the exclusion of the world of, e.g., the number series or arithmetic as relating to it.

Nevertheless we shall not take this path; it does not lead toward our goal which we can also characterize as *the acquisition of a new region of being never before delimited in its own peculiarity* – a region which, like any other genuine region, is a region of *individual* being. What that means we shall learn, more particularly, from the findings that follow.

We shall proceed, first of all, with a direct demonstrable showing and, since the being that we want to demonstrably show is nothing else than what we shall designate, for essential reasons, as "pure mental processes," "pure consciousness" with its pure "correlates of consciousness" and, on the other hand, its "pure Ego" we shall start with *the* Ego, *the* consciousness, and *the* mental processes which are given to us in the natural attitude.

I, the actual human being, am a real Object like others in the natural world. I effect cogitationes, acts of consciousness in both the broader and narrower sense and these acts, as belonging to this human subject, are occurrences within the same natural actuality. And likewise all my other mental processes, out of the changing stream of which the specific Ego-acts flash in so specifically peculiar a manner, pass over into one another, become connected in syntheses, become incessantly modified. In a *broadest sense,* the expression *consciousness* comprehends (but then indeed less suitably) *all* mental processes. "In the natural attitude," as we are even in our scientific thinking, by virtue of extremely firm habits which have never been contravened, we take all these findings of psychological reflection as real worldly occurences, just as mental processes in the lives of animate beings. So natural is it for us to see them only as such that now, when already acquainted with the possibility of an altered attitude and searching for the new Object-province, we do not even note that it is from these very spheres of mental processes that the new province arises by virtue of the new attitude. As a consequence, it follows that instead of keeping our regard turned toward those spheres, we turned it away from them and sought the new Objects in the ontological realms of arithmetic, geometry, and the like – where, after all, nothing genuinely new could be attained.

We shall therefore keep our regard fixed upon the sphere of consciousness and study what we find immanently within *it.* First of all, without as yet effecting the phenomenological judgment-exclusions, we shall subject it to a systematic, though by no means exhaustive, *eidetic* analysis. What we absolutely need is a certain universal insight into the essence of *any consciousness whatever* and also, quite particularly, of consciousness in so far as it is, in itself, by its essence consciousness of "natural" actuality. In these studies we shall go as far as is necessary to effect the insight at which we are aiming, namely the insight *that consciousness has, in itself, a being of its own which in its own absolute essence, is not touched by the phenomenological exclusion.* It therefore remains as the *"phenomenological residuum,"* as a region of being which is of essential necessity quite unique and which can indeed become the field of a science of a novel kind: phenomenology.

The "phenomenological" ἐποχή will deserve its name only by means of this insight; the fully conscious effecting of that ἐποχή will prove itself to be the operation necessary to *make "pure" consciousness, and subsequently the whole phenomenological region, accessible to us.* Precisely that makes it comprehensible why this region and the novel science correlated with it remained necessarily unknown: In the natural attitude nothing else but the natural world is seen. As long as the possibility of the phenomenological attitude had not been recognized, and the method for bringing about an originary seizing upon the objectivities that arise with that attitude had not been developed, the phenomenological world had to remain unknown, indeed, hardly even suspected.

Concerning our terminology we may add the following. Important motives, grounded in the epistemological problematic, justify our designating "pure" consciousness, about which we shall have so much to say, *as transcendental consciousness* and the operation by which it is reached the *transcendental* ἐποχή. As a method this operation will be divided into different steps of "excluding," "parenthesizing," and thus our method will assume the characteristic of a step-by-step reduction. For this reason we shall, on most occasions, speak of *phenomenological reductions* (but also, with reference to their collective unity, we shall speak of *the* phenomenological reduction) and, accordingly, from an epistemological point of view, we shall refer to transcendental reductions. It should be added that these terms and *all* our others must be understood exclusively in the senses that *our* expositions prescribe for them and not in any others which history or the terminological habits of the reader may suggest.

§34.   The Essence of Consciousness as Theme

We begin with a series of observations which we shall make without troubling ourselves with any phenomenological ἐποχή. We are directed to the "external world" in a natural manner and, without relinquishing the natural attitude, we effect a psychological reflection on our Ego and its mental living. Quite as we should if we had heard nothing of the new sort of attitude, we engross ourselves in the *essence of the "consciousness of something,"* in which, for example, we are conscious of the factual existence of material things, animate organisms, human beings, the factual existence of technical and literary works, and so forth. We follow our universal principle that every individual event has its essence, which can be seized upon in eidetic purity and, in this purity, must belong to a field of possible eidetic research. Accordingly, the general natural fact, "I am," "I think," "I have a world over against me," and the like, has its essential content with which we shall now busy ourselves exclusively. We therefore effect, as examples, any single mental processes whatever of consciousness and take them as they themselves are given to us in the natural attitude, as real human facts; or else we presentiate such mental processes to ourselves in memory or in freely inventive phantasy. On the basis of such examples which, let us presuppose, are perfectly clear, we seize upon and fix, in an adequate ideation, the pure essences that interest us. In the process, the single facts, the facticity of the natural world taken universally, disappear from our theoretical regard – as they do wherever we carry out a purely eidetic research.

Let us limit our theme still more narrowly. Its title runs: consciousness or, more distinctly, *any mental processes whatever of consciousness* in an extraordinarily broad sense, the exact limitation of which fortunately does not matter. Such a limitation does not lie at the beginning of analyses of the sort which we are carrying on here, but is a late result of great labors. As the starting point, we take consciousness in a pregnant sense and one which offers itself first, which we can designate most simply by the Cartesian term *cogito,* by the phrase "I think." As is well known, cogito was understood so broadly by Descartes that it comprised every "I perceive, I remember, I phantasy, I judge, I feel, I desire, I will," and thus all egoical mental processes which are at all similar to them, with their countless flowing particular formations. The Ego itself, to which they are all related or which, in very different manners, lives "in" them actively, passively or spontaneously, which "comports" itself receptively and otherwise in them, shall be at first left "out of consideration; more particularly, the Ego in every sense" shall be left out of consideration. Later on the Ego shall be dealt with thoroughly. For now, enough is left that gives support to analysis and the apprehension of essences. In that connection, we shall find ourselves immediately referred to those comprehensive concatenations of mental processes that compel a broadening of the concept, mental process of consciousness, beyond this sphere made up of cogitationes in the specific <Cartesian> sense.

We consider mental processes of consciousness *in the entire fullness of the concreteness* within which they present themselves in their concrete context – *the stream of mental processes* – and which, by virtue of their own essence, they combine to make up. It then becomes evident that every mental process belonging to the stream which can be reached by our reflective regard has an *essence of its own* which can be seized upon intuitively, a "content" which allows of being considered *by itself in its ownness*. Our concern is to seize upon and to universally characterize this own content of the cogitation in its *pure* ownness by excluding everything which does not lie in the cogitatio with respect to what the cogitatio is in itself. It is equally our concern to characterize the *unity of consciousness* required, and therefore necessarily required, *purely by what belongs to the cogitationes as their own* such that they could not exist without that unity.

§35. The Cogito as "Act." Non-actionality Modification

Let us begin with examples. Lying in front of me in the semi-darkness is this sheet of paper. I am seeing it, touching it. This perceptual seeing and touching of the sheet of paper, as the full concrete mental awareness *of* the sheet of paper lying here and given precisely with respect to these qualities, appearing to me precisely with this relative obscurity, with this imperfect determinateness in this orientation, is a cogitatio, a mental process of consciousness. The sheet of paper itself, with its Objective determinations, its extension, its Objective position relative to the spatial thing called my organism, is not a cogitatio but a cogitatum; it is not a mental process of perception but something perceived. Now something perceived can very well be itself a mental process of consciousness; but it is evident that such an affair as a material physical thing, for example, this sheet of paper given in the mental process of perception, is by essential necessity not a mental process but a being of a wholly different mode of being.

Before we investigate that further, let us multiply the examples. In perceiving proper, as an attentive perceiving, I am turned toward the object, for instance, the sheet of paper; I seize upon it as this existent here and now. The seizing-upon is a singling out and seizing; anything perceived has an experiential background. Around the sheet of paper lie books, pencils, an inkstand, etc., also "perceived" in a certain manner, perceptually there, in the "field of intuition"; but, during the advertence to the sheet of paper, they were without even a secondary advertence and seizing-upon. They were appearing and yet were not seized upon and picked out, not posited singly for themselves. Every perception of a physical thing has,

in this manner, a halo of *background-intuitions* (or background-seeings, in case one already includes in intuiting the advertedness to the really seen), and that is also a *"mental process of consciousness"* or, more briefly, "consciousness," and, more particularly, *"of"* all that which in fact lies in the objective "background" seen along with it. Obviously in saying this we are not speaking of that which is to be found "Objectively" in the Objective space which may belong to the seen background; we are not speaking of all the physical things and physical occurrences which valid and progressing experience may ascertain there. We speak exclusively of the halo of consciousness which belongs to the essence of a perception effected in the mode of "advertence to the Object" and, furthermore, of what is inherent in the essence proper of this halo. In it, however, there is the fact that certain modifications of the original mental process are possible which we characterize as a free turning of "regard" – not precisely nor merely of the physical, but rather of the *"mental regard"* [*"geistigen Blickes"*] – from the sheet of paper regarded at first, to the objects appearing, therefore intended to "implicitly" before the turning of the regard but which become explicitly intended to (either "attentively" perceived or "incidentally heeded") *after* the regard is turned to them.

Physical things are intended to not only in perception but also in memories and in presentations similar to memories as well as in free phantasies. All this, sometimes in "clear intuition," sometimes without noticeable intuitedness in the manner of "obscure" objectivations; in such cases they hover before us with different "characteristics" as actual physical things, possible physical things, phantasied physical things, etc. Of these essentially different mental processes obviously everything is true that we adduced about mental processes of perception. We shall not think of confusing the *objects intended to in* these modes of consciousness (for example, the phantasied water nymphs) with the mental processes themselves of consciousness which are consciousness *of* those objects. We recognize then that, to the essence of all such mental processes – these always taken in full concreteness – there belongs that noteworthy modification which converts consciousness in the *mode of actional* [*aktueller*] advertence into consciousness in the *male of non-actionality* [*Inaktualität*] and conversely. At the one time the mental process is, so to speak, "explicit" consciousness of its objective something, at the other time it is implicit, merely *potential*. The objective something can be already appearing to us as it does not only in perception, but also in memory or in phantasy; however, we are *not yet "directed" to it with the mental regard,* not even secondarily – to say nothing of our being, in a peculiar sense, "busied" with it.

In the sense pertaining to the sphere of the Cartesian examples we note something similar in no matter what other cogitationes: with respect to all mental processes of thinking, feeling, or willing, except that, as the next section will show, the "directedness to," the "advertedness to," which distinguishes actionality [*Aktualität*] does not (as in the preferred – because the simplest – examples of sensuous objectivations) coincide with that heeding of Objects of consciousness which *seizes upon and picks them out.* It is likewise obviously true of all such mental processes that the actional ones are surrounded by a "halo" of non-actional mental processes; the *stream of mental processes can never consist of just actualities.* Precisely these, when contrasted with non-actualities, determine with the widest universality, to be extended beyond the sphere of our examples, the *pregnant* sense of the expression *"cogito,"* "I have *consciousness* of something," "I effect an *act* of consciousness." To keep this fixed concept sharply separated, we shall reserve for it exclusively the Cartesian terms, cogito and cogitationes – unless we indicate the modification explicitly by some such adjunct as "non-actional."

We can define a *"waking"* Ego as one which, within its stream of mental processes, continuously effects consciousness in the specific form of the cogito; which naturally does not mean that it continually gives, or is able to give at all, predicative expression to these mental processes. There are, after all, brute animal Ego-subjects. According to what is said above, however, it is of the essence of a waking Ego's stream of mental processes that the continuously unbroken chain of cogitationes is continually surrounded by a medium of non-actionality which is always ready to change into the mode of actionality, just as, conversely actionality is always ready to change into non-actionality.

Husserl, E. (1930/1948), Selections from *Experience and Judgment*

From (1973) *Experience and Judgment*. Translated by S. Churchill. Evanston, IL: Northwestern University Press: 339–54. Originally published after his death as (1948) *Erfahrung und Urteil: Untersuchungen zur Genealogie der Logik*. Hamburg: Classen & Goverts.

The Acquisition of Pure Generalities by the Method of Essential Seeing [*Wesenserschauung*]

§86. The contingency of empirical generalities and a priori necessity

Empirical generalities, we said, have an extension of actual and really possible particulars. Acquired at first on the basis of the repetition of like and then merely similar objects given in actual experience, these generalities refer not only to this limited and, so to speak, denumerable extension of actual particulars, from which they have been originally acquired, but as a general rule they have a *horizon* which presumptively exhibits a broader experience of particulars which can be acquired in free arbitrariness by opening up this presumptive horizon of being. When it is a question of the realities of the infinite pre-given world, we can imagine *an arbitrary number of particulars capable of being given later on,* which likewise includes this empirical generality as a *real possibility.* The extension is then an infinitely open one, and still the unity of the empirically acquired species and the higher genus is a "contingent" one. This means that a contingently given particular object was the point of departure of the formation of the concept, and this formation led beyond the likewise contingent likenesses and similarities – contingent because the member acting as the point of departure for the comparison was contingent, given in actual experience. The concept opposed to this contingency is that of *a priori necessity.* It will be necessary to show how, in contrast to these empirical concepts, pure concepts are formed, concepts whose constitution does not thus depend on the contingency of the element actually given as the point of departure and its empirical horizons. These concepts do not envelop an extension which, as it were, is open merely *after the event,* but beforehand, a priori. This envelopment beforehand signifies that they must be capable of *prescribing rules to all empirical particulars.* With empirical concepts, infinity of extension implies only that I can imagine an arbitrary number of like particulars without its actually being evident whether, in the progress of actual experience, this presumptively posited "again and again" might perhaps undergo a cancellation, whether this being able to continue might one day actually reach a limit. With pure concepts, on the other hand, this infinity of actually being-able-to continue is *given with self-evidence,* precisely because, *before* all experience, these concepts prescribe rules for its later course and, consequently, rule out a sudden change, a cancellation. This idea of *a priori* generality and necessity will become even clearer in the course of our presentation.

§87. The method of essential seeing

a. Free variation as the foundation of essential seeing

From the preceding has already become clear that, for the acquisition of pure concepts or concepts of essences, an empirical comparison cannot suffice but that, by special arrangements, the universal which first comes to prominence in the empirically given must from the outset be freed from its character of contingency. Let us attempt to get a first concept of this operation. It is based on the modification of an experienced or imagined objectivity, turning it into an arbitrary example which, at the same time, receives the character of a guiding "model," a point of departure for the production of an infinitely open multiplicity of variants. It is based, therefore, on a *variation*. In other words, for its modification in pure imagination, we let ourselves be guided by the fact taken as a model. For this it is necessary that ever new similar images be obtained as copies, as images of the imagination, which are all concretely similar to the original image. Thus, by an act of volition we produce free variants, each of which, just like the total process of variation itself, occurs in the subjective mode of the "arbitrary." It then becomes evident that a unity runs through this multiplicity of successive figures, that in such free variations of an original image, e.g., of a thing, an *invariant* is necessarily retained as the *necessary general form*, without which an object such as this thing, as an example of its kind, would not be thinkable at all. While what differentiates the variants remains indifferent to us, this form stands out in the practice of voluntary variation, and as an absolutely identical content, an invariable *what*, according to which all the variants coincide: *a general essence*. We can direct our regard toward it as toward the necessarily invariable, which prescribes limits to all variation practiced in the mode of the "arbitrary," all variation which is to be variation of the same original image, no matter how this may be carried out. The essence proves to be that without which an object of a particular kind cannot be thought, i.e., without which the object cannot be intuitively imagined as such. This general essence is the *eidos*, the *idea* in the Platonic sense, but apprehended in its purity and free from all metaphysical interpretations, therefore taken exactly as it is given to us immediately and intuitively in the vision of the idea which arises in this way. Initially, this givenness was conceived as a givenness of experience. Obviously, a mere imagining, or rather, what is intuitively and objectively present in it, can serve our purpose just as well.

For example, if we take a sound as our point of departure, whether we actually hear it or whether we have it present as a sound "in the imagination," then we obtain the *eidos* sound as that which, in the course of "arbitrary" variants, is necessarily common, to all these variants. Now if we take as our point of departure another sound-phenomenon in order to vary it arbitrarily, in the new "example" we do not apprehend *another eidos* sound; rather, in juxtaposing the old and the new, we see that it is *the same*, that the variants and the variations on both sides join together in a single variation, and that the variants here and there are, in like fashion, *arbitrary particularizations of the one eidos*. And it is even evident that in progressing from one variation to a new one we can give this progress and this formation of new multiplicities of variation the character of an arbitrary progress and that, furthermore, in such progress in the form of arbitrariness the same *eidos* must appear "again and again": the same general essence "sound in general."

b. The arbitrary structure of the process of the formation of variants

That the *eidos* depends on a freely and arbitrarily producible multiplicity of variants attaining coincidence, on an open infinity, does not imply that an *actual* continuation to infinity is required, an actual production of all the variants – as if only then could we be sure that the *eidos* apprehended at the end actually conformed to all the possibilities. On the contrary, what matters is that the variation as a process of the formation of variants should itself have a *structure of arbitrariness*, that the process should be accomplished in the consciousness of an arbitrary development of variants. This does not mean – even if we break off – that we intend an actual multiplicity of particular, intuitive variations which lead into one another, an actual series of objects, offering themselves in some way or other and utilized arbitrarily, or fictively produced in advance; it means, rather, that, just as each object has the character of *exemplary arbitrariness*, so the multiplicity of variations likewise always has an arbitrary character: it is a matter of indifference what might still be joined to it, a matter of indifference what, in addition, I might be given to apprehend in the consciousness that "I could continue in this way." This remarkable and truly important consciousness of "and so on, at my pleasure" belongs essentially to every multiplicity of variations. Only in this way is given what we call an "infinitely open" multiplicity; obviously, it is the same whether we proceed according to a long process, producing or drawing arbitrarily on anything suitable, thus extending the series of actual intuitions, or whether we break off prematurely.

c. The retaining-in-grasp of the entire multiplicity of variations as the foundation of essential seeing

In this multiplicity (or, rather, on the groundwork of the open process of the self-constitution of variation, with the variants actually appearing in intuition) is grounded as a higher level *the true seeing of the universal as eidos*. Preceding this seeing, there is the transition from the initial example, which gives direction and which we have called a model, to ever new images, whether these are due to the aimless favor of association and the whims of passive imagination (in which case we only seize upon them arbitrarily as examples) or whether we have obtained them by our own pure activity of imaginative invention from our original model. In this transition from image to image, from the similar to the similar, all the arbitrary particulars attain overlapping coincidence in the order of their appearance and enter, in a purely passive way, into a synthetic unity in which they all appear as modifications of one another and then as arbitrary sequences of particulars in which the same universal is isolated as an *eidos*. Only in this continuous coincidence does something which is the same come to congruence, something which henceforth can be seen purely for itself. This means that it is *passively preconstituted* as such and that the seeing of the *eidos* rests in the *active intuitive apprehension* of what is thus preconstituted – exactly as in *every* constitution of objectivities of the understanding, and especially of general objectivities.

Naturally, the presupposition for this is that the multiplicity *as such* is present to consciousness as a *plurality* and never slips completely from our grasp. Otherwise, we do not attain the *eidos* as the ideally identical, which only *is* as *hen epi pollon*. If, for example, we occupy ourselves with the inventive imagining of a thing or a figure, changing it into arbitrarily new figures, we have something always new, and always only one thing: the last-imagined. Only if we retain in grasp the things imagined earlier, as a multiplicity in an open process, and only if we look toward the congruent and the purely identical, do we attain the *eidos*. Certainly, we need not ourselves actively and expressly bring about the overlapping coincidence, since, with the successive running-through and the retaining-in-grasp of what is run through, it takes place of itself in a purely passive way.

d. The relation of essential seeing to the experience of individuals. The error of the theory of abstraction

The peculiar character of essential seeing on the basis of variation will become still clearer if we contrast it with the intuitive experience of individual objects. Over against the specific *freedom* of variation, there is in all experience of the individual a wholly determined *commitment*. This means that when we receptively experience an individual on the basis of a passive pregivenness, when we turn toward it in order to apprehend it, when we take it in as existing, we thereby take our stand, so to, speak, on the ground of this apperception. By it, horizons are, prescribed for further possible experiences which will take place on this ground, pregiven from the first step. Everything which we further experience must be brought into a context of unanimity if it is to count as an object for us; failing this, it is canceled, nullified, is not taken in receptively as actual; unanimity must prevail on the ground of a unity of experience, a ground already prescribed for each individual object of experience; every conflict is excluded or, rather, leads to a cancellation. Every *experience in the pregnant sense*, which includes activity, at least of the lowest level, thus signifies *"taking a stand on the ground of experience."*

The same thing holds for *imagination* insofar as we imagine within a context such that the individual imaginings are to be linked together in the unity of one act of imagination. Here, in the mode of the quasi, is repeated all that has already been said about actual experience. We have a quasi-world as a unified world of imagination. It is the "ground" on which we can take our stand in the course of a unified act of imagination – only with this difference: that it is left to our free choice to decide how far we will allow this unity to extend; we can enlarge such a world at our pleasure, whereas fixed boundaries are set to the unity of an actual world by what was given previously.

In contrast to this constraint in the experience of the individual object, the specific *freedom of essential seeing* becomes intelligible to us: in the free production of the multiplicity of variations, in the progress from variant to variant, we are not bound by the conditions of unanimity in the same way as in the progress of experience from one individual object to another on the ground of the unity of experience. If, for example, we envisage to ourselves an individual house now painted yellow, we can just as well think that it could be painted blue or think that it could have a slate instead of a tile roof or, instead of this shape, another one. The house is an object which, in the realm of the possible, could have other determinations in place of, and incompatible with, whatever determinations happen to belong to it within the unity of a representation. This house, the same, is thinkable as *a* and as *non-a* but, naturally, if as *a*, then not *at the same time* as *non-a*. It cannot be both simultaneously; it cannot be actual while having *each* of them at the same time; but at any moment it can be *non-a* instead of *a*. It is, therefore, thought as an identical something in which opposite determinations can be exchanged. "Intuitively," in the attainment of this self-evidence, the existence of the object is certainly bound to the possession of one *or* the other of the opposing predicates and to the requirement of the exclusion of their joint possession; however, an *identical substrate* of concordant attributes is evidently present, except that its *simple* thesis is not possible, but only the *modified* thesis: if this identical something determined as a exists, then *a* belongs to it in the canceled form *non-a*, and conversely. To be sure, the identical substrate is not an individual pure and simple. The sudden change is that of an individual into a second individual incompatible with it in coexistence. An individual pure and simple is an existing individual (or one capable of existing). However, what *is seen as* unity *in the conflict is not an individual* but a concrete hybrid unity of individuals mutually nullifying and coexistentially exclusive: a unique consciousness with a unique content, whose correlate signifies concrete unity founded in conflict, in incompatibility. This remarkable hybrid unity is at the bottom of essential seeing.

The old theory of abstraction, which implies that the universal can be constituted only by abstraction on the basis of individual, particular intuitions, is thus in part unclear, in part incorrect. For example, if I construct the general concept tree – understood, of course, as a pure concept – on the basis of individual, particular trees, the tree which is present in my mind is not posited in any way as an individually determined tree: on the contrary, I represent it in such a way that it is the same in perception and in the free movement of imagination, that it is not posited as existing or even called into question, and that it is not in any way held to be an individual. The particular, which is at the bottom of essential seeing, *is not in the proper sense an intuited individual as such*. The remarkable unity which is at the bottom here is, on the contrary, an "individual" in the exchange of "nonessential" constitutive moments (those appearing, as complementary moments, outside the essential moments, which are to be apprehended as identical).

e. Congruence and difference in the overlapping coincidence of multiplicities of variation

What has already been said implies the following: with the *congruence* present in the coincidence of the multiplicities of variation there is connected, on the other hand, a *difference* in various aspects. If, for example, we pass from a given red color to a series of any other red colors whatsoever – whether we actually see them or whether they are colors floating "in the imagination" – we obtain the *eidos* "red," which, as the necessarily common, is what is congruent in the alteration of the "arbitrary" variants, while the different extensions in the coincidence, instead of being congruent, on the contrary come to prominence in conflict.

The *idea of the difference*, therefore, is only to be understood *in its involvement with the idea of the identically common element which is the eidos*. Difference is that which, in the overlapping of the multiplicities, is not to be brought into the unity of the congruence making its appearance thereby, that which, in consequence, does not make an *eidos* visible. To say that a unity, of congruence is not attained means that in the coincidence the different elements are in conflict with one another. Consider, for example, an identical color; at one time it is the color of this extension and shape, at another time of that. In the overlapping, the one conflicts with the other, and they mutually supplant each other.

But, on the other hand, it is clear that *things cannot enter into conflict which have nothing in common*. In our example, not only is an identical color already presupposed; it is even more important that, even if the one colored object were square, they still could not enter into conflict if both were not extended figures. Thus, every difference in the overlapping with others and in conflict with them points toward a new universal to be brought out (in our example, shape) as the universal of the superimposed differences which have momentarily come into the unity of conflict. This point will be of great importance for the theory of the hierarchical structure of ideas up to the highest regions.

By way of summary, we survey the three principal steps which pertain to the process of ideation:

1. The productive activity which consists in running through the multiplicity of variations.
2. The unitary linking in continuous coincidence.
3. The active identification which brings out the congruent over against the differences.

f.   Variation and alteration

One point still requires clarification. We speak of *variation* and of variants, not of *alteration* and phases of alteration. In fact, the two concepts are essentially different, despite a certain affinity.

An alteration is always alteration of a real thing, understood in a completely general sense as a temporal existent, something which endures, which continues through a duration. Every real thing is subject to change and is only in alteration or nonalteration. Nonalteration is only a limiting case of alteration. Alteration signifies a continual being-other or, rather, a becoming-other and yet being the same, individually the same, in this continual becoming-other: the alteration of a color, its fading, and so on, is an example of this. A real thing changes as this individual real thing; its state changes, but it retains its individual identity in this change of state. Nonalteration, on the other hand, implies: being the same in duration but, in addition, remaining continually the same in every phase of duration. With alteration, the state of being in duration and through the phases of duration is a state of being-other, or becoming-other, in each new phase, i.e., certainly remaining individually the same but, at the same time, not remaining continually the same.

When we direct our attention to the *phases* of the duration of the real thing and to that which occupies these phases, we have a multiplicity of figurations of the same thing: the same thing now, the same then, and so on, and, correspondingly, from phase to phase, the same as like or unlike. But when we change the orientation of our regard, directing our attention to the one enduring thing which presents itself in the phases, which "gradates" itself through time as the same, we experience the unity, the identity, which alters or does not alter, which continues and endures through the flux of multiplicities of figurations. This unity is not the universal of the individual temporal phases, any more than these are its variants. This unity is precisely what constitutes the unity of the individual which endures and which, as enduring, changes or remains the same. *In all alteration, the individual remains identically the same.* On the other hand, variation depends precisely on this: that we drop the identity of the individual and change it imaginatively into another possible individual.

On the other hand, it pertains to the alteration of an individual that we can also deal with its phases as variants (although by changing our point of view). Then we see that *no alteration is possible in which all the phases of the alteration not belong together generically.* A color can change only into a color and not, e.g., into a sound. From this it is clear that every possible alteration is accomplished within a highest genus, which it can never contravene.

§88.   The meaning of the phrase: "seeing" generalities

We speak of an essential "seeing" and, in general, of the seeing of generalities. This way of talking still requires justification. We use the expression "to see" here in the completely broad sense which implies nothing other than the *act of experiencing things oneself,* the fact of having seen things themselves, and, on the basis of this self-seeing, of having similarity before one's eyes, of accomplishing, on the strength of it, that mental overlapping in which the common, e.g., the red, the figure, etc., "itself" emerges – that is, attains intuitive apprehension. This, naturally, does *not* mean a *sensuous seeing.* One cannot see the universal red as one sees an individual, particular red; but the extension of the expression "seeing," which not without reason is customary in ordinary language, is unavoidable. With this, we wish to indicate that we appropriate, *directly and as itself,* a common and general moment of as many examples as desired, seen one by one, in a manner wholly analogous to the way in which we appropriate an individual particular in sensuous perception; although, to be sure, the seeing is more complex here. It is a seeing resulting from the actively comparative overlapping of congruence. This is true of every kind of intuitive apprehension of commonalities [*Gemeinsamkeiten*] and generalities, though where a pure *eidos* is to be seen as an *a priori*, this seeing has its special methodological form – precisely that which has been described, namely, that indifference with regard to actuality which is generated in variation, whereby what presents itself as actual acquires the character of an arbitrary example, an indifferent point of departure of a series of variations.

§89. The necessity of an explicit exclusion of all positing of being for the purpose of attaining pure generality

It might now be though that our description of essential seeing makes the task appear too difficult and that it is unnecessary to operate with the multiplicities of variation, which are stressed as allegedly fundamental, and likewise with the functions of imagination which participate therein in so peculiar a way. Would it not be enough to say that any arbitrary red here and red there, any arbitrary, pregiven plurality of red things, pertaining to experience or to any other representation, furnishes the possibility of an essential seeing of the *eidos* red? What would be necessary to describe is only the activity of running through what is given in overlapping coincidence and bringing the universal into view. However, it should be noted here that the word "arbitrary" in the context of our remarks must not be taken as a mere manner of speaking, or as constituting a nonessential attitude on our part, but that *it belongs to the fundamental character of the act of seeing ideas.*

But if in such a way of talking there is the notion that a determinate plurality of similar objects is enough to enable us to obtain a universal by a comparative coincidence, it is necessary to emphasize the following once more: certainly we obtain for this red here and that red there an identical and general element present in both, but precisely only as what is common to this and that red. We do not obtain pure red in general as *eidos*. To be sure, taking account of a third red or several, whenever they present themselves to us, we can recognize that the universal of the two is identically the same as the universal of the many. But in this way we always obtain only commonalities and generalities relative to empirical extensions; the possibility of progress *in infinitum* is still not given intuitively by this. However, as soon as we say that every arbitrary like moment, newly to be taken

account of, *must* yield the same result, and if we repeat once more: the *eidos* red is *one* over against the infinity of possible particulars which belong to this and any other red capable of being in coincidence with it then we are already in need of an infinite variation in our sense as a foundation. This variation provides us with what belongs to the *eidos* as its inseparable correlate, the so-called *extension of the eidos*, of the "purely conceptual essence," as the infinity of possible particulars which fall under it as its "particular exemplifications" and, Platonically speaking, are found with it in a relation of participation; every conceivable particular in general is referred to the essence, participates in it and in its essential moments. How the *totality* of the particulars which fall under the pure universal belong correlatively to it as its extension we will discuss forthwith.

First of all, it is necessary to point out that *even totally free variation is not enough* to actually give us the universal as pure. Even the universal acquired by variation must not yet be called *pure* in the true sense of the word, i.e., free from all positing of actuality. Although the relation to the contingent example, actually existing as a point of departure, is already excluded by the variation, a relation to actuality can still cling to the universal, and in the following way: For a pure *eidos*, the factual actuality of the particular cases by means of which we progress in the variation is completely irrelevant. And this must be taken literally. The actualities must be treated as possibilities among other possibilities, in fact as arbitrary possibilities of the imagination. This treatment is achieved only when every connection to pre-given actuality is most carefully excluded. If we practice variation freely but cling secretly to the fact that, e.g., these must be arbitrary sounds *in the* world, heard or able to be heard by men on earth, then we certainly have an essential generality as an *eidos* but one *related to our world of fact* and bound to this universal fact. It is a secret bond in that, for understandable reasons, it is imperceptible to us.

In the natural development of universal [*universalen*] experience, the unity of which is continually being realized, the experienced world is granted to us as the universal permanent ground of being and as the universal field of all our activities. As the firmest and most universal of all our habitualities, the world is valid and remains in its actual validity for us, no matter what interests we may pursue; like all interests, those involving eidetic cognition are also related to it. With all exercise of imagination, like the one which we have already considered, set in motion by the supposition of possible particulars, chosen arbitrarily and falling under a concept attained empirically, and so also with every imaginative variation involving the intention of seeing ideas, the world is coposited; every fact and every *eidos* remains related to the factual world, belonging to this world. Because of its universality, we, of course, do not notice in the natural attitude this hidden positing of the world and this bond to being.

Only if we become conscious of this bond, *putting it consciously out of play,* and so also free this broadest surrounding horizon of variants from all connection to experience and all experiential validity, do we achieve perfect purity. Then we find ourselves, so to speak, in a pure world of imagination, a *world of absolutely pure possibility.* Every possibility of this kind can then be a central member for possible pure variations in the mode of the arbitrary. From each of these possibilities results an absolutely pure *eidos,* but from any other only if the series of variations of the one and the other are linked together in a *single* series in the manner described. Thus for colors and for sounds a different *eidos* emerges; they are different in kind, and this with respect to what is purely intuited in them.

A pure *eidos,* an essential generality, is, e.g., the species red or the genus color, but only if it is apprehended as a pure generality, thus free from all presupposition of any factual existent whatsoever, any factual red or any real colored actuality. Such is also the sense of the statements of geometry, e.g., when we designate the circle as a kind of conic section, that is, when we apprehend it in an eidetic intuition; we are then not speaking of an actual surface as an instance belonging to a real actuality of nature. Accordingly, *a purely eidetic judging "in general,"* such as the geometrical, or that concerned with ideally possible colors, sounds, and the like is, in its generality, *bound to no presupposed actuality.* In geometry, we speak of conceivable figures, in eidetic color-theory of conceivable colors, which constitute the extension of purely seen generalities.

The whole of mathematics also operates with concepts originally created in this way; it produces its immediate eidetic laws (axioms) as truths which are "necessary and universal in the strict sense," "admitting of no possible exception" (Kant). It sees them as general [*generelle*] essence-complexes [*Wesensverhalte*], producible in an absolute identity for every conceivable

exemplification of its pure concepts – for those rigorously circumscribed multiplicities of variations or *a priori* extension – and, as *such,* self-evidently cognizable. From them, in a deductive intuition (*a priori* "self-evidence" of a necessary inference), mathematics then produces its theories and derived "theorems," again as ideal identities, perceptible in the arbitrary repetition of the activity which produced them.

§90. Pure generality and a priori necessity[1]

We now turn to the problem, already touched upon above, of the *extension of pure generalities* and to the problems, closely linked to this, concerning the relation of pure possibility and empirico-factual actuality.

In conformity with its origin in the method of free variation and the consequent exclusion of all positing of actual being, pure generality naturally can have no *extension consisting of facts,* of empirical actualities which bind it [to experience], but only an *extension of pure possibilities.* On the other hand, eidetic generality must always be posited in relation to admitted actualities. Every color occurring in actuality is certainly, at the same time, a possible color in the pure sense: each can be considered as an example and can be changed into a variant. Thus, in the realm of arbitrary freedom we can lift all actuality to a plane of pure possibility. But it then appears that even arbitrary freedom has its own peculiar constraint. What can be varied, one into another, in the arbitrariness of imagination (even if it is without connection and does not accord with the understanding of a reality conceivable in the imagination) bears in itself a necessary structure, an *eidos,* and therewith *necessary laws* which determine what must necessarily belong to an object in order that it can be an object of this kind. This necessity then also holds for everything factual: we can see that everything which belongs inseparably to the pure *eidos* color, e.g., the moment of brightness, must likewise belong to every actual color.

The universal truths, in which we merely display what belongs to pure essential generalities, precede all questions bearing on facts and the truths which concern them. Hence, these essential truths are called *a priori;* this means, *by reason of their validity, preceding all factuality,* all determinations arising from

---

[1] On this point, see also *Ideas,* pp. 15f.; ET, pp. 53 f. [**Original note**]

experience. Every actuality given in experience, and judged by the thinking founded on experience, is subject, insofar as the correctness of such judgments is concerned, to the unconditional norm that it must first comply with all the *a priori* "conditions of possible experience" and the possible thinking of such experience: that is, with the conditions of its pure possibility, its representability and positability as the objectivity of a uniformly identical sense.

Such *a priori* conditions are expressed for nature (for the actuality of physical experience) by the mathematics of nature with all its propositions. It expresses them "*a priori*," i.e., without dealing with "nature" as a fact. The reference to facts is the business of the *application*, which is always possible *a priori* and is self-evidently intelligible in this possibility. And now we can say in general: *judging actualities according to the laws of their pure possibility*, or judging them according to "laws of essences," *a priori* laws, *is a universal and absolutely necessary task which must be carried out for all actuality*. What is easy to make clear in the example of mathematical thinking and mathematical natural science is valid in a completely general way for *every objective sphere*. To each belongs the possibility of an *a priori* thinking, consequently an *a priori* science having the same functional application as this science – insofar as we give the a *priori* everywhere the same strict sense, the only one which is significant. There is not the slightest reason to consider the methodological structure of *a priori* thinking, as we have exhibited it in its general essential features in mathematical thinking, as an exclusive property of the mathematical sphere.[2] Indeed, in view of the general essential relationship of actuality and possibility, of experience and pure imagination, even to admit such a limitation would be completely absurd. From *every* concrete actuality, and every individual trait actually experienced in it or capable of being experienced, a path stands open to the realm of ideal or pure possibility and consequently to that of

---

[2] In this connection, however, it should be emphasized that the method of mathematical thinking of essences is, as a *method of idealization*, in important points to be distinguished from the intuition of essences in other subjects, whose fluid types cannot be apprehended with exactitude; this analogy thus holds only in the most general respects. On this difference, see also Edmund Husserl, *Crisis*, esp. pp. 16ff., 48ff.; ET, pp. 17ff., 48ff. [Original note]

a priori thinking. And in conformity with this completely general method, the method of formation of pure individual possibilities, as well as of the infinite "extensions" of the possibilities which merge into one another in the transformations of variation, is everywhere the same, and thus naturally also the originally intuitive formation of pure essential generalities pertaining to them: "ideas" (essences, pure concepts) and laws of essences.

§91. The extension of pure generalities

a. The totality of the pure extension of a concept affords no individual differentiation

Pure generalities have an extension of pure possibilities; on the other hand, they also have reference to empirical actuality as far as they "prescribe rules" to every actual thing. However, this is not to be understood as if, in addition to their extension of pure possibilities, they had an extension of actualities. This remarkable relation will become clear to us if we contrast a *pure conceptual extension* and a possible *empirical extension*.

To the extension of the pure concept "man" belong all men whom I can imagine, whether or not they are also to be found in *the* world, whether or not they are possible in the unity of this world, whether or not they are put in relation to it. They then occur in imaginings, which possibly are completely disconnected, and in other intuitions as being representable in themselves, and they constitute the explication of "a" man. It is just the same in the case of temporal durations. The extension of the idea "temporal duration" encompasses all temporal durations: those which are imaginable in a disconnected way and those which are actually experienced or capable of being experienced, as well as all temporal durations in the *one* time, namely, actual time. This *totality of the extension* of the concept of temporal duration affords *no individuation of the species* "temporal duration," just as the totality of imagined colors which belong to the smallest eidetic difference of color are not individual colors in the actual sense, are not individuations of this lowest species.

The species "duration" is specified insofar as within different intuitions, positing or not positing, interconnected or not interconnected, one can conduct a comparison of size. But then we come across the remarkable thing that within the *same* imagining and the arbitrary amplifications which pervade the unity of it and its world of imagination, and, accordingly, also within the unity of one experience, *a further differentiation* takes place, which is *not specific* and which cannot be taken out of this world; hence, if we compare the corresponding differences of one and another imaginary world, we can affirm neither identity nor nonidentity concerning them.

This is certainly true of all objective determinations, such as color, etc. But we see that it is *mediately* true of them in virtue of their temporal (and then, further, of spatial) differentiations, which are possible only in a "world." What ultimately differentiates the smallest difference of color within a world, i.e., individuates it, is the *hic et nunc,* thus the ultimate spatiotemporal difference, which on its part still also has its own specific differentiations.

There is individual differentiation only within a "world": actual individual differentiation in an actual world, possible individual differentiation in a possible one.

b. Differentiation of possibility and differentiation of actuality

How the *totality of pure conceptual extension* must be understood follows from what has been said. It refers to *pure possibilities* as its *particularizations. This logico-conceptual particularization is not a particularization of something objectively identifiable;* otherwise expressed, the logical requirement of individuality, which is the requirement of an object as an identical substrate of predicates and of objective truths (subject to the principle of noncontradiction), is not fulfilled by the particularization of a conceptual extension but is subject to the conditions of time. This means that for individual particularization we are subject to the requirement of a possibility of confirmation by a continuous connection of actual and possible (capable of being connected to actual) intuitions. *The totality of the pure extension of the concept* is not the totality of (real) objects in the world, is not an empirical totality, a totality in the *one* time.

For every essence we must therefore distinguish *two kinds of differentiations:*

1. *Differentiations according to possibility,* differentiation in the form of disconnected possibilities, referring back to disconnected imaginings or experiences giving them.
2. Differentiation within the framework of the unity of an interconnected actuality or quasi-actuality

or, better, *differentiation within the framework of a possible actuality* whose form is *one and the same* time. All such differentiations of an essence are constituted within an infinity of possible acts, which, however, are bound together insofar as they have a connection among themselves.

The universe of free possibilities in general is a *realm of disconnectedness;* it lacks a unity of context. However, every possibility which is singled out of this realm signifies at the same time the idea of a whole of interconnected possibilities, and to this whole necessarily corresponds a *unique* time. Each such whole defines a world. But two worlds of this kind are not connected with each other; their "things," their places, their times, have nothing to do with one another; it makes no sense to ask whether a thing in this world and one in that equally possible world are the same or not the same: only privative nonidentity and all relations of comparison – to call briefly to mind what was established in Part I – find an application here.

§92. The hierarchical structure of pure generalities and the acquisition of the highest concrete genera (regions) by the variation of ideas

In our investigations, pure generalities, essences of wholly different levels, have already come into prominence. For, obviously, the essences which we said determine the necessary laws for a whole sphere of objects are distinguished from those of the lowest kinds, like, for example, the *eidos* red. In other words, just as we have already been able to establish that there exists a *hierarchical structure* in the order of empirical generality, rising from lower generalities to those ever higher, so also there is naturally one for pure generalities. Which, then, are the highest, in the apprehension of which the activity of essential seeing culminates?

We start from the fact that, from one and the same example as a directive image, one can attain, by means of a free variation, pure essences which are very different. This is true in spite of the fact that all the multiplicities of variation in which an *eidos* is attained in an original seeing are linked to a unique multiplicity and, in some measure, are only aspects of a multiplicity unique in itself. For the linking of series of variations in a unique multiplicity can have a very different sense. Starting from an arbitrary red and continuing in a series of variations, we obtain the *eidos* red. If we had taken another red as our exemplary point of departure, we would certainly have obtained by intuition another multiplicity of variations; but it immediately becomes apparent that this new multiplicity belongs in the open horizon of the and-so-forth of the first, just as the first belongs in the horizon of the latter; the *eidos* is one and the same. Likewise, naturally, if we had varied an arbitrary green and had attained the *eidos* green. On the other hand, it should be noted that, in a certain way and in spite of their differences, the two series of variations, namely, that which gives the red and that which gives the green, are in their turn to be linked in an encompassing multiplicity of variations – in a unique multiplicity which no longer gives the *eidos* red or the *eidos* green but the *eidos* color in general. In the first case we have as our goal the attainment by variation of the seeing of red; for this, we must keep directing ourselves toward red; in other words, we must, despite the arbitrary nature of the activity of variation in other respects, confine ourselves to *one* direction: if at the beginning of the variation a common red lights up for us, we can then immediately arrest it and intend nothing other than red in general, therefore that identical red which any additional variation whatsoever would give us. If we are confronted with a green, we reject it as not belonging to this series of variations, as entering into conflict with the seen red which continues to be intended. If, on the other hand, we direct our interest on the fact that the variant green, which has just been rejected, is in conflict with all the variants of red and yet has something in common with them, therefore a point of coincidence, this commonality apprehended as a pure *eidos* can determine the variation: then, the multiplicities of variation for red and green, as also for yellow, etc., belong together reciprocally; the universal is now color.

Thus we could have this attitude from the start, *in the mode of a complete absence of commitment,* therefore without being committed to vary any universal already illuminated and to seek out the universal which lies beyond all the generalities which present themselves to be seen and then are limiting: in our example, the universal which lies beyond the generalities red, blue, yellow, etc., as the highest generality. For this, it is merely required that the variation, no matter how it may proceed, be simply a variation, that is, be joined together in general, in a thoroughly unified synthesis of coincidence, with a pervasive universal. *Such is the way to the constitution of the highest essential generalities as highest genera.* These are generalities which can have none higher than themselves. On the other hand, they have at the same time the property of being *contained in all the particular generalities* which it was necessary to produce in this total variation – because they belong to the limited spheres of variation of the latter – as *that which is ideally common to them.* The ideas red, green, and so forth, have an ideal participation in the idea color.

We can also say: ideas, pure generalities, can themselves function as variants in their turn, from them, one can then on a higher level intuit a universal, an *idea from ideas,* or idea of ideas, its extension is constituted by ideas, and only mediately by their ideal particulars.

In our example, the variation led to a highest abstract genus, to an *abstract essence.* For such is color; it is not an independent object, not an independent real thing existing for itself. It is extended, distributed over an extension; and extension belongs essentially to what is extended – above all, to a surface. But even this is nothing for itself but points to a body as that of which it is the limit. Thus we are finally led to a concrete object, here a spatial thing, of which the color is an abstract moment. To be sure, no process of variation from a given color leads to such an object. *Variation which sets out from the abstract always leads only to the abstract.*

But in the case of variation, we can start out *from the beginning from a concrete, independent object.* Thus, for example, by the variation of this fountain pen we come to the genus "useful object." But we can also drop this limitation and discover ever new possibilities of variation; we can, for example, imagine the fountain pen changed into a stone, and there is still something common which runs through them: both are spatially extended, material things. We have thus come to the highest genus "thing," which as the highest genus of *concreta* we call a *region.* Another region, for example, is the region "man" as a corporeal and mental essence. Regional essences have no other, higher generalities above them, and they set a fixed, unsurpassable limit to all variation. *A fundamental concept of a region cannot be converted into another by variation.* As a possible further operation, there is, at most, formalization, by which two concepts are apprehended under the formal category "something in general." But formalization is something essentially different from variation. It does not consist in imagining that the determinations of the variants are changed into others; rather, it is a disregarding, an emptying of all objective, material determinations.[3]

The higher generalities are obtained by variation of ideas. This implies that *the seeing of ideas is itself an analogue of simple experience,* insofar as it is a consciousness, to be sure, a higher and actively productive one, in which a new kind of objectivity, the universal, attains self-givenness. That which we can accomplish, beginning with experience, under the name "ideation" we can also bring about beginning with any other consciousness of a different sort, provided that it realizes something analogous, namely, brings a kind of objectivity to consciousness in original selfhood. Every form of ideation does this of itself; the idea seen is called seen here because it is not intended or mentioned vaguely and indirectly by means of empty symbols or words but is precisely apprehended directly and in itself (cf. also §88). Thus, from the basis which furnishes us with any kind of intuitive apprehending and having, we can always practice ideation, essentially by the same method.

Hence we not only can vary things of experience and thereby attain concepts of things as essential generalities, but we also "experience" sets which we have collected independently, real states of affairs, internal and external relations, whose seeing requires an activity which relates them, and so on. In this way we also obtain pure and general ideas of collections, of relations, and of every kind of state of affairs, in that, starting from the intuitive activities in which they attain givenness, we constitute precisely for all such objectivities multiplicities of variation which bring out the necessary and general essence. For the ideas obtained in this fashion we can then proceed in the same way, and so on. *We obtain therewith ideas of the "formal region": object-in-general.* It includes the ideas of the forms of possible objectivities.

§93. The difficulties of obtaining the highest genera, demonstrated in the obtaining of the region "thing"

The obtaining of the highest concrete genus, however, is not so simple as perhaps it might seem after our previous descriptions. A simple variation does not

---

[3] On this difference between generalization and formalization, cf. also *Ideas,* pp. 26f.; ET, pp. 64f.
[Original note]

provide access to it if we have not also taken methodological precautions that it be actually universal and actually take account of everything which belongs to the complete concept of a concrete region.

a. The method of establishing the example to be varied

If, to obtain the region "natural thing," we take as a point of departure either an exemplary thing of factual actuality or an already purely possible thing of pure imagination in order to carry out free variation on it, it is necessary not to overlook that the establishment of the example to be varied already demands an intricate method.

If we set out from an object of perception, it is certainly "given originally" to us in perception, but in principle only imperfectly; a systematic disclosure of the objective sense in an ongoing intuition is first required; we must first procure for ourselves a complete intuition of this thing. But we cannot freely institute an actual experience going to infinity of everything that this thing in truth is (*if* it is); on principle, what we obtain in the unity of an actual experience is something self-given imperfectly and from "one side"; what comes to self-possession as a *thing* is surrounded by a presumptive horizon, an internal horizon and an external horizon. We can at best proceed only to the unfolding of this horizon, which, with its systems of disjunctive possibilities, is a horizon of what is anticipated as possible, making clear to ourselves how subsequent experience could advance (what, in several mutually incompatible ways, it could be), how, in consequence, the thing could appear, and how it would be realized intuitively in this sequence as the same, as the unity of all these concordant appearances in the course of harmonious experience. We already stand, therefore, in a system of possible variation, we pursue one line of the possible harmonious experiences and their content of appearance, and let ourselves be continually guided by the initial perception with the objective sense established in it – but established only in such a way that this sense, with its actually and properly intuitive content, prescribes the style of the subsequent content of intuitive experience in conformity with the horizon, in the mode of a general determinability which is not an arbitrary determinability but one according to *rule.*

But, that this is true, we ourselves know only from variations and the contemplation of essences. If this is missing, then we naively follow the path from actual experience to a possible one; we naively accomplish what is intelligible to us when we talk obscurely of rendering intuitive the way in which this thing could be in an anticipation of its appearance, and which it must be for the progress of an experience to be implemented somehow or other. This possible experience is conceived here as a taking cognizance-of, as unfolding in deliberate individual apprehensions, with corresponding individual determinations (pre-conceptual determinations). We can then carry out free variation, at first by retaining (in the consciousness of free arbitrariness and the purely general) the initial contents of the perception and by throwing into relief the universal of the style being examined. But we can also drop the commitment to the initial content insofar as we change the initial perception into pure possibility and think this possibility itself

as varying freely, indeed as arbitrary and capable of being pursued in conformity with all the horizons of sense, including the systems resulting from them of the possible arrangement of experience in the style of harmonious experience of the same. In orienting regard, not toward subjective acts, but toward what is experienced in them as a thing, toward the thing experienced as always remaining identical and toward its various properties, there arises, in the variation and in the continuous self-coincidence in the universal, the *self-same in general*, in the general determinations which accrue to it in general. The generality which belongs to the fact, and to every possible fact (particular case) not fact but as far as it can be represented as at all the same and as a modification of the exemplary fact, is a pure generality, referred to pure possibilities.

Max Scheler (1874–1928)

Editors' introduction

Max Scheler is in many ways the forgotten phenomenologist. During his lifetime his philosophy was widely discussed in European intellectual circles and the breadth of his influence was impressive. It included Walther Rathenau (the industrialist, public intellectual and foreign minister in the Weimar Republic who was assassinated by right-wing extremists in 1922 because of his Jewish ancestry), Thomas Mann (the novelist and Nobel Laureate), the psychiatrist Kurt Schneider, and an entire school of sociology ('sociology of knowledge'). Scheler was also greatly praised by his philosophical colleagues.[1] Yet, compared to Husserl and Heidegger, the secondary literature on him is small[2] and his name is rarely mentioned in current philosophical discussions. He wrote on a very wide array of topics including psychopathology (see p. 241–250) and influenced a generation of European psychiatrists who were trying to take a phenomenological approach to psychopathology (see Parts II and III).

Scheler's philosophy is hard to summarize, not least because of the complexity of his writing style and the various kinds of writings he produced. He also changed some of his core views throughout his life. However, a thread running throughout his work is the question 'What is the human being?' Much of his work aimed to show that answering this question meant addressing what he considered to be key metaphysical issues (Scheler 2009b). In the following we address some of his dominant themes.

Scheler's conception of phenomenology

Though Scheler was not a student or follower of Husserl he sympathized with Husserl's point of departure and considered himself allied to the phenomenological movement (Spiegelberg 1965, pp. 228–31) Early on, he was much less convinced than Husserl of the possibility of there being a programmatic phenomenology or a 'rigorous science' and, foreshadowing Heidegger, he positioned himself against the idea that knowledge is, or ought to be, constituted from consciousness in the manner of Husserl's transcendental reduction.

> A philosophy based on phenomenology must be characterized first of all by the most intensely vital and most immediate contact with the world itself, that is, with those things in the world with which it is concerned
>
> (Scheler 1973a, p. 138).

Like Bergson, he thought that knowledge of others could be direct and that living creatures (animals) had sympathetic knowledge of the other that involved no reflective consciousness. Self-knowledge, or reflective consciousness, Scheler thought was a late developmental achievement, which, in the human being, gave a form of knowledge that was entirely different to the forms of knowing which we share with the animal kingdom.

Later on, Scheler came to think that the phenomenological reduction could be thought of as a way of highlighting this non-animal kind of knowledge (for which he uses the German word *Geist*) – bringing it, as it were, into relief. But he thought that this required a more radical philosophical technique of

---

[1] Heidegger called him 'the strongest philosophical force in modern Germany, nay, in contemporary Europe and in contemporary philosophy as such'; see Heidegger (1984), 'The Metaphysical Foundations of Logic'. In *In memoriam Max Scheler*. Translated by Michael Heim. Bloomington, IN: Indiana University Press: 50–2. The Spanish philosopher Oretega y Gasset called him 'the first man of the philosophical paradise' in Jose Ortega y Gasset, *Obras Completas*, vol. IV, p. 510. Hans-Georg Gadamer simply recalled: 'he was completely incredible'; see Gadamer (1987, p. 27). **[Editors' note]**

[2] An introduction to his work in English has been written by the editor of his collected works, Manfred Frings; see Frings (1995). **[Editors' note]**

cancellation of interests and drives (a cancellation of what he called *Drang*) than the epoché and phenomenological reduction that Husserl outlined. He compared his concept of the phenomenological reduction to the Buddha's meditative technique and he thought it qualitatively transformed objects in the world – sheering them away from space and time and from their constraints (Scheler 2009a, pp. 37–8). For Scheler, later in his life, the phenomenological reduction (as reinterpreted by him) became an integral part of his philosophy. It was what the human being did, or could do, to obtain knowledge in the mode of *Geist* (spiritual knowledge).

Values and the stratification of the emotional life

Scheler saw the human as, first and foremost, an emotional being. He thought that Western philosophy overemphasized rationality, ignoring the central importance of emotions as forms of knowledge of real (e.g. other human beings) and ideal (e.g. values) entities. Following Blaise Pascal, he spoke of a 'logic of the heart' and in his early work (*Formalism in Ethics and Non-Formal Ethics of Values*, 1913–16; Scheler 1973b) he tried to extend phenomenology into the realm of human emotional life and discover its a priori structures. He thought of values as entities that existed objectively and were revealed by the intentionality of emotions.

Scheler thinks human emotions are directed toward the values of the sensory or useful, and when these have a positive valence emotions of agreeableness are experienced. The prototypical human where this value predominates is the 'bon vivant' or 'entrepreneur'. This, according to Scheler, is a value rank that is lowest in an objective value hierarchy and that humans share with animals. Next are emotions that are directed toward the noble or ignoble, which, when having positive valence, are emotions of vitality. Scheler thinks these emotions are also shared with the animal kingdom. The prototype where this value predominates is the 'hero'. Conversely, values of the Mind and the Holy are not experienced by animals, according to Scheler. When human beings feel beauty or truth or justice, Scheler thinks they are experiencing emotions that have Mind or mental values as their object. Feeling such values is typical, for example, for the sage. When humans feel awe or humility, bliss or despair they are emoting about the value rank of the Holy. For Scheler, the saint is the model human corresponding to this rank of emotion and value.

The values any given human feels will depend upon a raft of 'real' factors such as their socio-economic time and place and Scheler thinks there are laws to be found here: for example he thought that humans vary with respect to their chances of feeling mental values (differences in intelligence, leisure time, culture and education, for example, would be critical) but equal with respect to their chances of feeling holy values (he did not accept, for example, Nietzsche's teaching that poverty or suffering must distort the perception of higher values).

Scheler gives us a model of the human being as a being emotionally lured by, or directed toward, values which surround it. He outlined various essential laws, which he thought led to a stratification of emotional life, and various ways self-deception could occur. The main law of the value hierarchy was that the values further up the rank (values of the Mind and the Holy) are the least powerful: as human beings we are most effectively lured by, or directed toward, values, which we share with the animal world.

Knowing other minds

Much of Scheler's thinking here consists of countering what he thinks are mostly self-engendered problems in philosophies of mind which have insufficient appreciation of the phenomenon of 'life'. He thinks that the rationalist stream in Western thought has tended to believe that self-awareness is prior to knowledge of others. This, Scheler thinks, gets the order wrong. Humans, Scheler believes, live foremost within other's mental lives and, as it were, passively imbibe the mental lives of others. Self-knowledge is built up through a gradual process of separation from the mental life of others. Our knowledge is, as it were, 'with' others before it is 'ours'. If this were not the case, according to Scheler, we would fail to be able to account for a range of ordinary experience – including experiences we share with animals.

Scheler also thinks that the empiricist stream in Western thought has tended to regard knowledge of others as inferred, or derived, from the sensory data of other people's bodies. This, he thinks, presupposes a mode which is associated with unusual, artificial and learnt stances toward others like that of a medical scientist toward a patient. It gets, according to Scheler, the phenomenological facts wrong. The knowledge of others occurs against a background of one vast field of expression (the body being the principal organic field) in which particular expressive unities stand out. The body does not stand out to us originally as an object (this requires a particular kind of representational work which, according to Scheler, we perform rarely). So, for example, we don't ordinarily interpret the redness of the cheek via a scientific route (a knowledge that would implicate the dilation of capillaries secondary to changes in autonomic nervous system activity implicating a change in the other's emotional state). This, says Scheler, is completely different from the immediate vicarious knowledge given to us in expressive unities: the shame of the blush, the entreaty of the outstretched hands, the threat of the clenched fist.

Philosophical anthropology

A few weeks before his death in 1928 Scheler wrote: 'The question, "what is the human being and what is his place in being?" has occupied me more fundamentally than any other question I have dealt with' (Scheler 2009, p. 3). Heidegger conceptualized the human in *Being and Time* as that being for whom being is a question. Both philosophers saw the human as an opening on being in general. Heidegger with his 'analytic of Dasein' distanced philosophical anthropology from the human sciences, approaching it through the Presocratics and poetry. Scheler's approach was more positive toward the sciences. He sought to clarify what he saw as the preconditions of the different human sciences (e.g. biological, psychological, economic, sociological, cultural). He thought this would help prevent the sciences making claims that went beyond what was metaphysically possible for them. For Scheler this would assist the development of knowledge of the spheres of being which converged in the human and their laws. In his model these spheres included the sphere of the body as inanimate object (any perspective on the human presupposing inert matter – i.e. the perspective of physics or chemistry), the sphere of the lived body (any perspective presupposing the human as living and expressive), the sphere of the other (any perspective presupposing the social world), the sphere of the psyche (any perspective presupposing drives, instincts, associative memory, practical intelligence

and the ability to make choices) and the sphere of spirit (any perspective presupposing culture). He saw philosophical anthropology as an open activity existing in relation to the human sciences capable of yielding knowledge of the human being as a whole. He died whilst he was actively advancing this project and only glimpses of his vision are available. We include a few excerpts but refer the interested reader to other translated writings.[3]

---

[3] In the Preface to his book (2009) *The Human Place in the Cosmos*. Translated by M. Frings. Evanston, IL: Northwestern University Press. Scheler writes: 'If the reader wants to get to know the stages of the development of my views on the immense subject under discussion, I would recommend the readings of my work given below in the following sequence.' Scheler lists:

1. (1973) On the ideas of man. Trans. C. Nabe. *Journal of the British Society for Phenomenology* 9(3).

2. (2007) *Ressentiment*. Trans. W. W. Holdheim. Milwaukee, WI: Marquette University Press.

3. Specific sections of (1973) *Formalism in Ethics and Non-Formal Ethics of Values*. Evanston, IL: Northwestern University Press. Translated by M. Frings and R. L., Funk. 'especially the elaboration on the experience of reality and those on perception in part III. Concerning my rejection of naturalistic theories about the human being, see part V, sections 4 & 5; concerning the stratification of emotional life, see part V, section 8; concerning "person", see part VI, A. Also consult the index under "man", "physical", "psychic", and so on'.

4. Relevant sections concerning the specifics of our emotive life in (1954) *The Nature of Sympathy*. Trans. P. Heath. London: Routledge and Kegan Paul.

5. The relationship between the human being and theories about history and society (1958) 'Man and History'. In *Philosophical Perpectives*. Trans. Haak. O. A. Boston, MA: Beacon, and (1980) *Die Wissenformen und die Gesellschaft*. London: Routledge and Kegan Paul. Of the works in this book *Erkenntnis und Arbeit* has not been translated but 'Problems of a sociology of knowlededge' has (Trans. M. Frings). Routledge & Kegan Paul (1980).

6. Humanity's potential for development Man in an era of Adjustment. In (1958) *Philosophical Perpectives*. Trans. O. A. Haak. Boston, MA: Beacon.

Scheler also makes reference to unpublished work in the foundations of biology, philosophical anthropology, theory of cognition and metaphysics. A collection of writings from his Nachlass including these themes is now published in English as *The Constitution of the Human Being* (2009b). [**Editors' note**]

Scheler sought a philosophical anthropology – a model of the human being as a whole – but he viewed his own seeking as an activity of 'becoming'; indeed he called his philosophy 'the philosophy of the open hand'. There seemed to be a tension between two qualities characterizing Scheler –that of a constant commitment to metaphysics and that of a restless revision of his own metaphysical commitments; but a tension of being (*Geist* and *Drang*) also characterized what he thought was the essence of the human – a being which houses two separate beings (*Geist* and *Drang*) which co-exist and interpenetrate. In the human '*Geist* and *Drang* are dovetailed' wrote Scheler (Scheler 2009a, p. 62). The spiritualization of life and the enlivening of spirit was for him a uniquely human task and responsibility. It was for Scheler the moral 'End' or final purpose but it was a becoming End or an unfinished purpose mirroring his concept of the 'God-in-becoming' that he thought was reciprocally related to each human being.

On phenomenology

Scheler, M. (1913/14), 'Phenomenology and the theory of cognition'

From (1973) *Selected Philosophical Essays.* Translated by D. Lachterman. Evanston, IL: Northwestern University Press: 136–201. Originally published as (1913/14) *Phänomenologie und Erkenntnislehre.* Now in vol. 10 of the *Collected Works.* Bonn, Germany: Bouvier Verlag.

It is the name of an attitude of spiritual seeing in which one can see [er-schauen] or experience [er-leben] something which otherwise remains hidden, namely, a realm of facts of a particular kind. I say "attitude" not "method". A method is a goal-directed procedure of thinking about facts, for example induction or deduction. In phenomenology, however, it is a matter, first of new facts, themselves, before they have been fixed by logic, and, second, of a procedure of seeing ... that which is seen and experienced is given only in the seeing and experiencing act itself, in its being acted out [*Vollzug*]; it appears in this act and only in it. It does not simply stand there and let itself be observed so that now this feature, now that, stands out in relief

*****

... in the presence of science the colors themselves, their pure content, turn into a mere X which

corresponds to this motion, this nervous process, this sensation. X, however, is not given itself. Thus draft after draft is drawn on red, so to speak. So long as we remain within science these drafts are negotiated in infinitely varied ways against other drafts which are drawn on red, but they are never redeemed.

Now phenomenology is, in principle, that mode of cognition ... which redeems all the drafts ... and the attitude phenomenological philosophy has toward a religious object or an ethical value is exactly the same as the one is has toward the color red.

Thus, what constitutes the unity of phenomenology is not a particular region of facts, such as, for example, mental or ideal objects, nature, etc., but only self-givenness in all possible regions.

This clearly shows that phenomenology has just as much and just as little to do with psychology as it has with mathematics, with logic, with physics, with biology, or with theology – and not a bit more.

*****

Phenomenological philosophy is distinguished from the prevalent forms of empiricism and rationalism by the fact that it is interested in the total mental experience which takes place in intentional acts, or in any of the forms of "consciousness of something", not only in the "representation" of objects. (The word "representation" is used here not in contrast to perception, but as signifying the unity of "theoretical" behavior.) In principle, the world is given in lived-experience as the "bearer of values" and as "resistance" as immediately as it is given as an "object".

*****

The phenomenological philosopher, thirsting for the lived-experience of being, will above all seek to drink at the very sources in which the contents of the world reveal themselves. His reflective gaze rests only on that place where lived-experience and its object, the world, touch one another. He is quire unconcerned whether what is involved here is the physical or the mental, number or God, or anything else. The "Ray" of reflection should try to touch only what is "there" in this closest and most living contact and only so far as it is there. In this sense, but only in this sense, phenomenological philosophy is the most radical empiricism and positivism.

Scheler, M. (1928), Selections from *Man's Place in Nature*

From (1971) *Man's Place in Nature*. Translated by H. Meyeroff. New York: Noonday Press. Originally published as (1928) *Die Stellung des Menschen im Kosmos*. Now in vol. 9 of the *Collected Works*. Bouvier Verlag: Bonn, Germany.

What does it mean to "de-actualise" the world or to "ideate" it? It does not mean, as Husserl believed, to suspend the existential judgment which is inherent in every natural act of perception ... No what it means is to suspend, at least tentatively, the experience of reality itself, or to annihilate the entire, indivisible, powerful impression of reality together with its affect-ive corollates. What it means is to remove the "anguish of earthly existence" which, as Schiller wrote, is over-come only "in those regions where the pure forms dwell". For all reality, because it is reality, and regard-less of what it is, is a kind of inhibiting, constraining pressure for every living being. Its corollate is "pure" anxiety, an anxiety without an object.

On feelings and value

Scheler, M. (1913–16), 'Feeling and feeling states'

From (1973) *Formalism in Ethics and Non-Formal Ethics of Values*. Translated by M. Frings and R. Funk. Evanston, IL: Northwestern University Press: 253–60. Originally published as (1913–16) *Der Formalismus in der Ethik und die Materiale Wertethik*. Now in vol. 2 of the *Collected Works*. Bonn, Germany: Bouvier Verlag.

Until recent times philosophy was inclined to a preju-dice that has its historical origin in antiquity. This prejudice consists in upholding the division between "reason" and "sensibility", which is completely inad-equate in terms of the structure of the spiritual.[4] This division demands that we assign everything that is not rational – that is not order, law, and the like – to sensibility. Thus our whole emotional life – and, for most modern philosophers, our conative life as well,

---

[4] The German word is *Geist* for which it is hard to find an exact equivalent in English. 'Spirit' or 'Mind' in the sense of 'life of the Mind' comes closest. It connotes all of cultural, artistic, intellectual, ethical and theological activity. [**Editors' note**]

even love and hate – must be assigned to "sensibility". According to this division, everything in the mind which is alogical, e.g., intuition, feeling, striving, loving, hating, is dependent on man's psychophysical organisation. The formation of the alogical becomes here a function of real changes in organisation during the evolution of life and history, and dependent on the peculiarities of the environment and all their effects. Whether there are original as well as essential differentiations in rank among the essences of acts and functions at the base of the alogical of our Mental life, that is, whether these acts and functions have an "originality" comparable to that of the acts in which we comprehend objects in pure logic – in other words, whether there is also a pure intuition and feeling, a pure loving and hating, a pure striving and willing, which is as independent of the psychophysical organisation of man as pure thought, and which at the same time possess their own original laws that cannot be reduced to law of empirical psychic life – this question is not even asked by people who share this prejudice.

*****

First, we must distinguish between the intentional "feeling of something" and mere feeling states ... There is original emotive intentionality. Perhaps this is most apparent when both a feeling and feeling it occur simultaneously, when a feeling is that toward which feeling is directed. Let us consider a feeling-state that is indubitably sensible, e.g., a sensible pain or state of pleasure, or a state that corresponds to the agreeableness of food, a scent, or a gentle touch, etc. Given such facts, such feeling-states, the kind and mode of feeling them is by no means yet determined. There are changing facts involved when I "suffer", "endure", "tolerate", or even "enjoy" "pain". What varies here isn't the function quality of feeling it ... is certainly not the state of pain. Nor is this variation to be found in general attention, with its levels of "noticing", "heeding", "noting", "observing", and "viewing". Pain observed is almost the opposite of pain suffered ... An individual can suffer the same degree of pain more or less than another individual.

Hence feeling-states and feeling [intentional feel-ing] are totally different ...

All specifically sensible feelings are, by their nature, states. They may be "connected" with objects through the simple contents of sensing, representing, or per-ceiving; or they may be more or less "objectless".

Whenever there is such a connection, it is always mediate. The subsequent acts of relating which follow the givenness of a feeling connect feelings with objects. This is the case, for instance, when I ask myself: "Why am I in this or that mood today?" "What is it that causes my sadness or joy?" ... I relate the object and the feeling-state in such cases through "thinking". The feeling itself is not originally related to an object, e.g., when I "feel the beauty of snow-covered mountain in the light of the setting sun" ...

However, the connection between intentional feeling and what is therein felt is entirely different from the above connection. This connection is present in all feeling of values(*). There is here an original relatedness, a directedness of feeling toward something objective, namely values ... This feeling ... has the same relation to its value-correlate as "representing" has to its "object", namely, an intentional relation ... feeling originally intends its own kind of objects, namely, "values". Feeling is therefore a meaningful occurrence that is capable of "fulfilment" and "non-fulfilment" (**).

*****

Let us call these feelings that receive values the class of intentional functions of feelings. It is not necessary for these functions to be connected with the objective sphere through the mediation of so-called objectifying acts of representation, judgement, etc. Such mediation is necessary only for feeling-states, not for genuine intentional feeling. During the process of intentional feeling, the world of objects "comes to the fore" by itself, but only in terms of its value-aspect. The frequent lack of pictorial objects in intentional feeling shows that feeling is originally an "objectifying act" that does not require the mediation of representation ... one overlooks these facts – indeed, even the task of setting them forth – if one assigns the entire sphere of feeling to psychology *originaliter*

*****

(*) Hence we distinguish:

1. ... feeling states ... e.g. suffering, enjoying. I wish to add that ... the feeling of the feeling-state itself can approximate a zero point. Very strong affectations of fright (e.g. on the occasion of an earthquake) often produce a virtually complete absence of feeling (Jaspers' General

Psychopathology, which I just received, gives some good descriptions of this.). In these cases sensitivity remains intact, and there is no reason to assume that the feeling-states are not present. What occurs ... is a marked increase in the intensity of the feeling[-state]; there is complete fulfilment by it, which makes us for a moment "feelingless" with respect to this feeling[-state]. We are put into a state of rigid and convulsive "indifference" toward it. In this case it is only when the feeling[-state] goes away, or when our complete fulfilment by it begins to disappear, that the feeling[-state] becomes an object of feeling proper [a feeling of feelings]. The rigid indifference begins to "dissolve", and we feel the feeling ...

2. The feeling of objective emotional characteristics of the atmosphere (restfulness of a river, serenity of the skies, sadness of a landscape), in which there are emotionally qualitative characteristics that can also be given as qualities of feeling, but never as "feelings", i.e. as experiences in relatedness to an ego. [i.e. they are intentional perhaps but not cognitive]

3. The feeling of values, e.g. agreeable, beautiful, good. It is here that feeling gains a cognitive function in addition to its intentional nature, whereas it does not do so in the first two cases.

(**) For this reason all "feeling of" is in principle "understandable", whereas pure feeling-states are subject only to observation and causal explanation.

On knowledge of other minds

Scheler, M. (1922), Selections from *The Nature of Sympathy*

From (1954) *The Nature of Sympathy*. Translated by P. Heath. London: Routledge: 9–12. Originally published as from *Wesen und Formen der Sympathie* (1922). Now in vol. 7 of the *Collected Works*. Bonn, Germany: Bouvier Verlag.

We shall not, at present, give any detailed account of those acts which serve to establish the existence of other people and their experiences ... But that 'experiences' occur there is given for us in expressive phenomena – again, not by inference, but directly, as a sort of primary 'perception'. It is in the blush that we perceive shame, in the laughter joy. To say that 'our only initial datum is the body' is completely erroneous. This is true only for the doctor or the scientist, i.e. for man in so far as he abstracts artificially from the expressive phenomena, which have an altogether primary givenness. It is rather that the same basic sense-data which go to make up the body for outward perception, can also construe, for the act of insight, the expressive phenomena which then appear, so to speak, as the 'outcome' of experiences within. For the relation here referred to is a symbolic, not a causal one.[5] We can thus have insight into others, in so far as we treat their bodies as a field of expression for their experiences. In the sight of clasped hands, for example, the 'please' is *given* exactly as the physical object is – for the latter is assuredly given as an object (including the fact that it has a back and a side), in visual phenomenon. However, the qualities (i.e. the character) of expressive phenomena and those of experiences exhibit connections of a unique kind, which do not depend at all on previous acquaintance with real experiences of our own, plus the other's expressive phenomena, such that a tendency to *imitate* the movements of the gesture seen would first have to reproduce our own earlier experiences. On the contrary, imitation, even as a mere 'tendency', already presupposes some kind of acquaintance with the other's experience, and therefore cannot explain what it is here supposed to do. For instance, if we (involuntarily) imitate a gesture of fear or joy, the imitation is never called forth simply by the visual image of the gesture; the impulse to imitate only arises when we have already apprehended the gesture as an expression of fear or joy. If this apprehension itself were only made possible, by a tendency to imitate and by the *reproduction*, thus evoked, of a previously experienced joy or fear (*plus* an empathic projection of what is reproduced into the other person), we should obviously be moving in a circle. And this applies also to the 'involuntary' imitation of gestures. It already presupposes an imitation of the inner intention of action, which could be realized by quite different bodily movements. We do not imitate the same or similar bodily movements in observed connections of the inorganic, e.g. in

inanimate nature, where they cannot be phenomena expressive of psychic experience. Further evidence against [this] theory of imitation lies in the fact that we can understand the experience of animals, though even in 'tendency' we cannot imitate their manner of expression; for instance when a dog expresses its joy by barking and wagging its tail, or a bird by twittering. The relationships between expression and experience have a *fundamental* basis of connection, which is independent of our specifically human gestures of expression. We have here, as it were, *a universal grammar*, valid for all languages of expression, and the ultimate basis of understanding all forms of mime and pantomime among living creatures. Only so are we able to perceive the *inadequacy* of a person's gesture to his experience, and even the contradiction between what the gesture expresses and what it is meant to express. ... The only way of explaining imitation, and the reproduction of a personal experience similar to that underlying a perceived expressive gesture, is that through this a genuine experience takes place in me, objectively similar to that which occurs in the other person whose expression I imitate. For such objective similarity of experience, however, there need be no present consciousness of the similarity, still less an intentionally directed act of 'understanding' or a reproduction of feeling or experience ... one who 'understands' the mortal terror of a drowning man has no need at all to undergo such terror, in a real, if weakened form ...

It also seems clear that what this theory[6] could explain for us, is the very opposite of genuine 'understanding'. This opposite is that infection by other's emotions, which occurs in its most elementary form in the behaviour of herds and crowds. Here there is actually a common making of expressive gestures in the first instance, which has the secondary effect of producing similar emotions, efforts and purposes among the people or animals concerned; thus, for instance, a herd takes fright on seeing signs of alarm in its leader, and so too in human affairs. But it is characteristic of the situation that there is a complete lack of mutual 'understanding'. Indeed the purer the case, inasmuch as a rudimentary act of understanding plays little or no part in it, the more clearly do its peculiar features emerge, namely that the participant

---

[5] We might also say that it is not the mere relation of a 'sign' to the presence of 'something', whereby the latter is subsequently inferred; it refers to a genuine, irreducible property of the sign itself. [**Original note**]

[6] Scheler is referring to Theodor Lipp's projective or imitative theory of empathy. [**Editors' note**]

takes the experience arising from him owing to his participation to be his own original experience, so that he is quite unconscious of the contagion to which he succumbs. This resembles those post-hypnotically suggested acts of will which are carried out without awareness of suggestion (unlike the obeying of commands, where one remains consciously aware that the other's will is not one's own); such acts indeed, are characteristically regarded by the agent as being his own, and so too the experiences arising through participation in a common gesture of expression are ascribed, not to others, but to oneself. For this reason, even in daily life, we distinguish between aping someone ('taking him off', for instance) and really understanding him, and point the contrast between them.

*****

But now let us enquire if the twofold starting-point ... is phenomenologically accurate: 1. that it is always our own self, merely, that is primarily given to us; 2. that what is primarily given in the case of others is merely the appearance of the body, its changes, movements, etc. and that only on the strength of this do we somehow come to accept it as animate and to presume the existence of another self.

Both assumptions commend themselves as self-evident, and both readily appeal to the fact that 'it could not be otherwise'. How indeed could we think any other thoughts, feel any other feelings than 'our own'? And how else should we come to know of the body? What else is there to perceive of him except his body? It is only from thence that our sense-organs receive stimuli, and only by means of such physical processes can there be any intercourse between individual minds.

Let us remember, however, that there is nothing of which the philosopher must be more wary than taking something to be self-evident, and then, instead of looking to seeing what is given, turning his attention to what 'can be given' according to some supposed realistic theory. For it will be evident that the foregoing assumptions involve a complete departure from the phenomenological standpoint, replacing it – and covertly at that – by a realistic one.[7]

1. For who can say that it is our own individual self and its experiences which are 'immediately given' in that mode of intuition, by which alone the mental, a self and its experiences, can possibly be apprehended, namely in inner intuition or perception? Where is the phenomenological evidence for this assertion?[8]

What is the meaning of the proposition that 'a man can only think his own thoughts and feel his own feelings?'. What is 'self-evident' about it? This only, that if once we postulate a real substratum for the experiences, of whatever kind, which I may happen to have, then all the thoughts and feelings which occur in me will in fact belong to this real substratum. And that is a tautology. Two real substrata, two soul-substances, for instance, or two brains, certainly cannot enter into one another, or switch from one to the other. But for the moment let us leave such questionable metaphysical hypotheses to one side. However, if we do seriously abandon these and all the presuppositions of realism in general, and stick to pure phenomenology, our proposition loses all semblance of being 'self-evident'. For nothing is more certain than that we think the thoughts of others as well as our own, and can feel their feelings (in sympathy) as we do our own. Are we not for ever distinguishing 'our own' thoughts from those we have read or which have been told to us? 'Our own' feelings from those we merely reproduce, or by which we have been infected (unconsciously, as we later realize)? 'Our own' will from that which we merely obey and which is plainly manifest to us at the time as the will of another, just as we distinguish our own true will from that which we are deceived into thinking our own, though it has been suggested to us by something else, in hypnosis, for instance? Even in these very trivial examples we find a string of 'possible' cases of what is supposed, on present assumptions, to be 'self-evidently' impossible. It may well be that our

---

[7] Scheler means that explanatory theories of psychology may covertly obfuscate phenomenological clarity. [Editors' note]

[8] The act of 'inner perception' is of a different polarity from that of 'outer perception' (and one in which there is no necessity for it to operate through sensory functions, let alone the sense organs). This distinction obviously has nothing to do with what is 'inside' or 'outside' for any given individual. 'Inner perception' is essentially concerned with apprehension of the mental, and it makes no difference to this whether perception is of oneself or another. On this subject cf. also see the essay on (1973c) 'The idols of self-knowledge'. [Original note]

thoughts are presented 'as' our own, and those of others as theirs, e.g. in merely understanding a piece of information. That is the normal case. But it may also happen that the thought of another is not presented as such, but as a thought of ours. Such is the case, for instance, in 'unconscious reminiscence' of things read or communicated. It also occurs when, imbued with a genuine tradition, we accept the thoughts of others, e.g. of our parents or teachers, as thoughts of our own: we then 'reproduce' such thoughts (or feelings) vicariously, without being explicitly conscious of the function of intellectual or emotional reproduction. And hence they appear to us as our own. It may also happen that one of our own thoughts or feelings is presented as belonging to someone else. Thus the mediaeval writers were often given to reading their own thoughts or those of their own time into the sources and documents of classical antiquity, thereby fathering Christian modes of thought upon Aristotle, for example. Whereas the tendency in modern times has been to take up ideas which have been unconsciously acquired and thought a thousand times, and put them forward as new and original, the older (mediaeval) habit was to extract ideas which actually were new and original from such authors as were invested with special authority. The latter represents the case of 'delusive empathy'. Just because the process of empathy is not explicit here, the individual's experience appears to him as having been derived from someone else.

It is possible, therefore, as these examples show, for the same experiences to be given both 'as our own' and 'as someone else's'; but there is also the case in which an experience is simply given, without presenting itself as our own or as another's, as invariably happens, for example, where we are in doubt as to which of the two it is.

*****

But how then is it possible to observe the mental life of another person? Let us now go on from the phenomenological fact that a mental experience may be presented in 'internal perception' regardless of whether it is 'my' experience or (characteristically) someone else's, to the question how such a thing is possible. For is not 'internal perception' necessarily also a perception of oneself? Is it possible to have internal perception of the self and the inner life of another person?

This question has hitherto received an unhesitatingly negative answer for the simple reason that no distinction has been drawn between the sphere of internal intuition (or those of internal perception, representation, feeling and the like), and the sphere of 'inner sense'. But 'internal intuition' can certainly not be defined by reference to its object, by saying that a person engaged in such intuition is perceiving 'himself'. For I can perceive myself in an external sense just as much as I can perceive anyone else. Every glance at my own body, every touch upon it, confirms the fact. If I touch my thumb with my middle finger, the double sensation still consists of one and the same sensory content at the surface of the two separate parts of the body. Thus internal perception represents a polarity among acts, such acts being capable of referring both to ourselves and to others. This polarity is intrinsically capable of embracing the inner life of others as well as my own, just as it embraces myself and my own experience in general, and not merely the immediate present. To be sure, certain conditions are required before the experiences of others can be presented to me in the act of internal intuition.

*****

It is a crucial objection to the view that mental life is essentially private that if its premises were correct, we ought equally to be led to the conclusion that Nature is also a private affair ... The only incorrigible certainty would be the existence of the solipsist's own momentary self. Now we actually approach such solipsism of the moment the more we confine our existence to our own body. And there is another conclusion of no less importance than this: anyone who denies our ability to perceive other selves and their experiences must equally be prepared to deny the perceptibility of matter.

2. But let us now turn to the other 'self evident' assumptions ... What else, it may be asked, can I be supposed to perceive of another man apart from his 'body' and the movements he makes?

Now to begin with, it only needs the simplest of phenomenological considerations to show that at any rate there is nothing self-evident about this. For we certainly believe ourselves to be directly acquainted with another person's joy in his laughter, with his sorrow and pain in his tears, with his shame in his blushing, with his entreaty in his outstretched hands, with his love in his look of affection, with his rage in the gnashing of his teeth, with his threats in the clenching of his fist, and with the tenor of this thoughts in the sound of his words. If anyone tells me that this is not 'perception', for it cannot be so, in view of the fact that a perception is simply a 'complex of physical sensations', and that there is certainly no sensation of another person's mind nor any stimulus from such a source, I would beg him to turn aside such questionable theories and address himself to the phenomenological facts. All he need do in the first place is to compare these examples with cases which actually exhibit what his theories lead him to accept a priori in the present instance, namely a conclusion amenable to proof. Thus, for example, the actions of a man with whom I have previously spoken, and whose feelings and intentions were, as I thought, plain to me, may yet compel me to the conclusion that either I have misunderstood him and deceived myself, or else that he has been lying or pretending to me. Here then I do actually draw conclusions about his state of mind. Again, by a similar inference from his looks to his thoughts and feelings, I may even prepare myself in advance, e.g. in dealing with someone whom I fear to be deranged or mad, or where I suspect dissimulation or an intention to deceive. I do this, in effect, wherever I find my internal and vicarious perception of his experiences unduly checked in any way, or where I am compelled for specific positive reasons, themselves derived (in the last resort) from perception, to postulate a discrepancy between inner experience and outer expression, an (involuntary or deliberate) breach of their symbolic interrelation – a relation which holds good regardless of the particular experiences or circumstances of the individual concerned. It is at this point only that I begin to draw conclusions. But it should not be forgotten in this that the material premises for these conclusions are based upon my elementary perception of the person concerned or other people; and they therefore presuppose these immediate perceptions. Thus I do not merely see the other person's eyes, for example; I also see that 'he is looking at me' and even that 'he is looking at me as though he wished to avoid my seeing that he is looking at me'. So too do I perceive that he is only pretending to feel what he does not feel at all, that he is severing the familiar bond between his experience and its natural expression, and is substituting another expressive movement in place of the particular phenomenon implied by his experience. Hence I can tell that he is lying, for example, not

merely by having proof that he must be aware that he is telling it differently, and that matters are other than he says they are; for in certain circumstances I can be directly aware of his lying itself, of the very act of lying, so to speak. Again, there is sense in my saying to somebody, 'That isn't really what you meant to say: you are expressing yourself badly', i.e. I grasp the meaning he has in mind, though here it certainly cannot be deduced from his words, since, otherwise I should not be in a position to correct them by reference to the meaning already given beforehand.

It may be argued, perhaps, that although such differences occur, they do not represent a difference between perception and inference, but only the contrast between a simple, primitive or 'unconscious' form of inference and a more elaborate and conscious one. But enough of such objections, fabricated in the interests of fallacious theory and capable of proving anything or nothing.[9]

Let us now go on to consider the claim that we can have no immediate perception of anything in other people except their bodies and physical movements.

Our immediate perceptions of our fellow-men do not relate to their bodies (unless we happen to be engaged in a medical examination), nor yet to the 'selves' or 'souls'. What we perceive are integral wholes, whose intuitive content is not immediately resolved in terms of external or internal perception. From this stage of givenness we can then go on, in the second place, to adopt the attitude of internal or external perception. But the fact that the individual bodily unity thus immediately presented should be associated, in general, with a possible object accessible both to internal and external perception, is founded upon the intrinsic connection between these intuitive contents, a connection which also underlies my own perception of myself. It is not acquired through

---

[9] It is easy to point to the psychological sources of this 'theory'. It comes down to us, historically speaking, as one of a number of theories typical of the Enlightenment (the contract theory of state, the conventional theory of language, etc.), which all conceive of the origins of the community in terms of an 'artificial society' in which distrust has become a permanent attitude. See Scheler (2007) *Ressentiment*. It may be noted that we often make inferences with regard to our own experiences also; as when we say; 'What sort of man can I be to have done that?', or when we seek to account for a mood of our own which in not intelligible in terms of our present circumstances. [**Original note**]

observation and induction from my own case. Such a connection holds good for the nature of all living organisms generally[10] ... If I adopt the approach of external perception, and rely upon the unities of appearance presented therein, they will enable me to form an impression of any part of the individual's body, however small; but in any combination of such unities I shall never come upon the unity of a smile, an entreaty, a threatening gesture and so on. Again, the shade of red which visibly covers the physical surface of a man's cheek can never present the unity of a blush, whose redness appears, as it were, as the outcome of the shame which I sense him to feel. If the cheek is red, merely, the same immediate appearance of redness might equally well betray over-heating, anger or debauchery, or be due to the light from a red lamp.

Perhaps this may give us a better understanding of the supposedly 'self-evident fact' that we can only perceive the bodies of other people.

On the human being

Scheler, M. (1914), 'On the idea of man'

From (1978) *Journal of the British Society for Phenomenology* **9**(3): 184–98. Translated by C. Nabe. Originally published as (1914) *Zur Idee des Menschen*. Now in vol. 3 of the *Collected Works*. Bonn, Germany: Bouvier Verlag.

Serious investigations into nature show only that man as *homo naturalis* is an animal, a small side road which life has taken within the class of vertebrates, i.e. within the primates. Therefore he has not at all "evolved" from the natural world, but rather man was an animal, is an animal and will forever remain an animal. But the seeker of God [the human being according to Scheler] with his essential predicates – this is a new essential class of things, a realm of "persons", which did not "evolve", just as colors, numbers, space and time, and other genuine essences did not "evolve". This realm [the realm of essences or 'Geist'] discloses itself at specific points of the living world and here comes into appearance. But *homo naturalis* did not "evolve" either from animals, precisely because he just was an animal, is and will remain an animal ... what foolish hubris drives Haeckel[11] to take his body and his "association centres" for something other than an animal body and an animal mind and dare to "look back "on the animal world as a "standpoint overcome"? But no it is not hubris, it is a wretched ressentiment which led to this formula. One must gradually perceive there to be an idea of man according to which he is the locus for the emergence and coming to light of an order of things essentially distinct from all nature; its name is spirit, culture and religion. But one falsifies this idea with a concept of "man" borrowed from anatomy, physiology and psychology, as a bad magician falsifies facts ... One calls it hubris, megalomania when man formerly traced his being and essence back to God. But one does not see that hubris and megalomania are at hand when one, without a view of God, dares to set oneself over against animals and imagines oneself to be "more", which has "evolved" out of them, instead of reaching the conclusion that one is an animal which become ill and 'lost its way'.[12]

*****

There is in man neither an impulse nor "law" that does not present itself in nature beneath him or in the realm of God, in "heaven" above him. Only as a "crossing-over" from one of these realms to the other,

---

[10] This also applies to the lower organisms. It is possible for a physiologist to give a completely 'mechanistic' explanation of the wrigglings of a severed worm, and to smile (like Jacques Loeb) at the notion that it is 'wriggling with pain' (since the headless portion also wriggles). But of course it is quite absurd to argue, from the possibility of this mechanico-causal explanation, that the movement is not also expressive of pain (by alleging that the worm cannot feel pain without its head). It would be as absurd as to argue that a man's blushing cannot be an expression of shame, since it can be explained mechanistically (as indeed it can) as a rush of blood to the cheeks. For what bearing does a mechanico-causal explanation have upon symbolic functions, such as the phenomena of expression? [**Original note**]

---

[11] German materialist biologist and naturalist of Scheler's times. [**Editors' note**]

[12] The concept of the human being as a 'sick animal' made sick by its excessive cerebral development was a Nietzschean idea discussed in German intellectual circles at Scheler's time. It has affinities with Freud's idea of civilization and its discontents. [**Editors' note**]

as a "bridge" and movement between them does man have his existence.

Scheler, M. (1928), Selections from *The Human Place in the Cosmos*

From (2009) *The Human Place in the Cosmos*. Translated by M. Frings. Evanston, IL: Northwestern University Press: 57–8. Originally published as (1928) *Die Stellung des Menschen im Kosmos*. Now in vol. 9 of the *Collected Works*. Bonn, Germany: Bouvier Verlag.

It is not the pairs of human lived body [Leib] and soul, or the objective body and a soul, or that of brains and soul in humans, that represent some sort of ontological dualism. The antithesis that we find in man, and subjectively experience as such, is one of a much higher and of a much more fundamental order: the antithesis of spirit [Geist] and life [Drang] . . .

When we take the "psychic" and the "physiological" to be two sides of one and the same process of life, to which correspond two ways of looking at the same process, the X which is *acting out* the two ways of looking at one and the same thing must be *superior* to the antithesis of body and soul. The X is nothing else but spirit which, as we saw, never becomes an object – but which, nevertheless, makes everything an object. Life is non-spatial, but it is in time . . . and what we call "spirit" is not only *trans-spatial* but also *trans-temporal*. Spirit's intentionality intersects, as it were, with the temporal course of life. Insofar as spirit needs *activity*, it is indirectly dependent on temporal life processes and is, so to speak, embedded in them.

Chapter

8

Martin Heidegger (1889–1976)

Editors' introduction

Martin Heidegger is credited as one of the greatest philosophers of the twentieth century and what is unarguable is the profound impact his thought has had on intellectual developments in the last 80 years. Further, as with Jaspers, Heidegger's own development as philosopher was inspired by his own reading of Husserl and Brentano, and how his interest in the *Logical Investigations* interacted in a novel way with his understanding of Aristotle.

As he puts it in 'My way to phenomenology' (Heidegger 1972, pp. 74–5):

I had learned from many references in philosophical periodicals that Husserl's thought was determined by Franz Brentano. Ever since 1907, Brentano's dissertation "On the manifold meaning of being since Aristotle" (1862) had been the chief help and guide of my first awkward attempts to penetrate into philosophy. The following question concerned me in quite a vague manner: If being is predicated in manifold meanings, then what is its fundamental meaning? What does Being mean? ... From Husserl's *Logical Investigations*, I expected a decisive aid in the questions stimulated by Brentano's dissertation. Yet my efforts were in vain because I was not searching in the right way. I realized this only very much later. Still, I remained so fascinated by Husserl's work that I read it again and again in the years to follow without gaining sufficient insight into what fascinated me.

Husserl came to Freiberg in 1916 as Heinrich Rickert's successor. Rickert had taken over Windelband's Chair in Heidelberg. Husserl's teaching took place in the form of a step-by-step training in phenomenological "seeing" which at the same time demanded that one relinquish the untested use of philosophical knowledge. But it also demanded that one give up introducing the authority of the great thinkers into the conversation. However, the clearer it became to me that the increasing familiarity with phenomenological seeing was fruitful for the interpretation of Aristotle's writings, the less could I separate myself from Aristotle and the other Greek

thinkers. Of course I could not see what decisive consequences my renewed occupation with Aristotle was to have. As I myself practised phenomenological seeing, teaching and learning in Husserl's proximity after 1919 and at the same time tried out a transformed understanding of Aristotle in a seminar, my interest leaned anew toward the Logical Investigations, above all the sixth investigation in the first edition (p. 78).

We will focus here on Heidegger's conception of phenomenology, covered in the selections from 'The Idea of Philosophy and the Problem of Worldview' and the 'Introduction to Phenomenological Research' and specifically how it differed from Husserl's, before turning to some of his key concepts that have been employed in existential – phenomenological psychiatry. These are illustrated in the readings from his best-known and most influential work, *Being and Time*.

Heidegger's conception of phenomenology

Heidegger's critique of Husserlian phenomenology was based around two interrelated ideas. Firstly, that Husserl's concerns were too theoretical and intellectual and neglected the practical, concrete elements of life. Secondly, he saw in Aristotle's philosophy a version of a 'proto-phenomenology' that was practically engaged. He was able to develop these insights, alongside his reading of Luther and Kierkegaard, into an account of Dasein, or being-there, in his most famous and influential work, *Being and Time*.

Heidegger's understanding of phenomenology turns on Aristotle's notion, from the *Nicomachean Ethics*, of *alētheuein* (unconcealing) and his conceptualisation of the essence of human life, which he calls 'Dasein' – usually translated as 'being-there' (Figal 2010). Dasein is hence a central point of reference for other entities and their concealment/unconcealment. Hence, as with Husserl, a phenomenon for Heidegger is 'that which appears'. But now, withdrawal, absence, hiddenness too become 'phenomena' for Heidegger and his phenomenology widens to include what Figal terms 'moments of a world, which can be experienced in their significance' (Figal 2010, p. 37). Phenomenology becomes linked to the process of discovery, production, and ultimately world formation. Heidegger justified this interpretation, in part, due to his etymological analysis of phenomenology: *phainomenon* meaning that which shows itself and *logos* as making something manifest (Polt 1999). As such, Heideggerian phenomenology remains descriptive yet is also concerned with how we, as Dasein, interpret Being through time and hence has been termed a transcendental, hermeneutical, phenomenological ontology (Polt 1999). Heidegger's overriding concern, in all his thinking, is to study Being, or Ontology. Hence, given the role of the Husserlian reduction in 'bracketing off' existence, it seems perverse for Heidegger to adapt Husserlian tools for his ontological project. Heidegger gets around this by rebutting the distinction between appearance and reality: a phenomenon is simply that which shows itself. Traditional subjects and disciplines take a domain of entities and study them as objects empirically, whereas Being itself is not such an entity in the world, alongside others. As Blattner puts it (Blattner 2006):

> Being is not such a domain, but rather the structure of anything that is. Being is not a feature or property of what is manifest, but rather a meaning-structure that is latent in any experience of anything, even experiences of imaginary things (which do not exist, but present themselves as if they did). We must, therefore, study being as we study the meaning of phenomena, namely phenomenologically' (p. 30).

Ontic and ontological

A key distinction in Heidegger's *Being and Time* is that between the 'ontic' and 'ontological'. This distinction is not only important in understanding Heidegger's views of science, phenomenology and ontology but in examining how his work has been used clinically, and how Heidegger himself critiqued that use. Polt offers us some useful definitions (Polt 1999):

- Ontology is a philosophical investigation of Being.
- Ontological means pertaining to Being.
- Ontical means pertaining to particular facts about entities, without regard to their Being (p. 34).

Ontical questions, facts about individual entities, can be answered by science; ontological questions can only be answered philosophically.

Related terms are Existential and Existentiell. The former is an understanding of the ontological structure of Dasein, Dasein's way of Being. In contrast, Existentiell is a specific individual's understanding of themselves and their way of being (Dreyfus 1991; Polt 1999). Hence, and this links to Heidegger's own critique of Binswanger, when we think of ourselves as clinicians, we may have an understanding that is Existentiell, we may understand our patients ontically and help them gain an Existentiell understanding of themselves. However, only when we study Dasein in general, using phenomenological ontology do we have an Existential understanding.

Being-there (Dasein)

Dasein is a term that Heidegger uses to try and avoid a Cartesian or Husserlian conception of subject or ego. For Heidegger, it denotes an everyday human being (Dreyfus 1991), a general and human way of being he refers to as 'being-there'. What is important about Dasein, as opposed to other entities, is that how it comports itself towards Being as an issue for itself. Hence, Dasein, in Division 1 of *Being and Time*, is the tool Heidegger uses to interrogate Being, or rather in laying out Dasein's stances to itself, others, and other entities, Dasein's understanding of Being can be revealed. Dasein means 'the self as the there (Da) of being (Sein), the place where an understanding of being erupts into being' (Stapleton 2010, p. 44). The term Dasein thus emphasizes its practical, immersive qualities, and its active engagement in the world and shared social practices, as opposed to more cognitive, rational properties dominant in the Cartesian and Husserlian traditions, properties that to focus on would fail, for Heidegger, to lead to an understanding of Being.

Care (Sorge)

Care, as an Existential category of Dasein, is meant, for Heidegger, to capture the necessarily wider, ontical particularities of what individual people care about. It is simply that which we concern ourselves about: our children, our spouse, our work and ambitions, our pleasure. However, care, crucially for Heidegger, is temporal. As beings that end in death, we are aware we have to plan ahead, our projects stretch before us in time. Care, ontologically, means 'the inevitability of concern, uncertainty, insecurity, projecting ahead and maintaining all aspects of our human engagements, as well as the desirability of responsibility and dedication. The inevitability for human beings indicates the ontological character of the term, Care, as distinct from instances of concern, solicitude, and organization' (Scott 2010, p. 60). Dasein is being-towards-death and it is Care that projects us into our finite future. It is perhaps worth emphasizing that Care is not necessarily maudlin or even goal-directed – it simply indicates that Dasein is at home in the world, amidst meaningful entities, and projecting itself into the future. Care, perhaps, is close to the response we have to something that is salient for us, or as Dreyfus puts it, 'making itself an issue' (Dreyfus 1991, p. 238). Care allows Heidegger to escape relativism: it is an invariant Existential of all Dasein, allowing a structural coherent whole in time. Care 'unifies the structural aspects of Dasein in the notion of a being that makes an issue of its being' (Dreyfus 1991, p. 243).

Ready-to-hand, present-to-hand (*Zuhanden, Vorhanden*)

An important way by which Heidegger demonstrates Dasein's engagement in the world, its care and its projects through time is through its use of equipment and how it encounters them as tools. Much like the body, tools, when used fluently and unreflectively, for Heidegger, drop out of experience. They become transparent, or rather, an invisible extension or means of Dasein's goals and projects. These tools are what Heidegger calls 'ready-to-hand' (*Zuhanden*). Although Heidegger's example of the hammer is well known, his concept of a ready-to-hand piece of equipment is wider than a tool as we might understand it: it includes this keyboard I am unaware of as I type, the classificatory systems of the WHO and APA I use unreflectively when engaged in clinical work, the language I speak without much thought. These are all tools and are defined in their value and utility. These entities that are 'ready-to-hand' are contrasted by Heidegger with those that are mere things, the 'present-at-hand' (*Vorhanden*). However, as alluded to in the examples above, not all 'ready-to-hand' objects are also 'present-at-hand' (for example, more conceptual tools like those in mathematics, logic, or those employed in classificatory systems) (Blattner 2006). To summarize the 'ready-to-hand' is a sort of entity, an entity defined by its involvement in our practices' (Blattner 2006, p. 53).

However, when my computer freezes, or my car doesn't start in the morning, that which was transparent and ready-to-hand becomes 'not to hand', unready-to-hand. And part of the phenomenology of the unready-to-hand being manifest lies in our frustration, the thwarting of our goals and plans, and it is this frustration, as to what the tool should be, that separates the unready-to-hand from the merely present-at-hand, yet lack of function, in our attempt to remedy, will tend to show the structure, mechanism, interrelations, etc. of the entity more sharply in our attempt to utilize it again. 'So, in breakdown experiences, the merely present makes an appearance, usually only to withdraw from the scene again, as my activity gets underway' (Blattner 2006, p. 59).

Thrownness (*Geworfenheit*)

This term, for Heidegger, tries to capture two features of Dasein that both describe his past but limit his forward projection. The first is the brute facticity of life: once we become self-aware we are already in a certain life, culture, society and with a family and history and there are constraints upon what we are and can be, what Heidegger refers to as 'nullities'. 'I find myself thrown into a world I did not make and into a life I did not ask for' (Kisiel 2010, p. 25).

However, it also carries the notion of being concerned and occupied with life: 'we are always already attuned to and disposed in the world' (Blattner 2006, p. 78). An absence of 'nullities' would also undercut this attunement to the world and lead Dasein into nihilistic meaninglessness. We take over the historical possibilities of our situation, of our facticity, and make them our own. 'Thrownness' also serves to emphasize Heidegger's shift from Husserl: away from 'an intentionally orientated consciousness to historically situated existence' (Kisiel 2010, p. 25).

Anxiety (*Angst*)

Thrownness reveals the contingency of the self and anxiety (*Angst*) is when this self-constituting becomes apparent to us. For Heidegger, anxiety is the collapse of meaning in our lives, with Care as other aspect: the demonstration of meaning and value for Dasein, and indicating the structure by which Dasein projects its projects into the finite future.

Because we cannot understand ourselves in anxiety, we cannot feel "at home" in the world . . . . Thus, Heidgegger characterizes the ambience or atmosphere

of anxiety as uncanniness or the mode of the not-at-home (unheimlich). We are, thus, alienated from the world, not because we do not know by what we are surrounded, but rather because the world offers us nothing in terms of which to make sense of own lives
(Blattner 2006, pp. 140–1).

As well as alienating us from equipment in the world, tools we use to pursue our goals, it also alienates us from others. *Angst* closes off the future as the lack of meaning and importance renders goals for the future incoherent. 'Anxiety discloses possibilities as irrelevant or insignificant' (Blattner 2006, p. 141). Blattner here draws parallels between anxiety and what we in psychopathology refer to as anhedonia, and further suggests that Heideggerian anxiety is an equivalent of what we would term depression, as well as panic attacks and agitation. However, despite these clinical parallels, anxiety is important for Heidegger due to its role ontologically in revealing how normally Dasein is preoccupied with meaning and future projects: anxiety is so stark as it reveals the normal state of affairs and the importance our own self-making. Anxiety doesn't disclose any deep truths about whom or what we are, or our ultimate purpose, but rather discloses that such issues are important for us, and that embedded social context is important. Contrary to existentialist glosses, Heidegger's *Dasein* is not a romantic isolationist hero, but one for whom anxiety reveals the routine importance of those to whom he is close to and the projects in which he is engaged.

Heidegger, M. (1919), 'The idea of philosophy and the problem of worldview,' War Emergency Semester

From (2000) *Towards the Definition of Philosophy*. London: Athlone Press (Continuum): 53–64. Originally given as a lecture in 1919. Originally published as (1987) *Zur Bestimmung der Philosophie*. Frankfurt am Main: Vittorio Klosterman.

Analysis of the Structure of Experience

§13. The Experience of the Question: 'Is There Something?'

Already in the opening of the question 'Is there ... ?' there is something. Our *entire* problematic has arrived at a crucial point, which, however, appears insignificant and even miserly. Everything depends on understanding and following this insignificance in its pure meaning, on fastening on to it and no longer thinking back to teleological method, ideal and material giving, psychical totality, material domain of things, and indeed – even especially so – the idea of primordial science and its method. We are standing at the methodological cross-road which will decide on the very life or death of philosophy. We stand at an abyss: either into nothingness, that is, absolute reification, pure thingness, or we somehow leap into *another world*, more precisely, we manage for the first time to make the leap [*Sprung*] into the world as such.

a) The Psychic Subject

We now know that a comprehensible series of problems and questions has led us to this insignificant and miserly question. If we forget this road, we deny our provenance *and ourselves*. If *we* were not at all first here, then there would be no such question. It is clear, therefore, that in the entire course of our deliberation we have withheld an essential element whose timely incorporation would have structured our problematic differently. We have not even arrived at the psychic totality in its completeness. We spoke of psychic processes without a common binding core, and of knowledge processes without a psychic subject in which these run their course. We moved within the insuperable perplexities of a 'psychology without soul'. It is by no means necessary that we should lose ourselves in metaphysics and think of the soul as substance, but we must round off the psychic context by way of its relation to the psychic subject. In this way the object and subject-matter of psychology will be complete and the difficulties resolved.

A psychic process in itself, isolated as a thing, explains nothing. Psychic processes like sensations, perceptions and memories, are explained as cognitive processes only when they occur in a *psychic subject which* knows. In this way bridges are now also made between psychic objects and the psychic subject, and the cognitive process is traced back to its origin.

Does this new positioning of the problem, presented *in this way*, bring us anything essentially new? Does the psychic subject explain anything? The material context of the psychic has certainly arrived at a point of unity of the subject-matter, but basically we have not left the material sphere. The problem has only been shifted within the psychic context of the subject-matter. Knowing as a psychic process is in no way explained when I acknowledge it as occurring in a psychic subject. One thing is put in relation to another thing, one psychic thing is connected to another, but the material context of the psychic itself is still highly problematic. What is it supposed to mean that one psychic thing is in another, and establishes a connection with something external to it? We are thrown from one thing to another, which like any thing remains mute.

We have made a hasty diversion, hoping to find a saving anchor in the neglected psychic subject. Once again we have given in to a stubborn habit of thought, without it occurring to us to explore the simple sense of the trivial question 'Is there something?' This question was deliberately chosen in order to minimize pre-judgements.

It was a restless disjointed course from one multiplicity of problems to another, a way which became ever more empty, finally dwindling to the barren question of a material context and its knowledge. We have gone into the aridity of the desert, hoping, instead of always *knowing* things, to intuit understandingly and to *understand intuitively*: '. . . and the Lord God let the *tree of life* grow up *in the middle of the garden* – and the tree of knowledge of good and evil' (Genesis 2: 9).

b)   The Interrogative Comportment. Various Senses of the 'There is'

We wish to respond to the simple sense of the question, to understand what it implies. It is a matter of hearing out the motives from which it lives. The question is lived, is experienced [*erlebt*]. I experience. I experience something vitally. When we simply give ourselves over to this experience, we know nothing of a process passing before us [*Vorgang*], or of an occurrence. Neither anything physical nor anything psychic is given. But one could immediately object: the experience is a process in me, in my soul, therefore obviously something psychic. Let us look at it carefully. This objection is not to the point, because it already reifies the experience rather than taking it as such, as it gives itself. No misunderstanding must creep into the word 'motive'. To hear out motives does not mean to search out causes of emergence or reifying conditions [*Bedingungen*], it does not mean to search out things which explain the experience in a thingly way and within a thingly context. We must understand the pure motives of the sense of the pure experience.

The term 'lived experience' [*Erlebnis*] is today so faded and worn thin that, if it were not so fitting, it

would be best to leave it aside. Since it cannot be avoided, it is all the more necessary to understand its essence.

In asking 'Is there something?' I comport myself by setting something, indeed anything whatsoever, before me as questionable. Let us here leave aside entirely the moment of question-ability: 'I comport myself.'

'I comport myself' – is this contained in the sense of the experience? Let us enact the experience with full vividness and examine its sense. To be sure, it would be no ill-conceived reification and substantification of the lived experience if I said that it contained something like 'I comport myself'. But what is decisive is that simple inspection [*Hinsehen*] does not discover anything like an 'I'. What I see is just that 'it lives' [*es lebt*], moreover that it lives towards something, that it is directed towards something by way of questioning, something that is itself questionable. What do 'questioning' and 'questionability' mean? Already here we are temporarily at a limit. What is the sense of the questioning comportment? If I bring this experience to givenness in its full sense and meaningful motives, can 'the essence of 'questionable' and 'questionability' be understood in an appropriate way? It is tempting to interpret the comportment of questioning in relation to a sought-after answer. Questioning comportment is motivated, one might say, by a desire to know. It arises from a drive for knowledge which itself originates from θαυμάζειν, astonishment and wonder.[1] If we were now to follow such interpretations and 'explanations', we would have to turn away from the simple sense of the experience; we would have to abandon the idea of holding on clearly to just what is given to us. We would have to venture into new and problematic contexts which would necessarily endanger the unadulterated authenticity of simple analysis. Let us therefore remain with the sense of the lived experience as such, keeping a firm hold on what it gives. It also gives that which, just on its own (in respect of questioning and questionability), cannot ultimately be understood. This is its ownmost meaning [*Eigensinn*] which it cannot explain by itself.

In this experience *something* is questioned in relation to anything whatsoever. The questioning has a definite content: whether *'there is'* a something, that is the question. The 'there is' [*es gibt*] stands in

---

[1] Aristotle, *Metaphysics* A 2, 982 b 11 f. **[Original note]**

question, or, more accurately, stands in questioning. It is not asked whether something moves or rests, whether something contradicts itself, whether something works, whether something exists, whether something values, whether something ought to be, but rather whether *there is* something. What does 'there is' mean?

There are numbers, there are triangles, there are Rembrandt paintings, there are submarines. I say that 'there is' still rain, today, that tomorrow 'there is' roast veal. A multiplicity of 'there is', each time with a different meaning, but in each case with an identical moment of meaning. Also this utterly flaccid meaning of 'there is', so to speak emptied of particular meanings, has precisely on account of its simplicity its manifold puzzles. Where can we find the meaningful motive for the meaning of 'there is'? Once again a new element of meaning refers the question and its content (there is) beyond itself.

It is asked whether there is *something*. It is not asked whether there are tables or chairs, houses or trees, sonatas by Mozart or religious powers, but whether there is *anything whatsoever*. What does 'anything whatsoever' mean? Something universal, one might say, indeed the most universal of all, applying to any possible object whatsoever. To say of something that it is something is the minimum assertion I can make about it. I stand over against it without presuppositions. And yet: the meaning of 'something', primitive as it appears to be, shows itself in accord with its sense as motivator of a whole process of motivations. This is already suggested by the fact that, in attempting to grasp the meaning of 'something in general', we return to individual objects with particular concrete content. Perhaps this reversion is necessary. In the final analysis it belongs to the meaning of 'something in general' to relate to something concrete, whereby the meaningful character of this 'relating' still remains problematic.

c) The Role of the Questioner

It was said above that the characterization which reads an '*I comport myself*' into the simple experience of the question is inappropriate and inapplicable, because in immediate observation I do not find anything like an 'I', but only an 'ex-perience [*Er-leben*] of something', a '*living towards something*'.

It will be objected that an 'I' does indeed belong to the sense of the question, i.e. that 'there is' means that it is given there, for *me the questioner*. Let us again immerse ourselves in the lived experience. Does this contain any kind of meaningful reference back to I myself, with this particular name and this age, I who stand here at the lectern? Examine the matter for yourself. Does there lie in the question 'Is there something?' a for me (Dr X) – a for me (candidate of philosophy, Y) – a for me (student of jurisprudence, Z)? Clearly not. Therefore, not only is no 'I' *immediately* apprehended, but in broadening out the sphere of intuition, thus abandoning any restriction to precisely *myself*, it is evident that the experience has no relation to any individual 'I'. Precisely because the question relates general to an 'I', it is without relation to my 'I'. These two phenomena necessarily motivate each other. *Just because the sense of the experience is without relation to my 'I' (to me as so and so), the still somehow necessary 'I' and I-relation are not seen in simple inspection.* As we shall show, this proposition is no mere tautology.

Yet the experience *is*, even when I avoid every kind of reification and insertion into a reifying context. It has a *now*, it is there – and is even somehow my experience. I am there with it, I experience it vitally, it belongs to my life, but it is still so detached from me in its sense, so absolutely far from the 'I', so absolutely 'I-remote' [*Ich-fern*].

I ask: 'Is there something?' The 'is there' is a 'there is' for an 'I', and yet it is not I to and for *whom* the question relates.

A wealth of quite new problem-connections is loosened up: problems to be sure, but on the other hand matters of immediate intuition that point to new contextures of meaning. However simply and primitively the interrogative experience gives itself, in respect of all its components it is peculiarly dependent. Nevertheless, from this experience a ground-laying and essential insight can now be achieved. (Characterization of the lived experience as event [*Ereignis*] – meaningful, not thing-like.)

Whatever course the further analysis might take, whatever questions might arise in respect of the analysis and its nature, it is crucial to see that we are not dealing with a reified context, and that the object of our examination is not merely an actually existing occurrence. The question is whether there is an object here at all. The living out of experience is not a thing that exists in brute fashion, beginning and ceasing to be like a process [*Vorgang*] passing by before us. The 'relating to' is not a thing-like part, to which some other thing, the 'something', is attached. The living and the lived of experience are not joined together in the manner of existing objects.

From this particular experience, the non-thingly character of all experiences whatsoever can be brought to full intuitive understanding.

§14. The Environmental Experience

We wish, however, and not simply for the sake of easing our understanding, to bring to mind a second experience, which to begin with stands in a certain contrast to the first. Bringing this contrast into view will at the same time advance the direction of our problem.

The content of the first experience, of the question 'Is there something?', resulted from following the assumption of a single exclusive reified context as existent (absolutization of thingliness). That could give the impression that the current state of our problematic prescribes a different experience for the purpose of analysis. This is not the case, and that it does not need to be the case, that there is rather a definite possibility of drawing every experience into the analysis as an example, makes itself plain. But this realm of selectability extends only to my experiences, the experiences that *I* have and *I* have had.

If we admit this, we add to our 'presuppositions' a very crude one. I bring a new experience to givenness not only for myself, but I ask you all, each isolated I-self who is sitting here, to do the same. Indeed we wish to a certain degree to enter into a unitary experience. You come as usual into this lecture-room at the usual hour and go to *your* usual place. Focus on this experience of 'seeing *your* place', or you can in turn put yourselves in my own position: coming into the lecture-room, I see the lectern. We dispense with a verbal formulation of this. What do 'I' see? Brown surfaces, at right angles to one another? No, I see something else. A largish box with another smaller one set upon it? Not at all. I see the lectern at which I am to speak. You see the lectern, from which you are to be addressed, and from where I have spoken to you previously. In pure experience there is no 'founding' interconnection, as if I first of all see intersecting brown surfaces, which then reveal themselves to me as a box, then as a desk, then as an academic lecturing desk, a lectern, so that I attach lectern-hood to the box like a label. All that is simply bad and misguided interpretation, diversion from a pure seeing into the experience. I *see* the lectern in one fell swoop, so to speak, and not in isolation, but as adjusted a bit too

high for me. I see – and immediately so – a book lying upon it as annoying to me (a book, not a collection of layered pages with black marks strewn upon them), I see the lectern in an orientation, an illumination, a background.

Certainly, you will say, that might be what happens in immediate experience, for me and in a certain way also for you, for you also see this complex of wooden boards *as* a lectern. This object, which all of us here perceive, somehow has the specific meaning 'lectern'. It is different if a farmer from deep in the Black Forest is led into the lecture-room. Does he see the lectern, or does he see a box, an arrangement of boards? He sees 'the place for the teacher', he sees the object as fraught with·meaning. If someone saw a box, then he would not be seeing a piece of wood, a thing, a natural object. But consider a Negro from Senegal suddenly transplanted here from his hut. What he would see, gazing at this object, is difficult to say precisely: perhaps something to do with magic, or something behind which one could find good protection against arrows and flying stones. Or would he not know what to make of it at all, just seeing complexes of colours and surfaces, simply a thing, a something which simply is? So my seeing and that of a Senegal Negro are fundamentally different. All they have in common is that in both cases something is seen. *My* seeing is to a high degree something individual, which I certainly may not – without further ado – use to ground the analysis of the experience. For this analysis is supposed to yield universally valid scientific results in conjunction with the elaboration of the problem.

Assuming that the experiences were fundamentally different, and that only my experience existed, I still assert that universally valid propositions are possible. This implies that these sentences would also be valid for the experience of the Senegal Negro. Let us put this assertion to one side, and focus once again on the experience of the Senegal Negro. Even if he saw the lectern simply as a bare something that is there, it would have a meaning for him, a moment of signification. There is, however, the possibility of showing that the assumption of the transplanted unscientific (not culture-less) Negro seeing the lectern as simply something is non-sensical but not contradictory, i.e. not impossible in a *formal-logical* sense. The Negro will see the lectern much more as something 'which he does not know what to make of'. The meaningful character of 'instrumental strangeness', and the meaningful character of the 'lectern', are in their essence absolutely identical.

In the experience of seeing the lectern something is given *to me* from out of an immediate environment [*Umwelt*]. This environmental milieu (lectern, book, blackboard, notebook, fountain pen, caretaker, student fraternity, tram-car, motor-car, etc.) does not consist just of things, objects, which are then conceived as meaning this and this; rather, the meaningful is primary and immediately given to me without any mental detours across thing-oriented apprehension. Living in an environment, it signifies to me everywhere and always, everything has the character of world. It is everywhere the case that *'it worlds'* [*es weltet*], which is something different from 'it values' [*es wertet*]. (The problem of the connection between the two belongs to the eidetic genealogy of primary motivations and leads into difficult problem spheres.)

§15. Comparison of Experiential Structures.
Process and Event

Let us again recall the environmental experience, my seeing of the lectern. Do I find in the pure sense of the experience, in my comportment on seeing the lectern, giving itself environmentally, anything like an 'I'? In this experiencing, in this living-towards, there is something of me: my 'I' goes out beyond itself and resonates *with* this seeing, as does the 'I' of the Negro in his own experience of 'something which *he* cannot make out'. *More precisely:* only through the accord of this particular 'I' does it experience something environmental, where we can say that 'it worlds'. Wherever and whenever 'it worlds' for me, *I* am somehow there. Now consider the experience of the question 'Is there something'? I do not find myself in this. The 'anything whatsoever', about whose 'there is' I ask, does not 'world'. The worldly is here extinguished, and we grasp every potential environing world as 'anything whatsoever'. This grasping, this firm fixing of the object as such, occurs at the cost of forcing back my own 'I'. It belongs to the meaning of 'anything whatsoever' that in its determination *I do not* as such come into accord with it: this resonating, this going out of myself, is prevented. The object, being an object as such, does not touch *me*. The 'I' that firmly fixes is no longer *I myself*. The firm fixing as an experience is still only a rudiment of vital experience; it is a devivification [*Entleben*]. What is

objectified, what is known, is as such removed [*entfernt*], lifted out of the actual experience. The objective occurrence, the happening as objectified and known, we describe as a *process;* it simply passes before my knowing 'I', to which it is related only by being-known, i.e. in a flaccid I-relatedness reduced to the minimum of life-experience. It is in the nature of the thing and thing-contexture to give themselves only in knowledge, that is, only in theoretical comportment and for the theoretical 'I'. In the theoretical comportment I am directed to something, but I do not live (as historical 'I') towards this or that worldly element. Let us once again contrast entire context's of experience, so that it does not appear that the 'opposition' pertains only to isolated experiences.

Let us place ourselves into the comportment of the astronomer, who in astrophysics investigates the phenomenon of sunrise simply as a process in nature before which he is basically indifferent, and on the other hand the experience of the chorus of Theban elders, which in Sophocles' *Antigone* looks at the rising sun on the first friendly morning after a successful defensive battle:

ἀκτὶς ἀελίου, τὸ κάλλιστον ἑπταπύλῳ φανὲν
Θήβᾳ τῶν προτέρων φάος

> Thou most beautiful glance of the sun,
> That upon seven-gated Thebes
> So long shines . . .[2]

This contrast does not solve but only initially poses the problem of the *how* of different modes of experience. But for the time being it will suffice for our purposes. How do we see the experiences? The questions of how such seeing is possible, of what it itself is, and whether it is not also theory (it is, after all, supposed to become science), will be set aside for the moment. Let us try to understand both experiences and see if we can regard them as processes, as objects which are re-presented, firmly fixed before us. But something does happen. In seeing the lectern I am fully present in my 'I'; it resonates with the experience, as we said. It is an experience proper to me and

---

[2] Sophocles, *Antigone* V. 100 *ff.*, in: *Sophoclis Tragoediae, cum praefatione Guilelmi Dindorfii*, Leipzig 1825, p. 172. German translation by Friedrich Hölderlin O Blick der Sonne, du schönster, der/Dem siebenthorigen Thebe/Seit langem scheint 2) in *Sämtliche Werke und Briefe,* ed. F. Zinkernagel, Leipzig 1915, vol. III, p. 374 f.
[Original note]

so do I see it. However, it is not a process but rather an *event of appropriation* [*Ereignis*] (non-process, in the experience of the question a residue of this event). Lived experience does not pass in front of me like a thing, but I appropriate [*ereigne*] it to myself, and it appropriates itself according to its essence. If I understand it in this way, then I understand it not as process, as thing, as object, but in a quite new way, as an event of appropriation. Just as little as I see something thing-like do I see an objectivated sphere of things, a Being, neither physical nor psychical Being. Attending strictly to the experience, I do not see anything psychical. Event of appropriation is not to be taken as if I appropriate the lived experience to myself from outside or from anywhere else; 'outer' and 'inner' have as little meaning here as 'physical' and 'psychical'. The experiences are events of appropriation in so far as they live out of one's 'own-ness', and life lives only in this way. (With this the event-like essence of appropriation is still not fully determined.)

Granted that I could make clear that my experiences are of a distinctive character, and are not thing-like or object-like beings, this evidence would have validity only for me and my experiences. How is a science supposed to be built upon this? Science is knowledge and knowledge has objects. Science determines and fixes objects in an objective manner. A science of experiences would have to objectify experiences and thus strip away their non-objective character as lived experience and event of appropriation.

Already when I speak of *two* of my experiences I have objectified them: the one and the other, both are a something. For every experience that I want to consider I must isolate and lift out, break up and destroy the contexture of the experience so that in the end and despite all efforts to the contrary, I have only a heap of things.

Heidegger, M. (1923–4), Selections from *Introduction to Phenomenological Research*

From (2005) *Introduction to Phenomenological Research*. Translated by Daniel O. Dahlstrom. Bloomington, IN: Indiana University Press. Originally published as (1994) *Gesamtausgabe*, vol. 17, *Einführung in die phänomenologische Forschung*. Edited by Friedrich-Wilhelm von Herrman. Frankfurt am Main: Vittorio Klosterman.

Preliminary Remark
The task of the lectures and the passion for questioning genuinely and rightly

The lectures have a twofold task: 1. Establishing and opening up the horizon within which specific *facts of the matter* are to be expected. Provisional orientation of the perspective, stripping away mistaken expectations. 2. Concretely working out the facts of the matter that have, step-by-step, been made more accessible; familiarity with the objects and with the way of dealing with them theoretically.

Before anything else, the following misguided expectations need to be stripped away: 1. No journalistic information about phenomenology, no divulging of some trick for perceiving essences. 2. More dangerous, because more entrenched: no foundation, no program or system, is given here; not even philosophy should be expected. It is my conviction that philosophy is at an end. We stand before completely new tasks that have nothing to do with traditional philosophy. This view is, however, only a clue. Only facts of the matter are of significance. Definition, classification, explication, and disputation are of secondary importance.

The task of the following considerations is threefold: 1. Elucidation of the *expression* "phenomenology"; 2. Representation of the *breakthrough* of phenomenological research in Husserl's *Logical Investigations*. 3. Representation of the *development* of phenomenology from this point on, to what extent it is maintained, to what extent it has taken a turn or in the end has been given up, as far as its decisive meaning is concerned.

History of the words: φαινόμενον and λόγος – two original words of Greek philosophy; from the transformation of their meanings, it becomes possible to understand how the specific meaning of phenomenology arose. Insofar as these words enunciate "existence," we move, with their clarification, within the history of Western humanity's existence and the history of its self-interpretation. From Husserl's self-interpretation of "phenomenology" immediately after the *Logical Investigations*, it becomes understandable how he conceives and further shapes the task of phenomenological research. As a way of showing what we are up to, we will fix on existence as our main theme; that is to say, world, dealings in it, temporality, language, one's own interpretation of existence, possibilities of interpreting existence.

No acquaintance with philosophical notions is presupposed. To the contrary, [there are only] three presuppositions: a passion for *questioning* genuinely and rightly.

The passion does not happen at will; it has its time and its tempo. A readiness must be there, the readiness that consists in: 1. concern for an instinctively certain mastery in regard to prejudice; 2. care about the process of becoming at home in a specific science; 3. being prepared for the fact that, when it comes to questioning in order to know, life would sooner help in questioning everything else than be of any help in questioning the soul's own inertia, the so-called theoretical consideration.

Ad 1. Not absence of prejudice, which is a utopia. The idea of having no prejudice is itself the greatest prejudice. Mastery in the face of each possibility of something establishing itself as prejudice. Not free from prejudices but free for the possibility of giving up a prejudice at the decisive moment on the basis of a critical encounter with the subject matter. That is the form of existence of a scientific human.

Ad 2. Lethargy towards knowledge is the consequence of science conceived as a collection of material that has already been worked over. This lethargy is characteristic of today's educated consciousness. One has to see that precisely this aspect is fatal. One no longer understands what is actually going on. This cowardice when it comes to questioning often adorns itself as religiosity. Ultimate questioning, questioning that confronts itself, appears as temerity to this religiosity. One flees in the face of a fundamental possibility of existence, a possibility that seems today, alas, to have lost its way. The *sciences* are one possibility of existence and of existence's critical confrontation with itself. If each person, in his place opposite his science, experienced in specific questions that he critically confronts himself and his world here, then he has understood what science means.

Ad 3. The readiness for the questioning consists in a certain *maturity of existence*: it has not lapsed into surrogates; it is also not a matter of finishing as soon as possible, but instead of holding out for years in uncertainty, of maturing from that uncertainty for the critical confrontation with the matters under investigation, of being free to reject every hasty answer. For this it is necessary to free oneself from a tradition which in Greek philosophy was genuine: scientific behaviour as theory. You need not think that you have to think what is thought here.

ΦΑΙΝΟΜΕΝΟΝ and ΛΟΓΟΣ in Aristotle and Husserl's Self-Interpretation of Phenomenology

Elucidation of the expression "phenomenology" by going back to Aristotle

The expression "phenomenology" first appears in the eighteenth century in Christian Wolff's School, in Lambert's *Neues Organon,* in connection with analogous developments popular at the time, like dianoiology and alethiology, and means a theory of illusion, a doctrine for avoiding illusion. A related concept is found in Kant. In a letter to Johann Heinrich Lambert, he writes: "It appears that a quite particular, although merely negative science (*phaenomenologia generalis*) must precede metaphysics, in which the validity and limits of the principia of sensibility are determined." Later "Phenomenology" is the title for Hegel's major work. In the Protestant theology of the nineteenth century, phenomenology of religions is conceived as a doctrine concerning the various manners of appearance of religions. "Phenomenology" also appears in Franz Brentano's lectures on metaphysics (based upon oral communication from Husserl). Why did Husserl choose this expression? Why is the doctrine about the avoidance of illusion named "phenomenology" in the eighteenth century, and how does φαινόμενον [phenomenon] come to have the meaning of "illusion"? Is there, then, in the expression φαινόμενον some motivation for using it to designate illusion? The term "appearance" must be left out of play since, as a purported translation of the Greek words, it creates confusion. Even, Περί ψυχής "On the soul," is misunderstood if one hangs on to the terms under discussion here. For Aristotle, perception, thinking, wanting are not experiences. Περί ψυχής is no psychology in the modern sense, but instead deals with the being of a human being (or of living beings in general) in the world.

Clarification of φαινόμενον on the basis of the Aristotelian analysis of perceiving the world by way of seeing

a) *φαινόμενον* as a distinctive manner of an entity's presence: existence during the day

Phenomenology is put together from λόγος and φαινόμενον. Φαινόμενον means: something that shows itself. Φαίνομαι, is the same as "to show itself," φαίνω the same as "to bring something to the light of day." The stem is φα, this is connected with Φῶς which is the same as light, daylightness. In a concrete text of scientific investigations it is necessary to establish what facts of the matter are meant by the words. We shall consider the fact of the matter apart from the word and then, on the basis of the text, establish the sense in which that fact of the matter is meant by the word. For this purpose we choose Aristotle's *De anima*, B (II), chapter 7 that deals with perceiving the world by way of *seeing*. It is necessary to keep every bit of knowledge from physics, physiology at bay since they lack Aristotle's focus. No explication with this sort of concreteness has ever been attempted again.

What is seeing, what is it that is perceived as such in seeing, how is what is accessible in seeing characterized with respect to its content and its perceptibility? Οὗ μὲν οὖν ἐστιν ἡ ὄψις τοῦτ' ἐστιν ὁρατόν. "What is perceivable in seeing is the visible"; something of this sort is characterized as colour. Colour is what is spread over something visible in itself. The respective coloring of an entity is perceived each time ἐν φωτί, in light, more precisely, in daylight [*im Hellen*].

Thus, the first thing to be made out is what *daylight* is. Daylight is apparently something that lets something else be seen through it, διαφανές [transparent]. This daylight is not of itself visible, but only by means of a colour, alien to it. Daylight is what allows something to be seen, namely, the actual colour (οἰκεῖον χρῶμα) of the things that I have in daylight: Aristotle discovered that daylightness is not a body

> (τί μὲν οὖν τὸ διαφανὲς καὶ τί τὸ φῶς, εἴρηται, ὅτι οὔτε πῦρ οὔθ' ὅλως σῶμα οὐδ' ἀπορροὴ σώματος ..., ἀλλὰ πυρὸς ἢ τοιούτου τινὸς παρουσία ἐν τῷ διαφανεῖ)

> (As for what the transparent [*Helle*] is and what light is, it has been explained that it is neither fire nor a body at all nor even the outflow of a body ... but presence of fire or some such thing in the transparent)

that it does not move, but is instead the heaven's actual manner of existing, allowing things to be seen, the day's being. Daylight is a *manner of presence* of [something] (παρουσία, ἐντελέχεια). Empedocles taught that light moves; καὶ οὐκ ὀρθῶς Ἐμπεδοκλῆς [but Empedocles was not right]. Trendelenburg saw in the Aristotelian doctrine a relapse; but this judgment shows that he did not understand Aristotle at all.

Αἴσθησις [perception] is the manner of existing of something living in its world. The manners of perceiving things are characterized by Aristotle by means of the *sort of thing perceived*, what is accessible in the perceiving. There are *three sorts* of αἰσθητά: 1. ἴδια, 2. κοινά, 3. συμβεβηκότα [things perceived: 1. special, 2. common, 3. incidentally at hand].

1. An ἴδιον is something accessible through one specific manner of perceiving and *only through that manner of perceiving*. It has the character of being ἀεὶ ἀληθές [always true].[24] Seeing, insofar as it exists, always uncovers only colour, hearing always uncovers only sound. 2. Κοινόν. There are characteristic ways of being that are not fitted to one specific manner of perceiving, e.g., κίνησις [change]. 3. συμβεβηκός is what is regularly perceived (κατὰ συμβεβηκὸς δὲ λέγεται αἰσθητόν, οἷον εἰ τὸ λευκὸν εἴη Διάρους υἱός [something perceptible is said to be incidentally at hand, for instance, if the white thing were Diaeres' son]). For, as a rule, I do not see colour, I do not hear sounds, but instead the singer's song, something that is encountered along with the immediate perceiving [*das im nächsten Vernehmen mitbegegnende*]. When it comes to the perceptibility of something κατὰ συμβεβηκός deception is possible and even the rule.

Aristotle determined colour, among other things, to be an ἴδιον. Daylight is the presence of fire. Daylight does not move. Only the sun moves, the presence of which is the daylight. Whoever says that daylight moves is speaking παρὰ τὰ φαινόμενα, he is speaking past what shows itself. Φαινόμενον is what shows itself of itself to be of a certain sort and is immediately here as such. Speaking in a Kantian fashion, daylight is the condition of the possibility of the perceptibility of colour. Precisely in this Kantian use of language, one can recognize the difference between what, in both cases, is understood by "condition." This is not to say, however, that Aristotle and Kant should be contrasted with one another as realists and idealists (there is no such contrast in Greek philosophy). What does "condition of the possibility of the perceptibility of colour" mean, what does "being a condition" mean for Aristotle? Colour is seen in daylight. The thing seen must be at daytime. Daylight is something that is part of the being of the world itself. Daylight is the sun's presence. The character of being for this manner of being-present is to let things be seen through it. Letting something be seen is the sun's manner of being. The perceptibility of things is subject to a condition, that of a specific manner of being of this world itself. "Being a condition" applies to a manner of being of the world itself. The sun's being on hand, precisely *what* we mean when we determine: *it is daytime*, is part of the existence in the world. By this means we speak of a fact of the matter that is part of the being of the world itself. The result of this is that φαινόμενον initially means nothing other than a *distinctive manner of an entity's presence*.

b) Φαινόμενον as anything that of itself shows itself in daylight or darkness

The concept φαινόμενον is not limited solely to the presence of things during the day. It is broader and designates anything showing itself of itself, whether it does so *in daylight* or *in darkness*.

What, now, is darkness? For someone arguing in an empty-headed way, it is obviously not difficult to determine what it is. Daylight is διαφανές, something that lets things be seen, darkness is an ἀδιαφανές, something that does not. But darkness also lets something be seen. There are visible things that are visible *only in the dark*:

> οὐ πάντα δὲ ὁρατὰ ἐν φωτί ἐστιν ἀλλὰ μόνον ἑκάστου τὸ οἰκεῖον χρῶμα· ἔνια γὰρ ἐν μὲν τῷ φωτὶ οὐχ ὁρᾶται, ἐν δὲ τῷ σκότει ποιεῖ αἴσθησιν, οἷον τὰ πυρώδη φαινόμενα.

> [Not everything is visible in light, but only the proper colour of each thing. For some things are not seen in light but produce perception in the dark, such as things that appear fire-like.]

Darkness is something that, in a quite specific way, lets things be seen. In order to establish the dark's difference from daylight, we must draw on a completely fundamental distinction of Aristotelian philosophy: the difference between ἐντελεχεία [actual being] and δυνάμει ὄν [potential being]. Darkness is a δυνάμει ὄν, something utterly positive. Since, in our doctrine of categories, we have not developed such primordial categories, we are unable to comprehend this peculiar structure. Insofar as darkness is a manner of "being away," it must be designated as στέρησις, as the absence of something that should actually be on hand. Darkness' being consists in being *potential* daylight. It would be talking past Aristotle, if one were to say: "Daylight is what lets things be seen; thus, darkness is what does not." The dark also lets things be seen.

The basic concepts of philosophy, such as they run their course in the historical development, are not some property or possession of philosophy that one can hold onto and that stands outside the development. They have become far more our own nemesis insofar as the consideration and interpretation of existing as a whole is pervaded by such concepts that amount to nothing more than a possession of words. They signify the great danger that one philosophizes today in words rather than about things.

Φαινόμενον and λόγος give expression to a fact of the matter. Later the motives in existence itself, on the basis of which φαινόμενον is able to take on the meaning of "illusion," will become intelligible – so, too, it will become understandable how a philosophy that has become superficial and coasts along in words grasps existing entities as an "appearance of something." Aristotle did not have so naive a metaphysics. And if one attempts today, with the word "appearance" in hand, to offer a critique of phenomenology, it is a groundless endeavour against which I can only protest (compare Rickert, *Logos*, 1923).

Φαινόμενον is what shows itself of itself as existing; it is encountered by life insofar as life stands towards its world in such a way that it sees the world, perceives it at all in the αἴσθησις. Ἴδια αἰσθητά [special perceptibles] are what are perceived in the strict sense of the term. On the other hand, κατὰ συμβεβηκός is perceiving immediately in such a way that from the outset something is originally here along with it. Only in this way are we able to see houses, trees, human beings. If I want to return to the ἴδια, then it is necessary to assume an isolated, artificial attitude. The expression φαινόμενον already designates what has been perceived κατὰ συμβεβηκός. If the sun shows itself, then it is here a foot wide, it does not appear so.

Now, the primordial nature of seeing for Aristotle is evident from the fact that he does not allow himself to be misled by the lack of an all-encompassing name for the things that only the night lets us see (thus for fireflies, etc.): ὁρατὸν δ' ἐστὶ χῶμα μέν, καὶ ὃ λόγῳ μὲν ἔστιν εἰπεῖν, ἀνώνυμον δὲ τυγχάνει ὄν [The visible is colour and what can be articulated in a statement, though it happens to be nameless]. What matters to him is merely the fact that these things are here, that they are seen and, on the basis of their factual content, lay claim to being taken as existing. The fact that there is no name for these things indicates, however, that our language (doctrine of categories) is a language of the day. This holds particularly for the Greek language and is connected in their case with the basic starting point of their thinking and their formation of concepts. One cannot remedy that by somehow constructing a doctrine of categories of the night. Instead we must go back to a point prior to this opposition in order to be able to understand why the day has this priority.

Thanks to the word-combination παρά τά φαινόμενα [beyond the phenomena], which recurs repeatedly in Aristotle, the particular character of the claim made by φαινόμενον and what is thereby seized upon emerges. If it is *explicitly* a matter of grasping existence, of retaining it, of securing what shows itself in itself, then we remain in the context of science. In this context the meaning of φαινόμενον comes to a head: what shows itself in itself, with the explicit claim of serving as the basis for all further questioning and explicating. What matters for science is σώζειν τά φαινόμενα [to save the phenomena]; what shows itself in itself is thereby pressed into a fundamental position. Something of this sort is possible in science. Science has the tendency to grasp and demonstrate existing entities in a way that does not leave anything uncovered. To be a scientific person is to be positioned in a specific manner over against the world's being. There are two determinations of this ἕξις [attitude], determinations that, in themselves, belong together: 1. familiarity with the things that are subject to the science, ἐπιστήμη τοῦ πράγματος [knowledge of the thing]; 2. a certain παιδεία [education], being educated in such a way that one knows how to conduct oneself in the field of scientific investigation. The individual who has the παιδεία can decide quite certainly whether someone who undertakes an investigation is prattling or whether what he is conveying emerges from the subject matter (καλῶς ἀποδίδωσιν [(whether) he conveys (it) well]). On the basis of such παιδεία one must decide what type of investigation is precisely suited to the object. With regard to the possibilities of the investigation, it has to be decided whether, like earlier thinkers, one should posit existing and the determinations of an object's being as secondary and speak primarily of the genesis or not. The answer is easy: only after one has fashioned the basis for the investigation, can one set out to answer the question of the origin and the "why" of the origin. The first thing that needs to be established in building a house is the εἶδος [form] and only then the ὕλη [matter]. Εἶδος means to make an impression. This making an impression is the house's being in its surroundings as a house, its look, "face." The φαινόμενον is the entity itself.

*****

Present-day phenomenology in Husserl's self-interpretation

Recapitulation of the facts of the matter gathered from the interpretation of Aristotle. Anticipation of the predominance of care about the idea of certainty and evidence over freeing up possibilities of encountering fundamental facts of the matter

To *recapitulate* the *result* of our analysis, it must be said that we have established: 1. Specific *facts of the matter* that point to the existence of the world and the existence of human life. The state of the matter has led us to a phenomenological characterization of the world and to a specific orientation of the one existing [*Daseiendem*] and it has done this in the sense of (a) a distinctive sort of being that shows itself in itself, and (b) the λόγος-character as an existing possibility of human life. There is a connection here insofar as the λόγος qua apophantic has the possibility of pointing out what shows itself. These facts of the matter, the existence of the world and of life, became so obvious that certain possibilities became apparent in them. 2. The existence of the world can abruptly turn around into something self-dissimulating, the λόγος can be of the sort that disguises existence. This connection reveals a fate that resides in existence itself, the fact that present there with its being is the possibility of deception and lies.

The aim of the interpretation up to this point has not been to make the development of a term [i.e., "phenomenology"] intelligible in some anecdotal form. The aim was instead to awaken interest in the matter, indeed, in such a way that the direction in which things were heading did not become transparent at first. We have to learn how to read and listen in the manner of waiting.

The background of the interpretation continues to be rooted in the matter at hand insofar as its concern is to make intelligible what is today known under the rubric "phenomenology." That can only mean: making intelligible the sort of *matters* treated in this discipline – what sort of matters present-day phenomenology claims to work on. In order to obtain this sorting, we need *a horizon of matters*. Against this horizon we will have to decide on the extent to which the *facts of the matter of present-day phenomenology* are still connected with what we have pointed out about the matter.

In order from the outset to characterize the development in which Aristotle shaped the basic constants of philosophical research, allow me to say the following. Subsequent developments in establishing the facts of the matter of philosophy and the motivation behind the various paths on which these facts were worked on have been *guided by the predominance of an empty and thereby fantastic idea of certainty and evidence.* This predominance of a specific idea of evidence predominates *over* every *genuine effort to free up the possibility of encountering the genuine matters of philosophy. Care about* a specific, *absolute knowledge,* taken purely as an idea, predominates over every question about the matters that are decisive. That is to say, the *entire development of philosophy reverses itself.* Beginnings of this development are already present in Aristotle and the Greeks and they are not accidental, e.g., the notion that the existence of the world as it presents itself is taken to be the specific world of illusion, so that in the future all decisive questions of philosophy are gathered purely from the idea of securing an absolute certainty, together with the tendency to surmount the existence of the world as something contingent. Let us add the observation that this development stems, not from a science's attempts to procure its distinctive manner of access to its subject matter, but instead from an idea that existence fabricates for itself, to a certain extent from an intelligence that has gone crazy.

Through the interpretation of the components of the term "phenomenology," we were confronted by quite definite facts of the matter of existence: the *world's being* and life as *being in a world.* In these two respects we saw at once that the world's being has the character of *showing itself* and that life's being entails a basic possibility of *speaking* about existence in such a way that being *is pointed out* by means of speech. The world's being and life's being have a quite *specific connection* with one another, thanks to *speaking's being.* The existence of the world in showing-itself in this way can turn around into a manner of *presenting-itself-as* something else. *Life is, in itself, capable of concealing the existing world.* Thus, both existence's possibilities and life's possibilities reveal existence to be endangered in a specific way, one that we expressed by saying that existence bears in itself the possibilities of deception and lies.

If we cling solely to the results of the analysis without reference to the theme "phenomenology," then we seem to have made no progress, but instead to be abruptly confronted with specific facts of the matter. However, to understand the connection, i.e., to understand the being and character of the matter that *phenomenology* works on, an orientation to a *horizon of the matter* is needed. I gave a clue for considering an utterly peculiar *reversal.* The predominance of care about the idea of an empty and thus fantastic certainty and evidence, prior to every attempt to free up the possibility of an encounter with specific, fundamental facts of the matter has led to shunting aside what was *originally* a *theme* of the consideration. Indeed, it has led to shunting it is worse, the choice of perspective was not guided by a certain *appropriation of the matters* at hand but instead by *a definite idea of science* – that the idea of a definite sort of knowledge determines the theme rather than, vice versa, that a definite composition of the matter indicates the possibilities of working on it scientifically.

By this means, a traditional idea of the introduction into science of any sort is fended off. [For this traditional idea,] it is not a matter of getting some empty cognizance of what the "object," what the "method" of the science in question is. The method is supposed to emerge during the critical confrontation with the subject matters. The traditional idea of determining and developing a research project works toward determining the "object": the object is such and such, this specific domain of science is [accordingly] worked on by means of specific methods. This sort of orientation is disregarded here.

But if we look closer and ask what we have gained up to this point in regard to the facts of the matter, something surprising presents itself. We have regarded existence in view of a peculiar sort of *self-showing.* We have learned nothing about the character of its *content* but instead have seemingly laid down an empty determination. We have not gathered what an object is. We have learned of a determination regarding *existence,* one that characterizes it in its *how: how it shows itself in itself* and *how,* based on this, *it hides itself.* It is just the same with the characterization of the λόγος. We have merely learned of the λόγος a specific, already characterized *manner of* its *being,* that of one time *pointing out* existence *itself,* then *disguising* it. This existence was not determined in terms of its content in the sense of a natural being or of an historical reality but instead in a seemingly empty way: only *how it exists.* By having emphasized these characteristic determinations of existence (namely, that what matters is *how* it exists), we have, in the interpretation, already gone beyond what was comprehensible to the Greeks in the context of their examination of existence.

If we compare this *how-character* [*Wie-Charakter*] of existence with others that the Greeks knew, then we see that they are concerned with *determinations of what* things are [*Was-Bestimmungen*]. There are various respects in which existence is characterized, respects rooted in the matter at hand: 1. Πράγματα, the things which "one" ["*man*"] has to deal with. The entity is accordingly addressed in this respect. 2. Χρήματα, the things insofar as they are used for needs that the existence of the world itself motivates and requires. 3. Ποιούμενα, the things in the world that are produced, that are made and are available as ἔργα [devices] for 1. and 2. 4. Φυσικά, the existing things of the world that are not produced but instead are in themselves, *coming to be* on the basis of their specific being but capable at the same time of being that out of which something can be produced (wood, iron) and thus having a relation to 3. 5. Μαθήματα, the sort of entities that have the specific lines of being able to be learned and concerning which there is a kind of knowing that can be communicated to everyone without their thereby having a practical relation to matters. 6. Within each of these characterizations and the being named by them, there are paradigmatic things which have the peculiar character of being that is designated atria. However, in order to see the connection of atria and the other concepts of being, it should be noted that this seemingly so abstract philosophical concept stands for possessions, property, what is lying around me at home, the "homestead" ["*Anwesen*"].

In *our* interpretation we did not encounter these categories of the world. We heard only of φαινόμενα. Οὐσία provides the basic character of the entity insofar as it is: *presence* [*Anwesenheit*]. It is also meant, implicitly, in the concepts of "thing" that have been noted. The *nearest sort of encounter* of the entity yields the φαινόμενα in terms of the formal *how-character* of that sort of encounter. Φαινόμενα then is precisely the being addressed in all these characters, but is this being only in *the* respect of *showing itself*. We have gathered this characteristic determination from the interpretation and established it for our further consideration. The closest sort of encounter of entities and the unfiltered grasp of them in this sort of encounter must in some way be *phenomenologically* decisive.

Consciousness as the theme of present-day phenomenology

We now have to pose the question: What is the *theme* or the *context of being, pertaining to the subject matter,* that is the object of *the* research that *today* is designated *phenomenology?* At the start allow me to give an utterly formal determination of it in connection, with the position that Husserl has advanced farthest up to now in the *Ideas to a Pure Phenomenology and Phenomenological Philosophy.* According to this text, phenomenology is the *descriptive eidetic science of transcendentally pure consciousness.* This determination is important for us simply as an indication that *consciousness* is the theme examined in phenomenology. For us the question arises: How does what is designated as consciousness come to enjoy the peculiar prerogative of providing the theme of a fundamental science such as phenomenology claims to be? Are we in-a position to make this peculiar prerogative intelligible? To make it intelligible on the basis of what we have become acquainted with up to now? And to do so in such a way that we show that the field of being that is named "consciousness" does not come to enjoy this position of priority accidentally or arbitrarily but instead that this prerogative of it is grounded in distinctive *possibilities* that *existence* bears within itself and that are already prefigured in Greek philosophy? If we succeed in demonstrating this, then we will see that these transformations [*Wandlungen*] themselves are grounded and motivated in our existence itself, and that the history that offers us such possibilities and transformations is not something contingent and remote that lies behind us and that we occasionally draw upon to illustrate our opinions. We will see, instead, that *in history's transformations* we encounter nothing other than *our own existence.*

For that reason, the present consideration is not an historical narration but a concrete look at quite *definite possibilities of our own existence.* If these are set forth and seen together with the aforementioned, we acquire with it the basis for a *fundamental differentiation* to be made at the beginning of our investigation.

a) Greek philosophy without a concept of consciousness

How does it become understandable that something like *consciousness* is philosophy's theme? This question becomes fundamental for us the moment we remind ourselves that the Greeks are unacquainted with consciousness or anything like consciousness. In Greek philosophy there is no concept of consciousness. At the same time, to be sure, it must be said that what, among other things, is conceived under *today's* specific, phenomenological concepts of consciousness is already found precisely among the Greeks. In the course of the analysis of perceiving, for example, Aristotle saw that we co-perceive a seeing itself as being [*Seiendes*]. We have an αἴσθησις [perception] of seeing. He asks himself what kind of perceiving it is that we perceive the seeing and the like with. So, too, in the case of νόησις, the question arises: Does the thinking [*Vermeinen*] that thinks the perceiving have the same character of being? Both questions are left undecided. From the standpoint of the specific facts of the matter of research today, we can call this a much more fundamental insight into this context than the rash decision underlying the orientation of modern psychology, namely, that the perception of seeing, that of thinking, and so forth are a matter of one and the same thing, the inner perception. However one intends to decide these things, perceiving how one conducts oneself has become a theme of the examination. What is perceived here should not be interpreted as an experience or mental existence in the modern sense. In spite of this fact, later Greek philosophy displays an acquaintance with what is today designated "consciousness" or "self-consciousness" – an acquaintance not on the path of philosophical reflection, but drawn instead from the natural experience of what we today call "conscience" [συνείδησις] in a very accentuated sense. Thus, it enters into the Christian consciousness of life and it undergoes a further explication in theology. But what was so designated is in no way an object of consideration. That something like consciousness would become a theme of an investigation is out of the question for the Greek and Christian consciousness.

b)   Phenomenology's breakthrough in Husserl's *Logical Investigations* and their basic tendency

In order to understand the thematic field's turn-around from *the entity that the world is* to the *entity that is consciousness of it,* it is necessary to sketch the features of the end-station, i.e., present-day phenomenology, as it becomes necessary for our examination. The research that we designate "phenomenology" appeared for the first time under the explicit title *Logical Investigations.* These investigations move within the framework of a traditional discipline called

"logic." From a purely personal standpoint, these themes were obvious ones for Husserl since he was driven from mathematical investigations to logical considerations in an effort to understand the distinctiveness of mathematical *thinking.* The *Logical Investigations* are not motivated by the ambition of working out anything like a new textbook in logic. Instead, the principal purpose is *to make the objects with which logic is preoccupied into the theme for once in such a way that research related to this is put into a position of being able actually to work on subject matters – that the specific objects of this discipline* are brought *to a specific intuition that identifies them.* "Intuition" here means simply: to make present to oneself the object in itself, just as it presents itself. The basic tendency of these *Logical Investigations* is to make this "presentation" one that is methodically secured. Such a tendency could only be genuinely effective through research that *discloses the subject matter.* The "results" of these investigations are so replete that they have born fruit in contemporary philosophy in a way that can no longer be measured today. Even the very ones "stimulated" by the investigations are only slightly conscious of the extent of their effect. The entire course of our examination starts from the *prospect of getting at the matters themselves,* working its way through a merely verbal knowledge to the things.

*****

Husserl's critique of naturalism

a)   Naturalization of consciousness

What does the critique look like and against whom is it directed? Against naturalism and historicism. We have to make clear to ourselves how in general the expression "naturalism" comes to be coined and what one has in mind when something is designated as such. Naturalism coincides with the discovery of nature. Analogously, historicism grew out of a discovery of history. The discovery of nature in question is the discovery of it as the object of a special science, the mathematical science of nature. Naturalism is a consequence of this discovery of nature. That is to say, the type of being and object in the context of nature becomes the guide to the content in comprehending *every sort* of being and objectivity. Accordingly, the *specific rigor of the mathematical science of nature* serves as the criterion for every domain of being and epistemic determination of it. The question is the extent to which a determinate *idea of a science and object* of this sort has in fact *expanded* to the thematic field of philosophy, in what sense the objective field of philosophy and its method are subjected to the idea of the mathematical science of nature.

The basic character of this science, apart from its rigor, is distinguished by the fact that its results can be formulated in laws. A law-likeness [*Gesetzmässigkeit*] that is scientific in the eminent sense is called "universally binding." The *binding character* of these propositions is so predominant and at the same time so imposing in human existence that it presents the genuine motive that leads to absolutizing the idea of this science. This nature is not something alien to philosophy since philosophy early on had a tendency to the sort of lawfulness [*Gesetzlichkeit*] that one can formulate as *a normative determination* [*Normierung*]. It is thus no accident that a science that has elevated itself to such rigorousness, as natural science has, makes this task its own and that the specific objects of philosophy succumb to natural science.

The first aspect of the effect of naturalizing philosophy lies in the fact that this same naturalist tendency leads to the *naturalization of consciousness*. (This juxtaposition of the idea and consciousness points back to *Descartes*.) How does it come to the naturalization precisely of consciousness, and what does that mean insofar as philosophy's task is to establish the sorts of lawfulness pertaining to modes of behaviour in terms of their meaningful connection? The task arises of acquiring the legitimate grounds for the fact that something like consciousness speaks of an object as actually being and identifies it as such. For this justification of the legitimacy of the claims and acts of consciousness, there is need for a study of these connections themselves. A critique of knowing is needed. Being that has the character of the soul or mind [*seelische Sein*], regarded as [part of] nature, is determined in the sense of *natural scientific categories*. The uniform organization of this misunderstanding is what one can designate as *experimental psychology*, insofar as it lays claim to being significant in a fundamental [*grundsätzlich*] way. It never entered into Husserl's mind to say something against experimental psychology as such. [What he does oppose is how] ideal laws are reinterpreted into the, sorts of lawfulness pertaining to sheer processes of consciousness. This is done not only in the domain of thinking, but also in the domain of voluntary action. The norms valid here are also reinterpreted into laws of psychological processes. Husserl explicitly stresses that the laws of formal logic make up the exemplary index of all ideality.

b) Naturalization of ideas

Next to the naturalization of consciousness, a further falsification of the idea of philosophy as rigorous science lies in the *naturalization of ideas*. For the explanation of the "idea," see the concrete investigations in the *Logical Investigations*, which are concerned with meanings These are seen as ideal unities in contrast to the multitude of acts that realize them in meaning something. This unity of the sense is an ideal unity of *validation*. On the basis of this ideal unity of propositions, completely determinate modes of lawfulness of their own sort arise. *The* philosophy that looks on everything as natural science reinterprets this specific lawfulness of the sense into a lawfulness of the *natural course* of the process of thinking the lawfulness of norms and ideas is reinterpreted into a lawfulness of the course of thinking. The idea, the lawfulness of ideas, is not seen at all. The critique at work in natural science is the sort of critique that is made in the course of achieving knowledge in natural science with its focus on the matters involved. As a critique in natural science, it is the sort that is bent on the facts of the matter under investigation. It is absurd, Husserl says, that the critical possibilities of an individual science should include the possibilities of investigating this science purely insofar as it is science. In the latter sort of investigation, a completely fundamental change of object has taken place. Mistaking this niveau is what enabled natural science to claim for itself the solution to epistemological problems and, as a result, to block the path to bringing the specific sort of object that "consciousness" is into view as such, and to clarifying from this vantage point the set of problems that knowledge and acting pose as being in their own right.

In the examination, the critique of naturalism was intentionally isolated from the critique of historicism. The latter will occupy us later and free up the view for a series of new facts of the matter.

Naturalism is, first, naturalism of ideas; second, naturalism of consciousness. [It is] the ideal connection of ideal laws which, when viewed with respect to life's modes of behavior, can be designated as various sorts of normative lawfulness to which the disciplines of theoretical science, axiology, and practical science correspond. The ultimate constant factors, in which these sorts of normative lawfulness are grounded, are ideas. It is characteristic of naturalism not to see the ideas, to be *blind to ideas.* Consciousness is the genuine theme of the critique, consciousness as a theme for epistemological treatment. There is a question whether the natural scientific method can in principle be expanded, the question of how it is in a position even merely to understand, let alone to justify the legitimacy of the exertions of consciousness.

c) Nature's being as experimental psychology's horizon

Let us ask: In what way does the critique seek to demonstrate that naturalism falsifies the impulse towards rigorously scientific philosophy? The clue to an answer is the following. If it turns out that natural science with its own means of positing objects and working in general cannot attain philosophy's field of problems, then any philosophy making use of this natural scientific method in any way is thereby doomed. *Experimental psychology is* nothing other than a scientific discipline that, in its manner of positing objects and idea of lawfulness, takes over the method of natural science.

A fourfold task presents itself: that of 1. characterizing the specific scientific status of mathematical natural science; 2. characterizing the scientific tendency of experimental psychology; 3. establishing philosophy's domain of problems; and 4. characterizing the discipline that treats this domain of problems satisfactorily (the scientific status is characterized with a view to the adequate way of seeing the type of object involved and then with a view to the type of treatment motivated by that way of seeing it).

The object of natural science is nature as physical nature, as the unity of a completely determinate, thingly being. As the basic character of this being, it is given that each thing in the sphere of being is perceivable as identically the same in a variety of diverse, direct perceptions. At the same time, this being of the natural thing is of the sort that this identifiable sameness of it is perceivable by a plurality of subjects. This thingly being is intersubjectively identifiable as being of a certain sort. Every one of these entities has, as one says, its determinate properties in the temporal and spatial expanse of things and stands at the same time in an entire complex of causal series. Each property of a thing is nothing other than a possibility, following under a causal law, of specifically regulated alterations of this thing in the context of nature as a whole. Thus, each thing is principally

determinable in the context of nature by going back to the functional connection of relations among things. This specific thingly unity is exhibited in appearances.

This distinctive *being of nature* is the unarticulated *horizon* into which the facts of the matter are gathered that *this psychology* vaguely and arbitrarily takes up from the tradition: fantasy, perception, representation. These basic phenomena do not themselves then become psychology's theme but instead, in connection with them, the facts of the matter are worked over in such a way that determinate regularities and law-likenesses are pinned down. These laws also bear within themselves the basic concepts from which they emerged, but with the same lack of intelligibility and differentiation. This basic deficiency of psychology is grounded in the predominance of the natural scientific manner of examination which looks for regularities of events and skips over the appearing thing. Psychology accordingly overlooks the fact that its specific domain is no such domain as that of natural science.

Today the objections made by Husserl already hold less since phenomenological work has penetrated into psychology and essential changes have become evident. Nevertheless, the changes are such that there is no hope at all of arriving at a new determination of psychology. The results of phenomenological work and use of terms have merely been taken over, but there 'is no purification of the science conducted from the standpoint of phenomenology.

d) The peculiar being of consciousness as the true object of philosophy and the method of discerning essences to acquire universally binding propositions

In contrast to *nature's being, consciousness* has this peculiarity, that there is nothing of the sort in it like an identity that is maintained in several direct experiences. This is principally excluded from the domain of mental being. Each perceptible experience is fundamentally [*grundsätzlich*] no longer the same, the moment it is allegedly perceived again. This nonidentifiability of an entity with the character of consciousness goes so far that it also holds for the same subject. The things of nature, by contrast, have an intersubjective identifiability. That is the concrete basis for the fact that the being of the mental is designated a "stream" and "flow." These are not trivial, popular labels; instead the reasons for them lie in the *peculiar manner of being of the mental* itself. This mental being that is thus characterized in regard to its perceptibility is principally the sort of being that does not exhibit itself via appearances; instead it is itself thus, as it appears, the object. Philosophy's object is never nature, but instead always a *phenomenon*. It is noteworthy that Husserl in the *Logical Investigations*, where he researches in a concrete, phenomenological fashion, directly rejects the use of the term "phenomenon." This peculiar being "consciousness" is a monadic unity, a unity that is characterized by the fact that it lies in a temporality that has a dually infinite horizon. Each entity of this domain of being can be pursued in the direction of an endless past and likewise in a futurity that is without end.

What *method* must correspond to the being of consciousness so that work on consciousness yields a *discipline* that leads to *universal* and *universally binding* propositions and an *absolute objectivity*? Insofar as this entity is a domain of being that is not nature but instead a phenomenon, the method cannot be that of natural scientific inquiry. Insofar as it is not nature, but has something like an essence, the sole method that leads to firm results is that of *discerning essences*. This method, and it alone, suffices for an examination of consciousness that gets at something other than a natural scientific, rule-like regularity and its determination; the sort of examination of consciousness that has the task of seeing *ideal connections* as ideal and bringing what it has seen into *binding propositions* of the science.

Clarification of the problems as purification and radicalization of their bias. The care about securing and justifying an absolute scientific status

In the face of this critical consideration, let us now ask: What motivates this critique, the manner in which it chooses its object and goes through it? How are we to characterize this critical method itself at all? Husserl speaks of the method as a *clarification of problems*.

The critique speaks *against* a *naturalization* in order to acquire *a genuine science of consciousness*. Insofar as this clarification is critique, the very *aim* and *idea of a scientific treatment of consciousness is made into something absolute*. The decision [involved in making the critique] is thus at the same time a decision *for* the relevant matter. In the course of this critique, what matters is to acquire the possibility of *a rigorous lawfulness*, the sort of lawfulness that is

rigorously objective, binding, and identifiable. The move toward genuine purification of the field of "consciousness" from every sort of matter of fact, a purification that is the basis of a philosophy as rigorous science – this move to a *universally binding character* is the already characterized *care about already known knowledge*.

An experience can never be iterated as the same for a subject. The genuine context of mental being is a succession of experiences, a succession regulated by a specific temporality and having a dually infinite horizon. In relation to the identifiability, one could say that it is intersubjectively identifiable insofar as a being proper to the soul [*ein seelisches Sein*] *can* be understood unambiguously by a plurality of subjects. But it may not be equated with the intersubjective identifiability of a thing of nature. This mental being [*dieses psychische Sein*] is conceived by psychology, as far as its manner of being is concerned, as coexisting with nature. Mental being is posited as grounded in the being of nature. Each lawfulness is the sort of lawfulness of something that is a matter of fact, and natural science has to do with various sorts of matters of facts. The question is whether there is anything like the possibility of making matter-of-factness as such intelligible by means of matters of fact.

We are not interested in the stance taken toward the being of nature and that of the soul. What interests us instead is the question of what *biases* [*Tendenzen*] are at work *in the critique of naturalism*, the question of what *care* guides both *the choice of the object and the critique*. We maintain first that the care out of which the choice of the object of the critique grows is *care about already known knowledge, care about securing knowledge* on the path of knowing the knowledge, *securing and justifying an absolute scientific status*. Naturalism is subjected to critique because its set of problems and method are bent on placing the normative lawfulness on a scientifically secured basis by means of an exact scientific treatment of consciousness. The *critique* is carried out in the manner of *clarifying the problems*. Problems are *taken up* and, with that, a specific *decision* is also made *about what is asked* and what the *tendency or bias* [*Tendenz*] *of the interrogation* is, a decision to *radicalize the bias* that is at work in what is taken up. What matters to Husserl is to bring the scientific bias to natural science radically to end. By taking up the critique as a clarification of the problems, the critique has decided *for* the scientific bias of naturalism. It is carried out in *a purification* in such a way that all the factors capable of endangering the acquisition of an *absolute evidence* and *certainty* are thrown out. This purification of the bias renders it absolute.

1. Hence, we next have to envision what *clarifying the problems* means, in order to see, from this vantage point, what the purification of the sets of problems and methods of the naturalistic philosophy looks like and how at every step *care about an absolute scientific status* is at work. 2. It is necessary to see how the *classification of the problems* is taken over in a positive sense from naturalism and how the specific inclination to it and to its method lies therein. 3. It is necessary to see how the *problem of knowing* takes centre stage and, indeed, the problem of *knowledge of physical nature*; it is necessary to see that this context of the problem thus provides the *horizon* for the theme of "consciousness." (4). It is necessary to see how in reference to certain *tendencies in history*, these tendencies are drawn upon in a positive way. . . .

Heidegger, M. (1927), 'The worldhood of the world'

From (2004) *Being and Time*. Translated by J. Macquarrie and E. Robinson. Oxford: Blackwell: 91–122. Originally published as (1927) *Sein und Zeit*. Tübingen: Max Niemeyer.

The Idea of the Worldhood of the World in General

Being-in-the world shall first be made visible with regard to that item of its structure which is the 'world' itself. To accomplish this task seems easy and so trivial as to make one keep taking for granted that it may be dispensed with. What can be meant by describing 'the world' as a phenomenon? It means to let us see what shows itself in 'entities' within the world. Here the first step is to enumerate the things that are 'in' the world: houses, trees, people, mountains, stars. We can *depict* the way such entities 'look', and we can give an *account* of occurrences in them and with them. This, however, is obviously a pre-phenomenological 'business' which cannot be at all relevant phenomenologically. Such a description is always confined to entities. It is ontical. But what we are seeking is Being. And we have formally defined 'phenomenon' in the phenomenological sense as that which shows itself as Being and as a structure of Being.

Thus, to give a phenomenological description of the 'world' will mean to exhibit the Being of those entities which are present-at-hand within the world, and to fix it in concepts which are categorial. Now the entities within the world are Things – Things of Nature, and Things 'invested with value' [*"wertbehaftete" Dinge*]. Their Thinghood becomes a problem; and to the extent that the Thinghood of Things 'invested with value' is based upon the Thinghood of Nature, our primary theme is the Being of Things of Nature – Nature as such. That characteristic of Being which belongs to Things of Nature (substances), and upon which everything is founded, is substantiality. What is its ontological meaning? By asking this, we have given an unequivocal direction to our inquiry.

But is this a way of asking ontologically about the 'world'? The problematic which we have thus marked out is one which is undoubtedly ontological. But even if this ontology should itself succeed in explicating the Being of Nature in the very purest manner, in conformity with the basic assertions about this entity, which the mathematical natural sciences provide, it will never reach the phenomenon that is the 'world': Nature is itself an entity which is encountered within the world and which can be discovered in various ways and at various stages.

Should we then first attach ourselves to those entities with which Dasein proximally and for the most part dwells – Things 'invested with value'? Do not these 'really' show us the world in which we live? Perhaps, in fact, they show us something like the 'world' more penetratingly. But these Things too are entities 'within' the world.

Neither the ontical depiction of entities within-the-world nor the ontological Interpretation of their Being is such as to reach the phenomenon of the 'world.' In both of these ways of access to 'Objective Being', the 'world' has already been 'presupposed', and indeed in various ways.

Is it possible that ultimately we cannot address ourselves to 'the world' as determining the nature of the entity we have mentioned? Yet we call this entity one which is "within-the-world". Is 'world' perhaps a characteristic of Dasein's Being? And in that case, does every Dasein 'proximally' have its world? Does not 'world' thus become something 'subjective'? How, then, can there be a 'common' world 'in' which, nevertheless, we *are*? And if we raise the question of the 'world', *what* world do we have in view? Neither the common world nor the subjective world, but *the worldhood of the world as such.* By what avenue do we meet this phenomenon?

'Worldhood' is an ontological concept, and stands for the structure of one of the constitutive items of Being-in-the-world. But we know Being-in-the-world as a way in which Dasein's character is defined existentially. Thus worldhood itself is an *existentiale*. If we inquire ontologically about the 'world', we by no means abandon the analytic of Dasein as a field for thematic study. Ontologically, 'world' is not a way of characterizing those entities which Dasein essentially is *not*; it is rather a characteristic of Dasein itself. This does not rule out the possibility that when we investigate the phenomenon of the 'world' we must do so by the avenue of entities within-the-world and the Being which they possess. The task of 'describing' the world phenomenologically is so far from obvious that even if we do no more than determine adequately what form it shall take, essential ontological clarifications will be needed.

This discussion of the word 'world', and our frequent use of it have made it apparent that it is used in several ways. By unravelling these we can get an indication of the different kinds of phenomena that are signified, and of the way in which they are interconnected.

1. "World" is used as an ontical concept, and signifies the totality of those entities which can be present-at-hand within the world.

2. "World" functions as an ontological term, and signifies the Being of those entities which we have just mentioned. And indeed 'world' can become a term for any realm which encompasses a multiplicity of entities: for instance, when one talks of the 'world' of a mathematician, 'world' signifies the realm of possible objects of mathematics.

3. "World" can be understood in another ontical sense – not, however, as those entities which Dasein essentially is not and which can be encountered within-the-world, but rather as that 'wherein' a factical Dasein as such can be said to 'live'. "World" has here a pre-ontological existentiell signification. Here again there are different possibilities: "world" may stand for the 'public' we-world, or one's 'own' closest (domestic) environment.

4. Finally, "world" designates the ontologico-existential concept of *worldhood*. Worldhood itself may have as its modes whatever structural wholes any special 'worlds' may have at the time; but it embraces in itself the *a priori* character of worldhood in general. We shall reserve the expression "world" as a term for our third signification. If we should sometimes use it in the first of these senses, we shall mark this with single quotation marks.

The derivative form 'worldly' will then apply terminologically to a kind of Being which belongs to Dasein, never to a kind which belongs to entities present-at-hand 'in' the world. We shall designate these latter entities as "belonging to the world" or "within-the-world" [*weltzugehörig oder innerweltlich*].

A glance at previous ontology shows that if one fails to see Being-in-the-world as a state of Dasein, the phenomenon of worldhood likewise gets *passed over*. One tries instead to Interpret the world in terms of the Being of those entities which are present-at-hand within-the-world but which are by no means proximally discovered – namely, in terms of Nature. If one understands Nature ontologico-categorially, one finds that Nature is a limiting case of the Being of possible entities within-the-world. Only in some definite mode of its own Being-in-the-world can Dasein discover entities as Nature. This manner of knowing them has the character of depriving the world of its worldhood in a definite way. 'Nature', as the categorial aggregate of those structures of Being which a definite entity encountered within-the-world may possess, can never make *worldhood* intelligible. But even the phenomenon of 'Nature', as it is conceived, for instance, in romanticism, can be grasped ontologically only in terms of the concept of the world – that is to say, in terms of the analytic of Dasein.

When it comes to the problem of analysing the world's worldhood ontologically, traditional ontology operates in a blind alley, if; indeed, it sees this problem at all. On the other hand, if we are to Interpret the world-hood of Dasein and the possible ways in which Dasein is made worldly [*Verweltlichung*], we must show *why* the kind of Being with which Dasein knows the world is such that it passes over the phenomenon of worldhood both ontically and ontologically. But at the same time the very Fact of this passing-over suggests that we must take special precautions to get the right phenomenal point of departure [*Ausgang*] for access [*Zugang*] to the phenomenon of worldhood, so that it will not get passed over.

Our method has already been assigned [*Anweisung*]. The theme of our analytic is to be Being-in-the-world, and accordingly the very world itself; and these are to be considered within the horizon of average everydayness – the kind of Being which is *closest* to Dasein. We must make a study of everyday Being-in-the-world; with the phenomenal support which this gives us, something like the world must come into view.

That world of everyday Dasein which is closest to it, is the *environment*. From this existential character of average Being-in-the-world, our investigation will take its course [*Gang*] towards the idea of worldhood in general. We shall seek the worldhood of the environment (environmentality) by going through an ontological Interpretation of those entities *within-the-environment* which we encounter as closest to us. The expression "environment" [*Umwelt*] contains in the 'environ' ["*um*"] a suggestion of spatiality. Yet the 'around' ["*Umherum*"] which is constitutive for the environment does not have a primarily 'spatial' meaning. Instead, the spatial character which incontestably belongs to any environment, can be clarified only in terms of the structure of worldhood. From this point of view, Dasein's spatiality, of which we have given an indication in Section 12, becomes phenomenally visible. In ontology, however, an attempt has been made to start with spatiality and then to Interpret the Being of the 'world' as *res extensa*. In Descartes we find the most extreme tendency towards such an ontology of the 'world', with, indeed, a counter-orientation towards the *res cogitans* – which does not coincide with Dasein either ontically or ontologically. The analysis of worldhood which we are here attempting can be made clearer if we show how it differs from such an ontological tendency. Our analysis will be completed in three stages: *(A)* the analysis of environmentality and worldhood in general; *(B)* an illustrative contrast between our analysis of worldhood and Descartes' ontology of the 'world'; *(C)* the aroundness [*das Umhafte*] of the environment, and the 'spatiality' of Dasein.

Analysis of Environmentality and Worldhood in General

The Being of the Entities Encountered in the Environment

The Being of those entities which we encounter as closest to us can be exhibited phenomenologically if we take as our clue our everyday Being-in-the-world, which we also call our *"dealings" in* the world and *with* entities within-the-world. Such dealings have already dispersed themselves into manifold ways of concern. The kind of dealing which is closest to us is as we have shown, not a bare perceptual cognition, but rather that kind of concern which manipulates things and puts them to use; and this has its own kind of 'knowledge'. The phenomenological question applies in the first instance to the Being of those entities which we encounter in such concern. To assure the kind of seeing which is here required, we must first make a remark about method.

In the disclosure and explication of Being, entities are in every case our preliminary and our accompanying theme [*das Vor- und Mitthematische*]; but our real theme is Being. In the domain of the present analysis, the entities we shall take as our preliminary theme are those which show themselves in our concern with the environment. Such entities are not thereby objects for knowing the 'world' theoretically; they are simply what gets used, what gets produced, and so forth. As entities so encountered, they become the preliminary theme for the purview of a 'knowing' which, as phenomenological, looks primarily towards Being, and which, in thus taking Being as its theme, takes these entities as its accompanying theme. This phenomenological interpretation is accordingly not a way of knowing those characteristics of entities which themselves are [*seiender Beschaffenheiten des Seienden*]; it is rather a determination of the structure of the Being which entities possess. But as an investigation of Being, it brings to completion, autonomously and explicitly, that understanding of Being which belongs already to Dasein and which 'comes alive' in any of its dealings with entities. Those entities which serve phenomenologically as our preliminary theme – in this case, those which are used or which are to be found in the course of production – become accessible when we put ourselves into the position of concerning ourselves with them in some such way. Taken strictly, this talk about "putting ourselves into such a position" [*Sichversetzen*] is misleading; for the kind of Being which belongs to such concernful dealings is not one into which we need to put ourselves first. This is the way in which everyday Dasein always *is*: when I open the door, for instance, I use the latch. The achieving of phenomenological access to the entities which we encounter, consists rather in thrusting aside our interpretative tendencies, which keep thrusting themselves upon us and running along with us, and which conceal not only the phenomenon of such 'concern', but even more those entities themselves *as* encountered of their own accord *in* our concern with them. These entangling errors become plain if in the course of our investigation we now ask which entities shall be taken as our preliminary theme and established as the pre-phenomenal basis for our study.

One may answer: "Things." But with this obvious answer we have perhaps already missed the prephenomenal basis we are seeking. For in addressing these entities as 'Things' *(res)*, we have tacitly anticipated their ontological character. When analysis starts with such entities and goes on to inquire about Being, what it meets is Thinghood and Reality. Ontological explication discovers, as it proceeds, such characteristics of Being as substantiality, materiality, extendedness, side-by-side-ness, and so forth. But even pre-ontologically, in such Being as this, the entities which we encounter in concern are proximally hidden. When one designates Things as the entities that are 'proximally given', one goes ontologically astray, even though ontically one has something else in mind. What one really has in mind remains undetermined. But suppose one characterizes these 'Things' as Things 'invested with value'? What does "value" mean ontologically? How are we to categorize this 'investing' and Being-invested? Disregarding the obscurity of this structure of investiture with value, have we thus met that phenomenal characteristic of Being which belongs to what we encounter in our concernful dealings?

The Greeks had an appropriate term for 'Things': πράγματα – that is to say, that which one has to do with in one's concernful dealings (πρᾶξις). But ontologically, the specifically 'pragmatic' character of the πράγματα is just what the Greeks left in obscurity; they thought of these 'proximally' as 'mere Things'. We shall call those entities which we encounter in concern *"equipment"*. In our dealings we come across equipment for writing, sewing, working, transportation, measurement. The kind of Being which equipment possesses must be exhibited. The clue for doing this lies in our first defining what makes an item of equipment – namely, its equipmentality.

Taken strictly, there 'is' no such thing as *an* equipment. To the Being of any equipment there always belongs a totality of equipment, in which it can be this equipment that it is. Equipment is essentially 'something in-order-to …' ["*etwas um-zu …*"]. A totality of equipment is constituted by various ways of the 'in-order-to', such as serviceability, conduciveness, usability, manipulability.

In the 'in-order-to' as a structure there lies an *assignment* or *reference* of something to something. Only in the analyses which are to follow can the phenomenon which this term 'assignment' indicates be made visible in its ontological genesis. Provisionally, it is enough to take a look phenomenally at a manifold of such assignments. Equipment – in accordance with its equipmentality – always is *in terms of* [*aus*] its belonging to other equipment: inkstand, pen, ink, paper, blotting pad, table, lamp, furniture, windows, doors, room. These 'Things' never show themselves proximally as they are for themselves, so as to add up to a sum of *realia* and fill up a room. What we encounter as closest to us (though not as something taken as a theme) is the room; and we encounter it not as something 'between four walls' in a geometrical spatial sense, but as equipment for residing. Out of this the 'arrangement' emerges, and it is in this that any 'individual' item of equipment shows itself. *Before* it does so, a totality of equipment has already been discovered.

Equipment can genuinely show itself only in dealings cut to its own measure (hammering with a hammer, for example); but in such dealings an entity of this kind is not *grasped* thematically as an occurring Thing, nor is the equipment-structure known as such even in the using. The hammering does not simply have knowledge about [*um*] the hammer's character as equipment, but it has appropriated this equipment in a way which could not possibly be more suitable. In dealings such as this, where something is put to use, our concern subordinates itself to the "in-order-to" which is constitutive for the equipment we are employing at the time; the less we just stare at the hammer-Thing, and the more we seize hold of it and use it, the more primordial does our relationship to it become, and the more unveiledly is it encountered as that which it is – as equipment. The hammering itself uncovers the specific 'manipulability' ["*Handlichkeit*"] of the hammer. The kind of Being which equipment possesses – in which it manifests itself in its own right – we call *"readiness-to-hand"* [*Zuhandenheit*]. Only because equipment has *this* 'Being-in-itself' and does not merely occur, is it manipulable in the broadest sense and at our disposal. No matter how sharply we just *look* [*nur nochhinseheni*] at the 'outward appearance' ["*Aussehen*]" of Things in whatever form this takes, we cannot discover anything ready-to-hand. If we look at Things just 'theoretically', we can get along without understanding readiness-to-hand. But when we deal with them by using them and manipulating them, this activity is not a blind one; it has its own kind of sight, by which our manipulation is guided and from which it acquires its specific Thingly character. Dealings with equipment subordinate themselves to the manifold assignments of the 'in-order-to'. And the sight with which they thus accommodate themselves is *circumspection*.

'Practical' behaviour is not 'atheoretical' in the sense of "sightlessness"). The way it differs from theoretical behaviour does not lie simply in the fact that in theoretical behaviour one observes, while in practical behaviour one *acts* [*gehandelt wird*], and that action must employ theoretical cognition if it is not to remain blind; for the fact that observation is a kind of concern is just as primordial as the fact that action has *its own* kind of sight. Theoretical behaviour is just looking, without circumspection. But the fact that this looking is non-circumspective does not mean that it follows no rules: it constructs a canon for itself in the form of *method*.

The ready-to-hand is not grasped theoretically at all, nor is it itself the sort of thing that circumspection takes proximally as a circumspective theme. The peculiarity of what is proximally ready-to-hand is that, in its readiness-to-hand, it must, as it were, withdraw [*zurückziehen*] in order to be ready-to-hand quite authentically. That with which our everyday dealings proximally dwell is not the tools themselves [*die Werkzeuge selbst*]. On the contrary, that with which we concern ourselves primarily is the work – that which is to be produced at the time; and this is accordingly ready-to-hand too. The work bears with it that referential totality within which the equipment is encountered.

The work to be produced, as the *"towards-which"* of such things as the hammer, the plane, and the needle, likewise has the kind of Being that belongs to equipment. The shoe which is to be produced is for wearing (footgear) [*Schuhzeug*]; the clock is manufactured for telling the time. The work which we chiefly encounter in our concernful dealings – the work that is to be found when one is "at work" on something [*das in Arbeit befindliche*] – has a usability which belongs to it essentially; in this usability it lets us

encounter already the "towards-which" for which *it* is usable. A work that someone has ordered [*das bestellte Werk*] is only by reason of its use and the assignment-context of entities which is discovered in using it.

But the work to be produced is not merely usable for something. The production itself is a using *of* something for something. In the work there is also a reference or assignment to 'materials': the work is dependent on [*angewiesen auf*] leather, thread, needles, and the like. Leather, moreover is produced from hides. These are taken from animals, which someone else has raised. Animals also occur within the world without having been raised at all; and, in a way, these entities still produce themselves even when they have been raised. So in the environment certain entities become accessible which are always ready-to-hand, but which, in themselves, do not need to be produced. Hammer, tongs, and needle, refer in themselves to steel, iron, metal, mineral, wood, in that they consist of these. In equipment that is used, 'Nature' is discovered along with it by that use – the 'Nature' we find in natural products.

Here, however, "Nature" is not to be understood as that which is just present-at-hand, nor as the *power of Nature*. The wood is a forest of timber, the mountain a quarry of rock; the river is water-power, the wind is wind 'in the sails'. As the 'environment' is discovered, the 'Nature' thus discovered is encountered too. If its kind of Being as ready-to-hand is disregarded, this 'Nature' itself can be discovered and defined simply in its pure presence-at-hand. But when this happens, the Nature which 'stirs and strives', which assails us and enthralls us as landscape, remains hidden. The botanist's plants are not the flowers of the hedgerow; the 'source' which the geographer establishes for a river is not the 'springhead in the dale'.

The work produced refers not only to the "towards-which" of its usability and the "whereof" of which it consists: under simple craft conditions it also has an assignment to the person who is to use it or wear it. The work is cut to his figure; he 'is' there along with it as the work emerges. Even when goods are produced by the dozen, this constitutive assignment is by no means lacking; it is merely indefinite, and points to the random, the average. Thus along with the work, we encounter not only entities ready-to-hand but also entities with Dasein's kind of Being – entities for which, in their concern, the product becomes ready-to-hand; and together with these we encounter the world in which wearers and users live, which is at the same time ours. Any work with which one concerns oneself is ready-to-hand not only in the domestic world of the workshop but also in the *public world*. Along with the public world, the *environing Nature [die Umweltnatur]* is discovered and is accessible to everyone. In roads, streets, bridges, buildings, our concern discovers Nature as having some definite direction. A covered railway platform takes account of bad weather; an installation for public lighting takes account of the darkness, or rather of specific changes in the presence or absence of daylight – the 'position of the sun'. In a clock, account is taken of some definite constellation in the world-system. When we look at the clock, we tacitly make use of the sun's position, in accordance with which the measurement of time gets regulated in the official astronomical manner. When we make use of the clock-equipment, which is proximally and inconspicuously ready-to-hand, the environing Nature is ready-to-hand along with it. Our concernful absorption in whatever work-world lies closest to us, has a function of discovering; and it is essential to this function that, depending upon the way in which we are absorbed, those entities within-the-world which are brought along [*beigebrachte*] in the work and with it (that is to say, in the assignments or references which are constitutive for it) remain discoverable in varying degrees of explicitness and with a varying circumspective penetration.

The kind of Being which belongs to these entities is readiness-to-hand. But this characteristic is not to be understood as merely a way of taking them, as if we were talking such 'aspects' into the 'entities' which we proximally encounter, or as if some world-stuff which is proximally present-at-hand in itself were 'given subjective colouring' in this way. Such an Interpretation would overlook the fact that in this case these entities would have to be understood and discovered beforehand as something purely present-at-hand, and must have priority and take the lead in the sequence of those dealings with the 'world' in which something is discovered and made one's own. But this already runs counter to the ontological meaning of cognition, which we have exhibited as a *founded* mode of Being-in-the-world. To lay bare what is just present-at-hand and no more, cognition must first penetrate *beyond* what is ready-to-hand in our concern. *Readiness-to-hand is the way in which entities as they are 'in themselves' are defined ontologico-categorially.* Yet only by reason of something present-at-hand, 'is there' anything ready-to-hand. Does it follow, however, granting this thesis for the nonce, that readiness-to-hand is ontologically founded upon presence-at-hand?

But even if, as our ontological Interpretation proceeds further, readiness-to-hand should prove itself to be the kind of Being characteristic of those entities which are proximally discovered within-the-world, and even if its primordiality as compared with pure presence-at-hand can be demonstrated, have all these explications been of the slightest help towards understanding the phenomenon of the world ontologically? In Interpreting these entities within-the-world, however, we have always 'presupposed' the world. Even if we join them together, we still do not get anything like the 'world' as their sum. If, then, we start with the Being of these entities, is there any avenue that will lead us to exhibiting the phenomenon of the world?

§16. How the Worldly Character of the Environment Announces itself in Entities Within-the-world

The world itself is not an entity within-the-world; and yet it is so determinative for such entities that only in so far as 'there is' a world can they be encountered and show themselves, in their Being, as entities which have been discovered. But in what way 'is there' a world ? If Dasein is ontically constituted by Being-in-the-World, and if an understanding of the Being of its Self belongs just as essentially to its Being, no matter how indefinite that understanding may be, then does not Dasein have an understanding of the world – a pre-ontological understanding, which indeed can and does get along without explicit ontological insights? With those entities which are encountered within-the-world – that is to say, with their character as within-the-world – does not something like the world show itself for concernful Being-in-the-world? Do we not have a pre-phenomenological glimpse of this phenomenon? Do we not always have such a glimpse of it, without having to take it as a theme for ontological Interpretation? Has Dasein itself, in the range of its concernful absorption in equipment ready-to-hand, a possibility of Being in which the worldhood of those entities within-the-world with which it is concerned is, in a certain way, lit up for it, *along with* those entities themselves?

If such possibilities of Being for Dasein can be exhibited within its concernful dealings, then the way lies open for studying the phenomenon which is thus lit up, and for attempting to 'hold it at bay', as it were, and to interrogate it as to those structures which show themselves therein.

To the everydayness of Being-in-the-world there belong certain modes of concern. These permit the entities with which we concern ourselves to be encountered in such a way that the worldly character of what is within-the-world comes to the fore. When we concern ourselves with something, the entities which are most closely ready-to-hand may be met as something unusable, not properly adapted for the use we have decided upon. The tool turns out to be damaged, or the material unsuitable. In each of these cases *equipment* is here, ready-to-hand. We discover its unusability, however, not by looking at it and establishing its properties, but rather by the circum-spection of the dealings in which we use it. When its unusability is thus discovered, equipment becomes conspicuous. This *conspicuousness* presents the ready-to-hand equipment as in a certain un-readi-ness-to-hand. But this implies that what cannot be used just lies there; it shows itself as an equipmental Thing which looks so and so, and which, in its readiness-to-hand as looking that way, has constantly been present-at-hand too. Pure presence-at-hand announces itself in such equipment, but only to with-draw to the readiness-to-hand of something with which one concerns oneself – that is to say, of the sort of thing we find when we put it back into repair. This presence-at-hand of something that cannot be used is still not devoid of all readiness-to-hand what-soever; equipment which is present-at-hand in this way is still not just a Thing which occurs somewhere. The damage to the equipment is still not a mere alteration of a Thing – not a change of properties which just occurs in something present-at-hand.

In our concernful dealings, however, we not only come up against unusable things within what is ready-to-hand already: we also find things which are missing – which not only are not 'handy' ["*handlich*"] but are not 'to hand' ["*zur Hand*"] at all. Again, to miss something in this way amounts to coming across something un-ready-to-hand. When we notice what is un-ready-to-hand, that which is ready-to-hand enters the mode of obtrusiveness. The more urgently [*Je dringlicher*] we need what is missing, and the more authentically it is encountered in its un-readiness-to-hand, all the more obtrusive [*um so aufdringlicher*] does that which is ready-to-hand become – so much so, indeed, that it seems to lose its character of readiness-to-hand. It reveals itself as something just present-at-hand and no more, which cannot be budged without the thing that is missing. The helpless way in which we stand before it is a deficient mode of concern, and as such it uncovers the Being-just-present-at-hand-and-no-more of something ready-to-hand.

In our dealings with the 'world' of our concern, the un-ready-to-hand can be encountered not only in the sense of that which is unusable or simply missing, but as something un-ready-to-hand which is *not* missing at all and *not* unusable, but which 'stands in the way' of our concern. That to which our concern refuses to turn, that for which it has 'no time', is something un-ready-to-hand in the manner of what does not belong here, of what has not as yet been attended to. Anything which is un-ready-to-hand in this way is disturbing to us, and enables us to see the *obstinacy* of that with which we must concern our-selves in the first instance before we do anything else. With this obstinacy, the presence-at-hand of the ready-to-hand makes itself known in a new way as the Being of that which still lies before us and calls for our attending to it.

The modes of conspicuousness, obtrusiveness, and obstinacy all have the function of bringing to the fore the characteristic of presence-at-hand in what is ready-to-hand. But the ready-to-hand is not thereby just *observed* and stared at as something present-at-hand; the presence-at-hand which makes itself known is still bound up in the readiness-to-hand of equip-ment. Such equipment still does not veil itself in the guise of mere Things. It becomes 'equipment' in the sense of something which one would like to shove out of the way. But in such a tendency to shove things aside, the ready-to-hand shows itself as still ready-to-hand in its unswerving presence-at-hand.

Now that we have suggested, however, that the ready-to-hand is thus encountered under modifi-cations in which its presence-at-hand is revealed, how far does this clarify the *phenomenon of the world*? Even in analysing these modifications we have not gone beyond the Being of what is within-the-world, and we have come no closer to the world-phenomenon than before. But though we have not as yet grasped it, we have brought ourselves to a point where we can bring it into view.

In conspicuousness, obtrusiveness, and obstinacy, that which is ready-to-hand loses its readiness-to-hand in a certain way. But in our dealings with what is ready-to-hand, this readiness-to-hand is itself understood, though not thematically. It does not vanish simply, but takes its farewell, as it were, in the conspicuousness of the unusable. Readiness-to-hand still shows itself, and it is precisely here that the worldly character of the ready-to-hand shows itself too.

The structure of the Being of what is ready-to-hand as equipment is determined by references or assignments. In a peculiar and obvious manner, the 'Things' which are closest to us are 'in themselves' ["*Ansich*"]; and they are encountered as 'in themselves' in the concern which makes use of them without noticing them explicitly – the concern which can come up against something unusable. When equipment cannot be used, this implies that the constitutive assignment of the "in-order-to" to a "towards-this" has been disturbed. The assignments themselves are not observed; they are rather 'there' when we concernfully submit ourselves to them [*Sichstellen unter sie*]. But *when an assignment has been disturbed* – when something is unusable for some purpose – then the assignment becomes explicit. Even now, of course, it has not become explicit as an ontological structure; but it has become explicit ontically for the circumspection which comes up against the damaging of the tool. When an assignment to some particular "towards-this" has been thus circumspectively aroused, we catch sight of the "towards-this" itself, and along with it everything connected with the work – the whole 'workshop' – as that wherein concern always dwells. The context of equipment is lit up, not as something never seen before, but as a totality constantly sighted beforehand in circumspection. With this totality, however, the world announces itself.

Similarly, when something ready-to-hand is found missing, though its everyday presence [*Zugegensein*] has been so obvious that we have never taken any notice of it, this makes a *break* in those referential contexts which circumspection discovers. Our circumspection comes up against emptiness, and now sees for the first time *what* the missing article was ready-to-hand *with*, and *what* it was ready-to-hand *for*. The environment announces itself afresh. What is thus lit up is not itself just one thing ready-to-hand among others; still less is it something

present-at-hand upon which equipment ready-to-hand is somehow founded: it is in the 'there' before anyone has observed or ascertained it. It is itself inaccessible to circumspection, so far as circumspection is always directed towards entities; but in each case it has already been disclosed for circumspection. 'Disclose' and 'disclosedness' will be used as technical terms in the passages that follow, and shall signify 'to lay open' and 'the character of having been laid open'. Thus 'to disclose' never means anything like 'to obtain indirectly by inference'.

That the world does not 'consist' of the ready-to-hand shows itself in the fact (among others) that whenever the world is lit up in the modes of concern which we have been Interpreting, the ready-to-hand becomes deprived of its worldhood so that Being-just-present-at-hand comes to the fore. If, in our everyday concern with the 'environment', it is to be possible for equipment ready-to-hand to be encountered in its 'Being-in-itself' [*in seinem "An-sich-sein"*], then those assignments and referential totalities in which our circumspection 'is absorbed' cannot become a theme for that circumspection any more than they can for grasping things 'thematically' but non-circumspectively. If it is to be possible for the ready-to-hand not to emerge from its inconspicuousness, the world *must not announce itself*. And it is in this that the Being-in-itself of entities which are ready-to-hand has its phenomenal structure constituted.

In such privative expressions as "inconspicuousness", "unobtrusiveness", and "non-obstinacy", what we have in view is a positive phenomenal character of the Being of that which is proximally ready-to-hand. With these negative prefixes we have in view the character of the ready-to-hand as "holding itself in"; this is what we have our eye upon in the "Being-in-itself" of something, though 'proximally' we ascribe it to the present-at-hand – to the present-at-hand as that which can be thematically ascertained. As long as we take our orientation primarily and exclusively from the present-at-hand, the 'in-itself' can by no means be ontologically clarified. If, however, this talk about the 'in-itself' has any ontological importance, some interpretation must be called for. This "in-itself" of Being is something which gets invoked with considerable emphasis, mostly in an ontical way, and rightly so from a phenomenal standpoint. But if some *ontological* assertion is supposed to be given when this is *ontically* invoked, its claims are not fulfilled by such a procedure. As the foregoing analysis has already made clear, only on the basis of the phenomenon of the world can the Being-in-itself of entities within-the-world be grasped ontologically.

But if the world can, in a way, be lit up, it must assuredly be disclosed. And it has already been disclosed beforehand whenever what is ready-to-hand within-the-world is accessible for circumspective concern. The world is therefore something 'wherein' Dasein as an entity already *was,* and if in any manner it explicitly comes away from anything, it can never do more than come back to the world.

Being-in-the-world, according to our Interpretation hitherto, amounts to a non-thematic circumspective absorption in references or assignments constitutive for the readiness-to-hand of a totality of equipment. Any concern is already as it is, because of some familiarity with the world. In this familiarity Dasein can lose itself in what it encounters within-the-world and be fascinated with it. What is it that Dasein is familiar with? Why can the worldly character of what is within-the-world be lit up? The presence-at-hand of entities is thrust to the fore by the possible breaks in that referential totality in which circumspection 'operates'; how are we to get a closer understanding of this totality?

These questions are aimed at working out both the phenomenon and the problems of worldhood, and they call for an inquiry into the interconnections with which certain structures are built up. To answer them we must analyse these structures more concretely.

§17. Reference and Signs

In our provisional Interpretation of that structure of Being which belongs to the ready-to-hand (to 'equipment'), the phenomenon of reference or assignment became visible; but we merely gave an indication of it, and in so sketchy a form that we at once stressed the necessity of uncovering it with regard to its ontological origin. It became plain, moreover, that assignments and referential totalities could in some sense become constitutive for worldhood itself. Hitherto we have seen the world lit up only in and for certain definite ways in which we concern ourselves environmentally with the ready-to-hand, and indeed it has been lit up only *with* the readiness-to-hand of that concern. So the further we proceed in understanding the Being of entities within-the-world, the broader and firmer becomes the phenomenal basis on which the world-phenomenon may be laid bare.

We shall again take as our point of departure the Being of the ready-to-hand, but this time with the purpose of grasping the phenomenon of *reference* or *assignment* itself more precisely. We shall accordingly attempt an ontological analysis of a kind of equipment in which one may come across such 'references' in more senses than one. We come across 'equipment' in *signs.* The word "sign" designates many kinds of things: not only may it stand for different *kinds* of signs, but Being-a-sign-for can itself be formalized as a *universal kind of relation,* so that the sign-structure itself provides an ontological clue for 'characterizing' any entity whatsoever.

But signs, in the first instance, are themselves items of equipment whose specific character as equipment consists in *showing* or *indicating.* We find such signs in signposts, boundary-stones, the ball for the mariner's storm-warning, signals, banners, signs of mourning, and the like. Indicating can be defined as a 'kind' of referring. Referring is, if we take it as formally as possible, a *relating.* But relation does not function as a genus for 'kinds' or 'species' of references which may somehow become differentiated as sign, symbol, expression, or signification. A relation is something quite formal which may be read off directly by way of 'formalization' from any kind of context, whatever its subject-matter or its way of Being.

Every reference is a relation, but not every relation is a reference. Every 'indication' is a reference, but not every referring is an indicating. This implies at the same time that every 'indication' is a relation, but not every relation is an indicating. The formally general character of relation is thus brought to light. If we are to investigate such phenomena as references, signs, or even significations, nothing is to be gained by characterizing them as relations. Indeed we shall eventually have to show that 'relations' themselves, *because of* their formally general character, have their ontological source in a reference.

If the present analysis is to be confined to the Interpretation of the sign as distinct from the phenomenon of reference, then even within this limitation we cannot properly investigate the full multiplicity of possible signs. Among signs there are symptoms [*Anzeichen*], warning signals, signs of things that have happened already [*Rückzeichen*], signs to mark something, signs by which things are recognized; these have different ways of indicating, regardless of what may be serving as such a sign. From such 'signs' we must distinguish traces, residues, commemorative monuments, documents, testimony, symbols, expressions, appearances, significations. These phenomena can easily be formalized because of their formal relational character; we find it especially tempting nowadays to take such a 'relation' as a clue for subjecting every entity to a kind of 'Interpretation' which always 'fits' because at bottom it says nothing, no more than the facile schema of content and form.

As an example of a sign we have chosen one which we shall use again in a later analysis, though in another regard. Motor cars are sometimes fitted up with an adjustable red arrow, whose position indicates the direction the vehicle will take – at an intersection, for instance. The position of the arrow is controlled by the driver. This sign is an item of equipment which is ready-to-hand for the driver in his concern with driving, and not for him alone: those who are not travelling with him – and they in particular – also make use of it, either by giving way on the proper side or by stopping. This sign is ready-to-hand within-the-world in the whole equipment-context of vehicles and traffic regulations. It is equipment for indicating, and as equipment, it is constituted by reference or assignment. It has the character of the 'in-order-to', its own definite serviceability; it is for indicating. This indicating which the sign performs can be taken as a kind of 'referring'. But here we must notice that this 'referring' as indicating is not the ontological structure of the sign as equipment.

Instead, 'referring' as indicating is grounded in the Being-structure of equipment, in serviceability for . . . . But an entity may have serviceability without thereby becoming a sign. As equipment, a 'hammer' too is constituted by a serviceability, but this does not make it a sign. Indicating, as a 'reference', is a way in which the "towards-which" of a serviceability becomes ontically concrete; it determines an item of equipment as for this "towards-which" [und bestimmt ein Zeug zu diesem]. On the other hand, the kind of reference we get in 'serviceability-for', is an ontologico-categorial attribute of equipment as equipment. That the "towards-which" of serviceability should acquire its concreteness in indicating, is an accident of its equipment-constitution as such. In this example of a sign, the difference between the reference of serviceability and the reference of indicating becomes visible in a rough and ready fashion. These are so far from coinciding that only when they are united does

the concreteness of a definite kind of equipment become possible. Now it is certain that indicating differs in principle from reference as a constitutive state of equipment; it is just as incontestable that the sign in its turn is related in a peculiar and even distinctive way to the kind of Being which belongs to whatever equipmental totality may be ready-to-hand in the environment, and to its worldly character. In our concernful dealings, equipment for indicating [Zeig-Zeug] gets used in a very special way. But simply to establish this Fact is ontologically insufficient. The basis and the meaning of this special status must be clarified.

What do we mean when we say that a sign "indicates"? We can answer this only by determining what kind of dealing is appropriate with equipment for indicating. And we must do this in such a way that the readiness-to-hand of that equipment can be genuinely grasped. What is the appropriate way of having-to-do with signs? Going back to our example of the arrow, we must say that the kind of behaving (Being) which corresponds to the sign we encounter, is either to 'give way' or to 'stand still' vis-à-vis the car with the arrow. Giving way, as taking a direction, belongs essentially to Dasein's Being-in-the-world. Dasein is always somehow directed [ausgerichtet] and on its way; standing and waiting are only limiting cases of this directional 'on-its-way'. The sign addresses itself to a Being-in-the-world which is specifically 'spatial'. The sign is not authentically 'grasped' ["erfasst"] if we just stare at it and identify it as an indicator-Thing which occurs. Even if we turn our glance in the direction which the arrow indicates, and look at something present-at-hand in the region indicated, even then the sign is not authentically encountered. Such a sign addresses itself to the circumspection of our concernful dealings, and it does so in such a way that the circumspection which goes along with it, following where it points, brings into an explicit 'survey' whatever aroundness the environment may have at the time. This circumspective survey does not grasp the ready-to-hand; what it achieves is rather an orientation within our environment. There is also another way in which we can experience equipment: we may encounter the arrow simply as equipment which belongs to the car. We can do this without discovering what character it specifically has as equipment: what the arrow is to indicate and how it is to do so, may remain completely undetermined; yet what we are encountering is not a mere Thing. The experiencing of a Thing requires a *definiteness* of its own [*ihre eigene Bestimmtheit*], and must be contrasted with coming across a manifold of equipment, which may often be quite indefinite, even when one comes across it as especially close.

Signs of the kind we have described let what is ready-to-hand be encountered; more precisely, they let some context of it become accessible in such a way that our concernful dealings take on an orientation and hold it secure. A sign is not a Thing which stands to another Thing in the relationship of indicating; it is rather *an item of equipment which explicitly raises a totality of equipment into our circumspection so that together with it the worldly character of the ready-to-hand announces itself.* In a symptom or a warning-signal, 'what is coming' indicates itself, but not in the sense of something merely occurring, which comes as an addition to what is already present-at-hand; 'what is coming' is the sort of thing which we are ready for, or which we 'weren't ready for' if we have been attending to something else. In signs of something that has happened already, what has come to pass and run its course becomes circumspectively accessible. A sign to mark something indicates what one is 'at' at any time. Signs always indicate primarily 'wherein' one lives, where one's concern dwells, what sort of involvement there is with something.

The peculiar character of signs as equipment becomes especially clear in 'establishing a sign' [*"Zeichenstiftung"*]. This activity is performed in a circumspective fore-sight [*Vorsicht*] out of which it arises, and which requires that it be possible for one's particular environment to announce itself for circumspection at any time by means of something ready-to-hand, and that this possibility should itself be ready-to-hand. But the Being of what is most closely ready-to-hand within-the-world possesses the character of holding-itself-in and not emerging, which we have described above. Accordingly our circumspective dealings in the environment require some equipment ready-to-hand which in its character as equipment takes over the 'work' of *letting* something ready-to-hand *become conspicuous.* So when such equipment (signs) gets produced, its conspicuousness must be kept in mind. But even when signs are thus conspicuous, one does not let them be present-at-hand at random; they get 'set up' [*"angebracht"*] in a definite way with a view towards easy accessibility.

In establishing a sign, however, one does not necessarily have to produce equipment which is not yet ready-to-hand at all. Signs also arise when one *takes as a sign* [*Zum-Zeichen-nehmen*] something that is ready-to-hand already. In this mode, signs 'get established' in a sense which is even more primordial. In indicating, a ready-to-hand equipment totality, and even the environment in general, can be provided with an availability which is circumspectively oriented; and not only this: establishing a sign can, above all, reveal. What gets taken as a sign becomes accessible only through its readiness-to-hand. If, for instance, the south wind 'is accepted' [*"gilt"*] by the farmer as a sign of rain, then this 'acceptance' [*"Geltung"*] – or the 'value' with which the entity is 'invested' – is not a sort of bonus over and above what is already present-at-hand in itself – *viz*, the flow of air in a definite geographical direction. The south wind may be meteorologically accessible as something which just occurs; but it is *never* present-at-hand *proximally* in such a way as this, only occasionally taking over the function of a warning signal. On the contrary, only by the circumspection with which one takes account of things in farming, is the south wind discovered in its Being.

But, one will protest, *that which* gets taken as a sign must first have become accessible in itself and been apprehended *before* the sign gets established. Certainly it must in any case be such that in some way we can come across it. The question simply remains as to *how* entities are discovered in this previous encountering, whether as mere Things which occur, or rather as equipment which has not been understood – as something ready-to-hand with which we have hitherto not known 'how to begin', and which has accordingly kept itself veiled from the purview of circumspection. *And here again, when the equipmental characters of the ready-to-hand are still circumspectively undiscovered, they are not to be Interpreted as bare Thinghood presented for an apprehension of what is just present-at-hand and no more.*

The Being-ready-to-hand of signs in our everyday dealings, and the conspicuousness which belongs to signs and which may be produced for various purposes and in various ways, do not merely serve to document the inconspicuousness constitutive for what is most closely ready-to-hand; the sign itself gets its conspicuousness from the inconspicuousness of the equipmental totality, which is ready-to-hand and 'obvious' in its everydayness. The knot which one ties in a handkerchief [*der bekannte "Knopf im Taschen-tuch"*] as a sign to mark something is an example of this. What such a sign is to indicate is always something with which one has to concern oneself in one's everyday circumspection. Such a sign can indicate many things, and things of the most various kinds. The wider the extent to which it can indicate, the narrower its intelligibility and its usefulness. Not only is it, for the most part, ready-to-hand as a sign only for the person who 'establishes' it, but it can even become inaccessible to him, so that another sign is needed if the first is to be used circumspectively at all. So when the knot cannot be used as a sign, it does not lose its sign-character, but it acquires the disturbing obtrusiveness of something most closely ready-to-hand.

One might be tempted to cite the abundant use of 'signs' in primitive Dasein, as in fetishism and magic, to illustrate the remarkable role which they play in everyday concern when it comes to our understanding of the world. Certainly the establishment of signs which underlies this way of using them is not performed with any theoretical aim or in the course of theoretical speculation. This way of using them always remains completely within a Being-in-the-world which is 'immediate'. But on closer inspection it becomes plain that to interpret fetishism and magic by taking our clue from the idea of signs in general, is not enough to enable us to grasp the kind of 'Being-ready-to-hand' which belongs to entities encountered in the primitive world. With regard to the sign-phenomenon, the following Interpretation may be given: for primitive man, the sign coincides with that which is indicated. Not only can the sign represent this in the sense of serving as a substitute for what it indicates, but it can do so in such a way that the sign itself always *is* what it indicates. This remarkable coinciding does not mean, however, that the sign-Thing has already undergone a certain 'Objectification' – that it has been experienced as a mere Thing and misplaced into the same realm of Being of the present-at-hand as what it indicates. This 'coinciding' is not an identification of things which have hitherto been isolated from each other: it consists rather in the fact that the sign has not as yet become free from that of which it is a sign. Such a use of signs is still absorbed completely in Being-towards what is indicated, so that a sign as such cannot detach itself at all. This coinciding is based not on a prior Objectification but on the fact that such Objectification is

completely lacking. This means, however, that signs are not discovered as equipment at all – that ultimately what is 'ready-to-hand' within-the-world just does not have the kind of Being that belongs to equipment. Perhaps even readiness-to-hand and equipment have nothing to contribute [*nichts auszurichten*] as ontological clues in Interpreting the primitive world; and certainly the ontology of Thinghood does even less. But if an understanding of Being is constitutive for primitive Dasein and for the primitive world in general, then it is all the more urgent to work out the 'formal' idea of worldhood – or at least the idea of a phenomenon modifiable in such a way that all ontological assertions to the effect that in a given phenomenal context something is *not yet* such-and-such or *no longer* such-and-such, may acquire a *positive* phenomenal meaning in terms of what it is *not*.

The foregoing Interpretation of the sign should merely provide phenomenal support for our characterization of references or assignments. The relation between sign and reference is threefold. 1. Indicating, as a way whereby the "towards-which" of a serviceability can become concrete, is founded upon the equipment-structure as such, upon the "in-order-to" (assignment). 2. The indicating which the sign does is an equipmental character of something ready-to-hand, and as such it belongs to a totality of equipment, to a context of assignments or references. 3. The sign is not only ready-to-hand with other equipment, but in its readiness-to-hand the environment becomes in each case explicitly accessible for circumspection. *A sign is something ontically ready-to-hand, which functions both as this definite equipment and as something indicative of* [*was ... anzeigt*] *the ontological structure of readiness-to-hand, of referential totalities, and of worldhood.* Here is rooted the special status of the sign as something ready-to-hand in that environment with which we concern ourselves circumspectively. Thus the reference or the assignment itself cannot be conceived as a sign of it is to serve ontologically as the foundation upon which signs are based. Reference is not an ontical characteristic of something ready-to-hand, when it is rather that by which readiness-to-hand itself is constituted.

In what sense, then, is reference 'presupposed' ontologically in the ready-to-hand, and to what extent is it, as such an ontological foundation, at the same time constitutive for worldhood in general?

§18. Involvement and Significance; the Worldhood of the World

The ready-to-hand is encountered within-the-world. The Being of this entity, readiness-to-hand, thus stands in some ontological relationship towards the world and towards worldhood. In anything ready-to-hand the world is always 'there'. Whenever we encounter anything, the world has already been previously discovered, though not thematically. But it can also be lit up in certain ways of dealing with our environment. The world is that in terms of which the ready-to-hand is ready-to-hand. How can the world let the ready-to-hand be encountered? Our analysis hitherto has shown that what we encounter within-the-world has, in its very Being, been freed for our concernful circumspection, for taking account. What does this previous freeing amount to, and how is this to be understood as an ontologically distinctive feature of the world? What problems does the question of the worldhood of the world lay before us?

We have indicated that the state which is constitutive for the ready-to-hand as equipment is one of reference or assignment. How can entities with this kind of Being be freed by the world with regard to their Being? Why are these the first entities to be encountered? As definite kinds of references we have mentioned serviceability-for-detrimentality [*Abtraglichkeit*], usability, and the like. The "towards-which" [*das Wozu*] of a serviceability and the "for-which" [*das Wofür*] of a usability prescribed the ways in which such a reference or assignment can become concrete. But the 'indicating' of the sign and the 'hammering' of the hammer are not properties of entities. Indeed, they are not properties at all, if the ontological structure designated by the term 'property' is that of some definite character which it is possible for Things to possess [*einer möglichen Bestimmtheit von Dingen*]. Anything ready-to-hand is, at the worst, appropriate for some purposes and inappropriate for others; and its 'properties' are, as it were, still bound up in these ways in which it is appropriate or inappropriate, just as presence-at-hand, as a possible kind of Being for something ready-to-hand, is bound up in readiness-to-hand. Serviceability too, however, as a constitutive state of equipment (and serviceability is a reference), is not an appropriateness of some entity; it is rather the condition (so far as Being is in question) which makes it possible for the character of such an entity to be defined by its appropriatenesses. But what, then, is "reference" or "assignment" to mean? To say that the Being of the ready-to-hand has the structure of assignment or reference means that it has in itself the character of *having been assigned or referred* [*Verwiesenheit*]. An entity is discovered when it has been assigned or referred to something, and referred as that entity which it is. *With* any such entity there is an involvement which it has *in* something. The character of Being which belongs to the ready-to-hand is just such an *involvement*. If something has an involvement, this implies letting it be involved in something. The relationship of the "with ... in ..." shall be indicated by the term "assignment" or "reference".

When an entity within-the-world has already been proximally freed for its Being, that Being is its "involvement". With any such entity as entity, there is some involvement. The fact that it has such an involvement is *ontologically* definitive for the Being of such an entity, and is not an ontical assertion about it. That in which it is involved is the "towards-which" of serviceability, and the "for-which" of usability. With the "towards-which" of serviceability there can again be an involvement: *with* this thing, for instance, which is ready-to-hand, and which we accordingly call a "hammer", there is an involvement in hammering; with hammering, there is an involvement in making something fast; with making something fast, there is an involvement in protection against bad weather; and this protection 'is' for the sake of [*um-willen*] providing shelter for Dasein – that is to say, for the sake of a possibility of Dasein's Being. Whenever something ready-to-hand has an involvement with it, *what* involvement this is, has in each case been outlined in advance in terms of the totality of such involvements. In a workshop, for example, the totality of involvements which is constitutive for the ready-to-hand in its readiness-to-hand, is 'earlier' than any single item of equipment; so too for the farmstead with all its utensils and outlying lands. But the totality of involvements itself goes back ultimately to a "towards-which" in which there is *no* further involvement: this "towards-which" is not an entity with the kind of Being that belongs to what is ready-to-hand within a world; it is rather an entity whose Being is defined as Being-in-the-world, and to whose state of Being, worldhood itself belongs. This primary "towards-which" is not just another "towards-this" as something in which an involvement is possible. The primary 'towards-which' is a "for-the-sake-of-which". But the 'for-the-sake-of' always pertains to the Being of *Dasein,* for which, in its Being, that very Being is essentially an *issue.* We have thus indicated the interconnection by which the structure of an involvement leads to Dasein's very Being as the sole authentic "for-the-sake-of-which"; for the present, however, we shall pursue this no further. 'Letting something be involved' must first be clarified enough to give the phenomenon of worldhood the kind of definiteness which makes it possible to formulate any problems about it.

Ontically, "letting something be involved" signifies that within our factical concern we let something ready-to-hand *be* so-and-so *as* it is already and *in order that* it be such. The way we take this ontical sense of 'letting be' is, in principle, ontological. And therewith we Interpret the meaning of previously freeing what is proximally ready-to-hand within-the-world. Previously letting something 'be' does not mean that we must first bring it into its Being and produce it; it means rather that something which is already an 'entity' must be discovered in its readiness-to-hand, and that we must thus let the entity which has this Being be encountered. This *'a priori'* letting-something-be-involved is the condition for the possibility of encountering anything ready-to-hand, so that Dasein, in its ontical dealings with the entity thus encountered, can thereby let it be involved in the ontical sense. On the other hand, if letting something be involved is understood ontologically, what is then pertinent is the freeing of *everything* ready-to-hand as ready-to-hand, no matter whether, taken ontically, it is involved thereby, or whether it is rather an entity of precisely such a sort that ontically it is *not* involved thereby. Such entities are, proximally and for the most part, those with which we concern ourselves when we do not let them 'be' as we have discovered that they are, but work upon them, make improvements in them, or smash them to pieces.

When we speak of having already let something be involved, so that it has been freed for that involvement, we are using a *perfect* tense *a priori* which characterizes the kind of Being belonging to Dasein itself. Letting an entity be involved, if we understand this ontologically, consists in previously freeing it for [*auf*] its readiness-to-hand within the environment. When we let something be involved, it must be involved in something; and in terms of this "in-which", the "with-which" of this involvement is freed.

Our concern encounters it as this thing that is ready-to-hand. To the extent that any *entity* shows itself to concern – that is, to the extent that it is discovered in its Being – it is already something ready-to-hand environmentally; it just is not 'proximally' a 'world-stuff' that is merely present-at-hand. .

As the Being of something ready-to-hand, an involvement is itself discovered only on the basis of the prior discovery of a totality of involvements. So in any involvement that has been discovered (that is, in anything ready-to-hand which we encounter), what we have called the "worldly character" of the ready-to-hand has been discovered beforehand. In this totality of involvements which has been discovered beforehand, there lurks an ontological relationship to the world. In letting entities be involved so that they are freed for a totality of involvements, one must have disclosed already that for which [*woraufhin*] they have been freed. But that for which something environmentally ready-to-hand has thus been freed (and indeed in such a manner that it becomes accessible *as* an entity within-the-world first of all), cannot itself be conceived as an entity with this discovered kind of Being. It is essentially not discoverable, if we henceforth reserve *"discoveredness"* as a term for a possibility of Being which every entity *without* the character of Dasein may possess.

But what does it mean to say that that for which entities within-the-world are proximally freed must have been previously disclosed? To Dasein's Being, an understanding of Being belongs. Any understanding [*Verständnis*] has its Being in an act of understanding [*Verstehen*]. If Being-in-the-world is a kind of Being which is essentially befitting to Dasein, then to understand Being-in-the-world belongs to the essential content of its understanding of Being. The previous disclosure of that for which what we encounter within-the-world is subsequently freed, amounts to nothing else than understanding the world – that world towards which Dasein as an entity always comports itself.

Whenever we let there be an involvement with something in something beforehand, our doing so is grounded in our understanding such things as letting something be involved, and such things as the "with-which" and the "in-which" of involvements. Anything of this sort, and anything else that is basic for it, such as the "towards-this" as that in which there is an involvement, or such as the "for-the-sake-of-which" to which every "towards-which" ultimately goes back – all these must be disclosed beforehand with a certain intelligibility [*Verständlichkeit*]. And what is that wherein Dasein as Being-in-the-world understands itself pre-ontologically? In understanding a context of relations such as we have mentioned, Dasein has assigned itself to an "in-order-to" [*um zu*], and it has done so in terms of a potentiality-for-Being for the sake of which it itself is – one which it may have seized upon either explicitly or tacitly, and which may be either authentic or inauthentic. This "in-order-to" prescribes a "towards-this" as a possible "in-which" for letting something be involved; and the structure of letting it be involved implies that this is an involvement which something *has* – an involvement which is *with* something. Dasein always assigns itself from a "for-the-sake-of-which" to the "with-which" of an involvement; that is to say, to the extent that it is, it always lets entities be encountered as ready-to-hand. *That wherein* [*Worin*] Dasein understands itself beforehand in the mode of assigning itself is *that for which* [*das Woraufhin*] it has let entities be encountered beforehand. *The "wherein" of an act of understanding which assigns or refers itself, is that for which one lets entities be encountered in the kind of Being that belongs to involvements; and this "wherein" is the phenomenon of the world.* And the structure of that to which [*woraufhin*] Dasein assigns itself is what makes up the *worldhood* of the world.

That wherein Dasein already understands itself in this way is always something with which it is primordially familiar. This familiarity with the world does not necessarily require that the relations which are constitutive for the world as world should be theoretically transparent. However, the possibility of giving these relations an explicit ontologicoexistential Interpretation, is grounded in this familiarity with the world; and this familiarity, in turn, is constitutive for Dasein, and goes to make up Dasein's understanding of Being. This possibility is one which can be seized upon explicitly in so far as Dasein has set itself the task of giving a primordial Interpretation for its own Being and for the possibilities of that Being, or indeed for the meaning of Being in general.

But as yet our analyses have done no more than lay bare the horizon within which such things as the world and worldhood are to be sought. If we are to consider these further, we must, in the first instance, make it still more clear how the context of Dasein's assigning-itself is to be taken ontologically.

In the *act of understanding* [*Verstehen*], which we shall analyse more thoroughly later ..., the relations indicated above must have been previously disclosed; the act of understanding holds them in this disclosedness. It holds itself in them with familiarity; and in so doing, it holds them *before* itself, for it is in these that its assignment operates. The understanding lets itself make assignments both in these relationships themselves and of them. The relational character which these relationships of assigning possess, we take as one of *signifying*. In its familiarity with these relationships, Dasein 'signifies' to itself: in a primordial manner it gives itself both its Being and its potentiality-for-Being as something which it is to understand with regard to its Being-in-the-world. The "for-the-sake-of-which" signifies an "in-order-to"; this in turn, a "towards-this"; the latter, an "in-which" of letting something be involved; and that in turn, the "with-which" of an involvement. These relationships are bound up with one another as a primordial totality; they are what they are as this signifying [*Bedeuten*] in which Dasein gives itself beforehand its Being-in-the-world as something to be understood. The relational totality of this signifying we call *"significance"*. This is what makes up the structure of the world – the structure of that wherein Dasein as such already is. *Dasein, in its familiarity with significance, is the ontical condition for the possibility of discovering entities which are encountered in a world with involvement (readiness-to-hand) as their kind of Being, and which can thus make themselves known as they are in themselves [in seinem An-sich].* Dasein as such is always something of this sort; along with its Being, a context of the ready-to-hand is already essentially discovered: Dasein, in so far as it *is*, has always submitted itself already to a 'world' which it encounters, and this *submission* belongs essentially to its Being.

But in significance itself, with which Dasein is always familiar, there lurks the ontological condition which makes it possible for Dasein, as something which understands and interprets, to disclose such things as 'significations'; upon these, in turn, is founded the Being of words and of language.

The significance thus disclosed is an existential state of Dasein – of its Being-in-the-world; and as such it is the ontical condition for the possibility that a totality of involvements can be discovered.

If we have thus determined that the Being of the ready-to-hand (involvement) is definable as a context of assignments or references, and that even worldhood may so be defined, then has not the 'substantial Being' of entities within-the-world been volatilized into a system of Relations? And inasmuch as Relations are always 'something thought', has not the Being of entities within-the-world been dissolved into 'pure thinking'?

Within our present field of investigation the following structures and dimensions of ontological problematics, as we have repeatedly emphasized, must be kept in principle distinct: 1. the Being of those entities within-the-world which we proximally encounter – readiness-to-hand; 2. the Being of those entities which we can come across and whose nature we can determine if we discover them in their own right by going through the entities proximally encountered – presence-at-hand; 3. the Being of that ontical condition which makes it possible for entities within-the-world to be discovered at all – the worldhood of the world. This third kind of Being gives us an *existential* way of determining the nature of Being-in-the-world, that is, of Dasein. The other two concepts of Being are *categories*, and pertain to entities whose Being is not of the kind which Dasein possesses. The context of assignments or references, which, as significance, is constitutive for worldhood, can be taken formally in the sense of a system of Relations. But one must note that in such formalizations the phenomena get levelled off so much that their real phenomenal content may be lost, especially in the case of such 'simple' relationships as those which lurk in significance. The phenomenal content of these 'Relations' and 'Relata' – the "in-order-to", the "for-the-sake-of", and the "with-which" of an involvement – is such that they resist any sort of mathematical functionalization; nor are they merely something thought, first posited in an 'act of thinking.' They are rather relationships in which concernful circumspection as such already dwells. This 'system of Relations', as something constitutive for worldhood, is so far from volatilizing the Being of the ready-to-hand within-the-world, that the worldhood of the world provides the basis on which such entities can for the first time be discovered as they are 'substantially' in themselves. And only if entities within-the-world can be encountered at all, is it possible, in the field of such entities, to make accessible what is just present-at-hand and no more. By reason of their Being-just-present-at-hand-and-no-more, these latter entities can have their 'properties' defined mathematically in

'functional concepts'. Ontologically, such concepts are possible only in relation to entities whose Being has the character of pure substantiality. Functional concepts are never possible except as formalized substantial concepts.

In order to bring out the specifically ontological problematic of worldhood even more sharply, we shall carry our analysis no further until we have clarified our Interpretation of worldhood by a case at the opposite extreme.

Heidegger, M. (1927), 'Fear as a mode of state-of-mind'

From (2004) *Being and Time*. Translated by J. Macquarrie and E. Robinson. Oxford: Blackwell: 179–82. Originally published as (1927) *Sein und Zeit*. Tübingen: Max Niemeyer.

There are three points of view from which the phenomenon of fear may be considered. We shall analyse: 1. that in the face of which we fear, 2. fearing, and 3. that about which we fear. These possible ways of looking at fear are not accidental; they belong together. With them the general structure of states-of-mind comes to the fore. We shall complete our analysis by alluding to the possible ways in which fear may be modified; each of these pertains to different items in the structure of fear.

That in the face of which we fear, the 'fearsome', is in every case something which we encounter within-the-world and which may have either readiness-to-hand, presence-at-hand, or Dasein-with as its kind of Being. We are not going to make an ontical report on those entities which can often and for the most part be 'fearsome': we are to define the fearsome phenomenally in its fearsomeness. What do we encounter in fearing that belongs to the fearsome as such? That in the face of which we fear can be characterized as threatening. Here several points must be considered. 1. What we encounter has detrimentality as its kind of involvement. It shows itself within a context of involvements. 2. The target of this detrimentality is a definite range of what can be affected by it; thus the detrimentality is itself made definite, and comes from a definite region. 3. The region itself is well known as such, and so is that which is coming from it; that which is coming from it has something 'queer' about it. 4. That which is detrimental, as something that threatens us, is not yet within striking distance [*in beherrschbarer Nähe*], but it is coming close. In such a drawing-close, the detrimentality radiates out, and therein lies its threatening character. 5. This drawing-close is within what is close by. Indeed, something may be detrimental in the highest degree and may even be coming constantly closer; but if it is still far off, its fearsomeness remains veiled. If, however, that which is detrimental draws close and is close by, then it is threatening: it can reach us, and yet it may not. As it draws close, this 'it can, and yet in the end it may not' becomes aggravated. We say, "It is fearsome". 6. This implies that what is detrimental as coming-close close by carries with it the patent possibility that it may stay away and pass us by; but instead of lessening or extinguishing our fearing, this enhances it.

In *fearing as such*, what we have thus characterized as threatening is freed and allowed to matter to us. We do not first ascertain a future evil (*malum futurum*) and then fear it. But neither does fearing first take note of what is drawing close; it discovers it beforehand in its fearsomeness. And in fearing, fear can then look at the fearsome explicitly, and "make it clear' to itself. Circumspection sees the fearsome because it has fear as its state-of-mind. Fearing, as a slumbering possibility of Being-in-the-world in a state-of-mind (we call this possibility 'fearfulness' ["*Furchtsamkeit*"]), has already disclosed the world, in that out of it something like the fearsome may come close. The potentiality for coming close is itself freed by the essential existential spatiality of Being-in-the-world.

That which fear fears *about* is that very entity which is afraid – Dasein. Only an entity for which in its Being this very Being is an issue, can be afraid. Fearing discloses this entity as endangered and abandoned to itself. Fear always reveals Dasein in the Being of its "there", even if it does so in varying degrees of explicitness. If we fear about our house and home, this cannot be cited as an instance contrary to the above definition of what we fear about; for as Being-in-the-world, Dasein is in every case concernful Being-alongside. Proximally and for the most part, Dasein is in terms of *what* it is concerned with. When this is endangered, Being-alongside is threatened. Fear discloses Dasein predominantly in a privative way. It bewilders us and makes us 'lose our heads'. Fear closes off our endangered Being-in, and yet at the same time lets us see it, so that when the fear has subsided, Dasein must first find its way about again.

Whether privatively or positively, fearing about something, as being-afraid in the face of something, always discloses equiprimordially entities within-the-world and Being-in – the former as threatening and the latter as threatened. Fear is a mode of state-of-mind.

One can also fear about Others, and we then speak of "fearing for" them [*Fürchten für sie*]. This fearing for the Other does not take away his fear. Such a possibility has been ruled out already, because the Other, for whom we fear, need not fear at all on his part. It is precisely when the other is *not* afraid and charges recklessly at what is threatening him that we fear most for him. Fearing-for is a way of having a co-state-of-mind with Others, but not necessarily a being-afraid-with or even a fearing-with-one-another. One can "fear about" without "being-afraid". Yet when viewed more strictly, fearing-about is "being-afraid-for-*oneself*". Here what one "is apprehensive about" is one's Being-with with the Other, who might be torn away from one. That which is fearsome is not aimed directly at him who fears with someone else. Fearing-about knows that in a certain way it is unaffected, and yet it is co-affected in so far as the Dasein-with for which it fears is affected. Fearing-about is therefore not a weaker form of being-afraid. Here the issue is one of existential modes, not of degrees of 'feeling-tones'. Fearing-about does not lose its specific genuiness even if it is not 'really' afraid.

There can be variations in the constitutive items of the full phenomenon of fear. Accordingly, different possibilities of Being emerge in fearing. Bringing-close close by, belongs to the structure of the threatening as encounterable. If something threatening breaks in suddenly upon concernful Being-in-the-world (something threatening in its 'not right away, but any moment'), fear becomes *alarm* [*Erschrecken*]. So, in what is threatening we must distinguish between the closest way in which it brings itself close, and the manner in which this bringing-close gets encountered – its suddenness. That in the face of which we are alarmed is proximally something well known and familiar. But if, on the other hand, that which threatens has the character of something altogether unfamiliar, then fear becomes *dread* [*Grauen*]. And where that which threatens is laden with dread, and is at the same time encountered with the suddenness of the alarming, then fear becomes *terror* [*Entsetzen*]. There are further variations of fear, which we know as timidity, shyness, misgiving, becoming startled. All modifications of fear, as possibilities of having a state-of-mind, point to the fact that Dasein as Being-in-the-world is 'fearful' ["*furchtsam*"]. This 'fearfulness' is not to be understood in an ontical sense as some tactical 'individualized' disposition, but as an existential possibility of the essential state-of-mind of Dasein in general, though of course it is not the only one.

Introduction

9

In this chapter we present some of the main efforts to outline the phenomenological approach in psychiatry. It is far from clear that the phenomenological movement ever settled on a single method or set of methods which could be applied to psychiatry. Husserl himself changed his views about method in phenomenology over the course of his life. However, what seemed to remain constant was a turning toward the transcendental Ego. This has led critics (e.g. Dennett 1991, p. 44) to criticize Husserl's approach by equating it to introspectionism. Regardless of the validity of these criticisms (see Ratcliffe 2009 and Cerbone 2003 for good accounts) the question arises about how phenomenology can be applied in psychiatry where the Ego, or consciousness, is not one's own but another's – and another's in whom the presumption of a consciousness similar to one's own cannot necessarily be made. Spiegelberg has usefully called the effort to apply phenomenology to other people's mental states 'phenomenology through vicarious experience' (Spiegelberg 1964).

Why should one want to develop a vicarious phenomenology? Perhaps the place to begin is Emil Kraepelin, a figure of central importance to modern psychiatry. In the following extract, Kraepelin describes an encounter with a young man with schizophrenia. It is played out in the third-person perspective. Kraepelin approaches the case like a neurologist. The case material is put into a public, impersonal space and reported upon with the detachment of an observer.

Gentlemen,– The patient I will show you to-day has almost to be carried into the room, as he walks in a straddling fashion on the outside of his feet. On coming in, he throws off his slippers, sings a hymn loudly, and then cries twice (in English), "My _ father, my real father!" He is eighteen years old, and a pupil of the Oberrealschule (higher grade modern secondary school), tall, and rather strongly built, with a pale complexion, on which there is very often a transient flush. The patient sits with his eyes shut, and pays no attention to his surroundings. He does not look up even when he is spoken to, but he answers, beginning in a low voice, and gradually screaming louder and louder. When asked where he is, he says, "You want to know that too; I tell you who is being measured and is measured and shall be measured. I know all that, and could tell you, but I do not want to." When asked his name, he screams, "What is your name? What does he shut? He shuts his eyes. What does he hear? He does not understand; he understands not. How? Who? Where? When? What does he mean? When I tell him to look, he does not look properly. You there, just look! What is it? What is the matter? Attend; he attends not. I say, what is it, then? Why do you give me no answer? Are you getting impudent again? How can you be so impudent? I'm coming! I'll show you! You don't turn whore for me. You mustn't be smart either; you're an impudent, lousy fellow, an impudent, lousy fellow, as stupid as a hog. Such an impudent, shameless, miserable, lousy fellow I've never met with. Is he beginning again? You understand nothing at all – nothing at all; nothing at all does he understand. If you follow now, he won't follow, will not follow. Are you getting still more impudent? Are you getting impudent still more? How they attend, they do attend," and so on. At the end he scolds in quite inarticulate sounds.

The patient understands perfectly, and has introduced many phrases he has heard before into his speech, without once looking up. He speaks in an affected way, now babbling like a child, now lisping and stammering, sings suddenly in the middle of what he is saying, and grimaces. He carries out orders in an extraordinary fashion, gives his hand with the fist clenched, goes to the blackboard when he is asked, but, instead of writing his name, suddenly knocks down a lamp, and throws the chalk among the audience. He makes all kinds of senseless movements, pushes the table away, crosses his arms, and turns round on his axis, chair and all, or sits balancing, with his legs crossed and his hands on his head. Catalepsy can also be made out. When he is to go away, he will not get up, has to be pushed, and calls out loudly, "Good-morning, gentlemen; it has not pleased me." The only physical disturbance worth noticing is a considerable acceleration of the pulse to 160 beats.

At first sight, the patient might perhaps be considered maniacal, but closer consideration reveals several features inconsistent with this view. The first of these is the patient's *inaccessibility*. Although he undoubtedly understood all our questions, he has not given us a single useful piece of information. His talk was indeed connected with our questions, but it contained no answer, but only a series of disconnected sentences, having no relation whatever either to the question or to the general situation. Again, the frequent *repetition of the same phrases* could very plainly be followed in his talk, which finally degenerated into *unmeaning abuse*, without the occurrence of any external cause or the appearance of strong excitement in the patient himself. We have already learned to recognise some of the symptoms – the negativism shown in his refusal to answer, and perhaps in his keeping his eyes continually shut, and also the stereotypism. A new feature is *confused speech*, quite incoherent talk, without the patient's being irrational or showing strong excitement – a symptom which is not found in this form of mania. Maniacal patients may certainly talk in a confused way, but, at the most, it is only transitorily and in the worst states of excitement, with loss of memory, that they lose the connection so completely. Even then it is almost always possible to get some kind of relevant answer from them. And we only meet with the gross obscenity of speech known as "coprolalia" in maniacal patients when they are very much irritated.

Other diagnostically important symptoms to be seen in our patient are *catalepsy*, sudden *impulsive actions*, *grimacing*, and *extraordinary, affected behaviour*. His remarkable attitude, his aimless movements, and the strange transformation of everyday actions, such as walking, speaking, and giving his hand, the so-called "mannerisms," are what principally distinguish his actions from the brisk and bustling activity of the maniac, which is so much more comprehensible to us who are sane. The senselessness of a maniacal patient's actions results from his great divertibility and the rapid succession of ever-fresh abortive impulses, but here the impulses themselves are quite aimless, and do not follow one another at all quickly, even though some particular impulse may be converted into action with violent suddenness. Hence, in mania actions bear the stamp of flightiness and precipitancy, but here of incomprehensibility and absurdity. There the mood is exuberant and unrestrained, while here, in spite of all external unrest, the absence of profound emotional excitement is obvious enough.

In accordance with these arguments, we will not hesitate to attribute the condition before us, not to maniacal-depressive insanity, but to *dementia praecox*, of which

we find the characteristic symptoms present here – viz., good comprehension, with atrophy of the emotions and various kinds of vitiations of the will ...

(Kraepelin 1906, pp. 79–81).

Let us now look at a response to this case from another psychiatrist – R. D. Laing – when he was at the peak of his romantic powers in 1964. Unlike Kraepelin's third-person perspective Laing adopts the second-person perspective. He wants to reach out and establish contact with the patient's world. Laing wants to understand the patient not observe him.

> Now there is no question that this patient is showing the 'signs' of catatonic excitement. The construction we put on this behaviour will, however, depend on the relationship we establish with the patient, and we are indebted to Kraepelin's vivid description which enables the patient to come, it seems, alive to us across 50 years and through his pages as though he were before us. What does this patient seem to be doing? Surely he is carrying on a dialogue between his own parodied version of Kraepelin, and his own defiant rebelling self. 'You want to know that too? I tell you who is being measured and is measured and shall be measured. I now all that, and I could tell you, but I do not want to.' This seems to be plain enough talk. Presumably he deeply resents this form of interrogation which is being carried out before a lecture-room of students. He probably does not see what it has to do with the things that must be deeply distressing him. But these things would not be 'useful information' to Kraepelin except as further 'signs' of a 'disease'.

> Kraepelin asks him his name. The patient replies by an exasperated outburst in which he is now saying what he feels is the attitude implicit in Kraepelin's approach to him: What is your name? What does he shut? He shuts his eyes ... Why do you give me no answer? Are you getting impudent again? You don't whore for me? (i.e. he feels that Kraepelin is objecting because he is not prepared to prostitute himself before the whole classroom of students), and so on ... such an impudent, shameless, miserable, lously fellow I've never met with ... etc.

> Now it seems clear that this patient's behaviour can be seen in at least two ways, analogous to the ways of seeing a vase or face. One may see his behaviour as 'signs' of a 'disease'; one may see his behaviour as expressive of his existence .... What is the boy's experience of Kraepelin? He seems to be tormented and desperate. What is he 'about' in speaking and acting in this way? He is objecting to being measured and tested. He wants to be heard ...

If one is adopting such an attitude towards a patient [the third person attitude], it is hardly possible at the same time to understand what he may be trying to communicate to us ... if I am sitting opposite you and speaking to you, you may be trying 1) to assess any abnormalities in my speech, or 2) to explain what I am saying in terms of how you are imagining my brain cells to be metabolizing oxygen, or 3) to discover why, in terms of past history and socio-economic background, I should be saying these things at this time. Not one of the answers that you may or may not be able to supply to these questions will in itself supply you with a simple understanding of what I am getting at

(Laing 1990, pp. 30–3).

Laing articulates succinctly a reaction to Kraepelin that one finds occurring even at the time Kraepelin was active. It amounts to the view that the third-personal stance misses the 'what it is like' of psychiatric phenomena and the fact that the phenomena come laden in meaning. In 1912 a Munich psychiatrist called Willhelm Specht founded the 'Journal of Pathopsychology' (*Zeitschrift für Pathopsychologie*). The journal positioned itself against an inappropriately neurological or psychological rendering of psychiatric phenomena which it held to be over-dominant in the psychiatry of the time. Both, it was thought, resulted in an attitude toward psychopathology in which the experience of the patient became of secondary interest. It was experience resulting from a disordered brain in the case of the somatic doctrine or experience resulting from unconscious libidinal processes in the case of the psychoanalytical doctrine influential at the time. In the journal's first issue there was an article by Max Scheler; in its second, one by Karl Jaspers. Jaspers sums up the sentiment later:

Historically looked at, the prevalence of the doctrine 'mental illnesses are cerebral illnesses' has had *helpful* as well as *harmful* effects. It has helped research into the brain. Every hospital has its anatomical laboratory, but it has harmed psychopathological research proper. Unwittingly many a psychiatrist has been overcome by the feeling that if only we had an exact knowledge of the brain, we would then know the psychic life and its disturbances. This has led psychiatrists to abandon psychopathological studies as unscientific, so that they have lost whatever psychopathological knowledge had been gained up to then

(Jaspers 1963a, p. 459).

Theories call for a certain simplicity whereas the understanding of meaning uncovers an infinite manifold. As it is Freud believed that practically everything psychic could be traced back to sexuality in a broad sense as if it were the sole and primary power

(Jaspers 1963a, p. 540).

Thus it seems vicarious phenomenology in psychiatry was a response to a real problem in psychiatry. When the observational/reductive methods of the natural sciences (including on this account Freud's attempt at extending those methods into the realm of meaning) were applied wholesale to mental illness, there was a sense that something important was being missed. What is interesting is that the response – right back in 1912 – had at its core Jaspers and Scheler. It didn't emerge as any simple application of Husserl's 'method'.

Both Jaspers and Scheler made contributions to the phenomenological approach in psychiatry. Jaspers made the more extensive and influential contributions. Scheler's contributions were more in the way of stimulus, for example his text on compensation hysteria, (please refer to p. 241), and through his students such as Schneider.

Jaspers developed a distinction between what he called 'the subjectivity of morbid psychic life' and 'meaningful connection in psychic life'. Only the former did he link to Husserl. The latter he thought derived from very different philosophical sources and he made particular mention of Dilthey (please refer to p. 6). In his philosophical memoir he explains how he proceeded:

My own studies and reflections on what was being said and done in psychiatry had shown me ways that were new at the time. The impulses for two main steps came from philosophers.

As a method I adopted and retained Husserl's phenomenology – which he initially called 'descriptive psychology' – discarding only its refinement to essence perception. It turned out to be possible and fruitful to describe the inner experiences of the sick as phenomena of consciousness. By the patient's own self-description, not only hallucinations but delusive experiences, modes of ego-consciousness and types of emotion could be defined well enough for positive recognition in other cases. Phenomenology became a research method.

The other influence was Dilthey's call for a psychology that would be "descriptive and analytical" rather than theoretically explicative. I accepted the challenge, termed the matter "understanding psychology", and worked out the procedures – long known in practice, and actually used by Freud in his peculiar fashion – which let us comprehend the genetic links of the psyche, the motivations and relationships of meaning, as distinguished from the phenomena of direct experience

(Jaspers 1963b, pp. 209–10).

What Jaspers called phenomenology was a procedural version of Husserl's methods of consciousness description. It had none of the philosophical ambitions of Husserl's phenomenology and Jaspers labelled it his 'static' method. It was the method to employ for arriving at basic psychopathological facts. These facts were seen as theory-neutral and value-neutral and were the things which psychiatry, as a science, had the job of explaining. An outline of this method is given in Jaspers' essay 'The phenomenological approach in psychopathology' which follows (please refer to p. 91).

In contrast to this Jaspers' 'understanding psychology' was a psychology of meaningful connections or motivational causation. Jaspers understood this form of causation as distinct from the form of causation which is non-psychic and not specific to animals and humans (i.e. the form of causation that also applies to nails and stone, etc.). The philosopher Edith Stein, an early participant in the phenomenological movement, expressed this psychic kind of causation in the following way in 1917:

> The foreign individual's body as such is given as a part of physical nature in causal relationships with other physical objects. He who pushes it imparts motion to it, etc. But these causal relationships are not all. As we know, the foreign physical body is not seen as a physical body, but as a living one. We see it suffer and carry out effects other than the physical. Pricking a hand is not the same as pounding a nail into a wall, even though it is the same procedure mechanically, namely driving a sharp object. The hand senses the pain if struck, and we see this ... We "see" this effect because we see the hand as sensitive, because we project ourselves into it empathically and so interpret every physical influence on it as a "stimulus" evoking a psychic response.

> Along with these effects of outer causes, we comprehend effects within the individual himself. For example, we may see a child actively romping about and then becoming tired and cross. We then interpret tiredness and the bad mood as the effects of movement ... Now, we may not infer the causal sequence from the data obtained, but also experience it empathically. For example, we comprehend interpsychic causality similarly when we observe the process of contagion of feelings in others while we ourselves are immune to the infectious material. Perhaps when the actor says: "You can hear nothing but sobbing and women weeping", we perceive a suppressed sob in all parts of the audience. And projecting ourselves into this soul-stirring spirit, we become seized by the mood portrayed. In this way we get an image of the causal process being enacted.

> Finally, we also perceive how an individual affects the outer world by every action that changes physical nature, by impulsive as well as willful ones. For example, when I observe the "reaction" to a stimulus when a stone flying toward someone is driven from its course by a "mechanical" resistance movement, I see a causal process into which psychic connecting links have been inserted. Projecting myself into the other, I interpret the object as a stimulus and experience the release of the counter-movement. I then experience the stone's diversion from its course as the effect of the reaction

(Stein 1989, pp. 71–2).

Jaspers thought that understanding this causation required a kind of lived, or embodied, cognition. Dilthey had called this *Verstehen* and argued it was essential to the methods of the historical and cultural sciences (Please refer to p. 6). Detached cognition in the mode of natural science would miss these meaningful connections which only showed themselves in the flow of life – a little bit like how we grasp the motivations of a character in a novel by following that character's development within the story. Jaspers labelled this 'genetic' method where by 'genetic' he meant pertaining to development over time, temporal evolution, rather than anything to do with genes or genetic material. His *General Psychopathology* contains approximately 150 pages of material under this category and variously includes précis of Jung, Freud, Nietzsche, Kierkegaard, Klages, etc. In what follows we give some extracts from the *General Psychopathology* where Jaspers tries to tell us what this method is (please refer to p. 101). To this day it remains intriguing but also far from clear.

Despite Jaspers' philosophical bent his methodological approach to psychopathology was cautious about philosophy.[1] The static method was a descriptive, fact-finding, endeavour adapted to the needs of a branch of medicine dealing in morbid subjectivity; his genetic method related to the interpretative methods of what we now call 'the social sciences'.

Max Scheler's contributions were much more philosophical. He saw psychopathology as existing in a fruitful interaction with the phenomenological movement.

---

[1] See Owen 2008 for a further examination of this issue. [Editors' note]

The influence of phenomenology on a few younger psychiatrists is especially exciting and reacts powerfully on the phenomenological philosophy itself

(Scheler 1973a, p. 151).

And he delighted in seeing psychiatrists making use of his phenomenological philosophy.

It has been a particular pleasure to me that the first edition of this book should have received considerable attention, not only from professional philosophers and psychologists, but also among exponents of the new phenomenological approach in psychiatry

(Scheler 1954, preface to 2nd edn).

Scheler himself wrote little on method but he seems to have seen psychopathology as a means of testing various philosophical theories of perception, mind and the human person in general. Crudely, his idea was that if a philosophical view on a matter showed itself as true only in pathological or exceptional cases then this was evidence that the philosophical view was false. One example he was fond of giving concerned associationist philosophies of mind. These philosophies, Scheler claimed, gave accurate accounts of mind as it undergoes cognitive decline in ageing.[2] This helps us see, Scheler thought, that they are not the sorts of philosophies of mind we should be after.[3]

In his essay 'The idols of self-knowledge', first published in Specht's journal as 'On self deceptions', Scheler

develops a novel account of perception by focusing on the phenomena of hallucinations and illusions. He contrasts his account with the philosophical theories of perception current in his day by, in effect, arguing that they fail to save the psychopathological phenomena.

The abundance of non-sensory factors contained in normal perception and the poverty of most philosophical theories of perception are seen in their proper light by means of the method of psychopathology applied here. . . . If this [method] is systematically applied we can, for the first time, hope . . . that the components of perception will be taken as what they are, in their fullness, and not as what they "could" or "should" be for the sake of some arbitrary theory of their genesis

(Scheler 1973b, p. 59).

The young group of psychiatrists Scheler refers to include many of the authors in this volume: Kurt Schneider, Karl Jaspers, Ludwig Binswanger, Henricus Rümke. All of these psychiatrists certainly took inspiration from Scheler although ultimately many of them decided Scheler's approach was unclear. An interesting methodological issue arises here concerning the use psychiatry and psychology makes of philosophy (or one philosopher's work in particular) as a basis for making sense of psychopathology. Overall, Jaspers was sceptical of this philosophical 'grounding' of psychopathology (although he himself, a psychiatrist, evolved into a philosopher and his own philosophy heavily influences later editions of his psychiatric textbook *General Psychopathology*). Jaspers thought that psychopathology ought to be held to the standards of science, that science aimed at value-neutrality and that science was separate from the aspirations of philosophy. Kurt Schneider (a pupil of both Scheler and Jaspers) ultimately sided with Jaspers on this matter and limited (at least overtly) the extent to which his psychopathology was philosophical. But he remained open-minded: 'In addition to somatogenesis and psychogenesis, there is a third theoretical possibility: namely, metagenesis, that is, some genuine "aberration" of the mind, without somatic or psychic foundation, and this, at any rate here and perhaps elsewhere, will have to remain an open question' (Schneider 1959, p. 10).

Another group of psychiatrists – particularly Eugene Minkowski and Ludwig Binswanger[4] – thought

---

[2] See, for example, Max Scheler (2009a) p. 18. [Editors' note]

[3] A similar approach is taken by Ernst Cassirer in 1929 in relation to brain injury patients. In 'Toward a pathology of the symbolic consciousness' (Cassirer 1957), Cassirer examines the phenomena of aphasia, agnosia and apraxia. Two points are worth making about Cassirer's approach. Firstly, as well as surveying the clinical literature, he visited a clinic (his cousin's Kurt Goldstein's (please refer to p. 132)) and interacted with brain injury patients personally. Secondly, he deliberately avoids discussion of neurobiological or psychological mechanisms. Following an appraisal of the phenomena, Cassirer argues that philosophies of language that are sceptical of the conceptual or cognitive value of language approximate to aphasia, agnosia and apraxia and therefore cannot be adequate. (We thank Dr Edward Skidelsky and Dr Nobert Andersch for bringing Cassirer's approach to psychopathology to our attention.) Something like this approach is also present in Merleau-Ponty's 1945 work *The Phenomenology of Perception* (Merleau-Ponty 2002) which draws substantively upon psychopathological case reports – some of them in this reader – to develop an adequate philosophical notion of the body. [Editors' note]

[4] This original group – the 'Zurich school' – also included Erwin Straus and Victor von Gebsattel. A useful account of the history of these phenomenological psychiatrists is given by Arthur Tatossian (1979). [Editors' note]

psychopathology ought to have closer ties to philosophy and to individual philosophers in particular. For Minkowski it was Bergson; for Binswanger this was Heidegger and then later Husserl. These 'structural' or 'existential' phenomenological approaches to psychopathology did not endeavour, as Jaspers had it, to find theory-neutral, value-neutral psychopathological facts; rather they sought to inquire into how psychopathology flows out of more basic disturbances in the human being as a whole – disturbances in the structure or the constitution of the human person. In Binswanger's case he thought he had found a fruitful theory of the human being in Heidegger's ontology of 'Dasein' or 'Existence' (please refer to Chapter 8, p. 49). So, for example, he thought that schizophrenia could be understood as a human being in which the two modes Heidegger termed *Vorhandenheit* and *Zuhandenheit* (please refer to Chapter 8, p. 50) had become disproportioned. In schizophrenia, the mode of *Zuhandenheit* become overborne or lost and *Vorhandenheit* dominated.

Minkowski kept close to Bergson's view of the human being as a dual entity comprising 'Intellect' and 'Intuition' (please refer to Chapter 5, pp. 10–11) and seemed less interested than Binswanger in developing a system as such. Minkowski thought we could improve our metaphorical understanding of nosological entities such as schizophrenia and depression by drawing upon Bergson's philosophy. Schizophrenia, according to Minkowski, could be understood as an atrophy of Intuition in Bergson's sense (a loss of contact with the flow or duration of life) and a hypertrophy of intellect (a coming to the fore of representational, static, geometrical capabilities). He called this a 'morbid dualism'. Depression was, Minkowowski thought, also a sort of morbid dualism but one in which disturbances in the flow of duration gave rise to a lived materialism (Minkowski 1970). These metaphysical characterizations Minkowski seems to take on the one hand as metaphors but on the other hand as basic disturbances, or 'generating disorders', from which the 'symptoms' of the mentally ill derive. For both Binswanger and Minkowski, a model of the human being as a whole (a philosophical *anthropology*) enabled a philosophical *psychopathology*. Following Scheler's stimulus, the philosophical anthropology came to react powerfully upon the psychopathology and the psychopathology (it was hoped) would come to react powerfully upon the development of philosophical anthropology. These approaches are complex,

rich and sometimes vague. They make extensive use of philosophical, literary and clinical case material. In what follows, we give Minkowski's Bergsonian approach (please refer to Chapter 12, pp. 102–116) in which he outlines his concept of a 'generating disorder' and shows us his phenomenological approach – interacting with patients over long periods of time and making use of various sources of information. He works with a case of de Clérambault's syndrome in which meaningful connections (in Jaspers' sense) and psychotic features (indicating more basic disturbances in mental life) are entangling. He tries to trace the changing presentations of the patient back to basic structural disturbances of lived time and lived space.

Following this we give an example of Binswanger's Heideggerian approach in which he reflects upon his existential take on psychiatry (please refer to Chapter 13, pp. 117–130). Binswanger seeks to illuminate different psychopathological states by casting them as different forms of 'being-in-the-world' or 'world designs' – Heideggerian concepts. He then tries to think through the implications of this approach for psychiatry. Minkowski and Binswanger share the phenomenological approach of Jaspers insofar as they are descriptive and careful to avoid interpretations in terms of psychological constructs or folk ideas (what Minkowski calls 'ideo-affective' aspects) but they diverge from Jaspers' belief in a theory-neutral and a value-neutral psychopathology – seeking rather to advance beyond description and press a knowledge exchange between psychiatry and philosophy.

In summary, the application of phenomenology to psychiatry occurred as a response to the exclusively third-person approach to psychopathology exemplified by psychiatrists such as Kraepelin. Karl Jaspers and Max Scheler were important early stimulators of the application of phenomenology to psychiatry. A key distinction arises, within this application, between the Jasperian approach which was basically sceptical about a philosophical psychopathology and a Schelerian approach which looked forward to a philosophical psychopathology but left only fragments of a methodology or a system. Philosophical psychopathology was then developed by Minkowski and Binswanger – the 'structural' and 'existential' approaches respectively – and this was done by making significant use of a single philosophical system (Bergson's in the case of Minkowski and Heidegger's in the case of Binswanger). The texts that follow outline Jaspers' approach and the structural and existential approaches.

10 Jaspers' approach 1: Static understanding – 'phenomenology'

Jaspers, K. (1912), 'The phenomenological approach in psychopathology'

From (1968) *British Journal of Psychiatry* **114**: 1313–23.
Translated by J. N. Curran. Originally published as (1912)
Die phänomenologische Forschungsrichtung in der
Psychopathologie. *Zeitschrift für die gesamte Neurologie
und Psychiatrie* 9: 391–408.

The Subjectivity of Psychic Events

In the examination of a psychiatric patient it is usual to distinguish between objective and subjective symptoms. Objective symptoms include all concrete events that can be perceived by the senses, e.g. reflexes, registrable movements, an individual's physiognomy, his motor activity, verbal expression, written productions, actions and general conduct, etc.; all measurable performances, such as the patient's capacity to work, his ability to learn, the extent of his memory, and so forth, also belong here. It is also usual to include under objective symptoms such features as delusional ideas, falsifications of memory, etc., in other words the rational contents of what the patient tells us. These, it is true, are not perceived by the senses, but only understood; nevertheless, this "understanding" is achieved through rational thought, without the help of any empathy into the patient's psyche.

Objective symptoms can all be directly and convincingly demonstrated by anyone capable of sense-perception and logical thought; but subjective symptoms, if they are to be understood, must be referred to some process which, in contrast to sense-perception and logical thought, is usually described by the same term, "subjective". Subjective symptoms cannot be perceived by the sense-organs, but have to be grasped by transferring oneself; so to say, into the other individual's psyche; that is, by empathy. They can only become an inner reality for the observer by his participating in the other person's experiences, not by any intellectual effort. Subjective symptoms include all those emotions and inner processes, such as fear, sorrow, joy, which we feel we can grasp immediately from their physical concomitants; these we thus take to "express" the underlying emotion. Then there are all those psychic experiences and phenomena which patients describe to us and which only become accessible to us at secondhand through the patient's own judgment and presentation. Lastly, subjective symptoms also include those mental processes which we have to infer from fragments of the two previous kinds of data, manifested by the patient's actions and the way he conducts his life.

It is usual to connect with this classification into objective and subjective symptoms a very definite contrast of values. According to this, only the objective symptoms offer certainty; they alone form a basis for scientific study, whereas subjective symptoms, though we cannot easily do without them for our preliminary assessments, are considered to be quite unreliable for making final judgments and unfruitful for the purpose of any further scientific investigation. There is a widespread desire to base our study of mental disorder on objective symptoms alone and ideally to disregard subjective symptoms altogether. This is a viewpoint which has its adherents – not all equally consistent – in psychology, just as it has in psychiatry. An "objective psychology" is set up in opposition to "subjective psychology". The former claims to concern itself with objective data only; its natural consequence is psychology without a psyche. The supporters of the latter (who, it should be said, have never failed to recognize the real but different values of the former) take into account self-observation, subjective analysis, the determination of the different modes of psychic life and of the specific nature of its phenomena, and ascribe value to such investigations even if they are made in the absence of any objective criteria. As examples of objective psychology we may cite the whole field of sense-perception, mnemometrics, performance curves and their components. The last will serve here to illustrate the fact that such investigations do lead quite systematically to the elimination of everything that can be called mental or psychic. It is not the feeling of fatigue but "objective fatigue" which is being investigated. All such concepts as fatiguability, the power of recovery, learning ability, practice, the effects of rest periods, etc., refer to performances that can be measured objectively, and it does not matter whether one is dealing here with a machine, a live but mindless organism, or a human being endowed with a mind. Nevertheless, those who claim to be purely objective investigators do quite frequently make a secondary use of subjective psychic phenomena to further their interpretations of objective performances and make comparisons possible – and, of course, they have every right to do so. But when this happens, they are making use of "subjective psychology", with which this paper is to deal. Now, there is no doubt that objective psychology produces results which are more obvious, more convincing, and easier for everyone to grasp than does subjective psychology. But whereas the difference in *degree* of certainty is simply quantitative, when it comes to the *kind* of certainty, the difference is qualitative and fundamental. This is so because subjective psychology always aims at the final realization of the concepts and ideas which form the inner representation of psychic processes, whereas objective psychology finds its ultimate aim in observation in undisputed fields such as sense-perception and the rational contents of thought and by such means as graphs and statistics.

The Systematic Study of Subjective Experience

What then are the precise aims of this much-abused subjective psychology? While objective psychology, by eliminating everything psychic, transforms itself into physiology, subjective psychology wishes to preserve this same psychic life as its object of study. It asks itself – speaking quite generally – what does mental experience depend on, what are its consequences, and what relationships can be discerned in it ? The answers to such questions are its special aims. But in approaching each problem subjective psychologists have to face the need to make clear both to themselves and to others what particular psychic experience is meant, for they are confronted with a manifold diversity of psychic phenomena which

cannot be surveyed or investigated as a whole but from which particular elements must be selected for investigation. So before real inquiry can begin it is necessary to identify the specific psychic phenomena which are to be its subject, and form a clear picture of the resemblances and differences between them and other phenomena with which they must not be confused. This preliminary work of representing, defining, and classifying psychic phenomena, pursued as an independent activity, constitutes phenomenology. The difficult and comprehensive nature of this preliminary work makes it inevitable that it should become for the time being an end in itself.

So long as such independent, systematic investigations had not been undertaken, this phenomenological approach remained limited to a number of unconnected opinions based on chance incidents or implications and *ad hoc* constructions; among these some useful pointers can certainly be found, but it is essential that they should be followed up by further research.

Within the sphere of psychological research E. Husserl has taken the first decisive step towards a systematic phenomenology, his predecessors in this having been Brentano and his school and Th. Lipps. In psychopathology, there have been a number of attempts to create a phenomenology,[1] though there has not yet been constituted a generally recognized field of research intended to prepare the ground systematically for the tasks of psychopathology proper. Since phenomenology does in fact offer a productive field of work in which everyone can take part, some programmatic exposition of its aims and methods seems indicated.

The Limitations of Empathy

In everyday life no one ever thinks in terms of isolated mental phenomena, whether his own or someone else's.

---

[1] Kandinsky's *Kritische und klinische Betrachtungen im Gebiete der Sinnestäuschungen*, Berlin, 1885, is almost entirely phenomenological in character. Oesterreich's *Die Phänomenologie des Ich in ihren Grundproblemen*, Leipzig, 1910, and Hacker's "Systematische Traumbeobachtungen", *Archiv f. Psych.* wl. 21.1, 1911, both conduct systematic phenomenological investigations into phenomena particularly vital for psychopathology. I have myself made efforts in this direction in two papers: "Zur Analyse der Trugwahrnehmungen" and "Die Trugwahrnehmungen". (Reprinted in *gesammelte Schriften zur Psychopathologie*, Springer-Verlag, Berlin. 1963). [**Original note**]

Our inward concern is always with that which is the object of our experience, not with the mental processes which accompany our experiencing. We understand other people, not through considering and analysing their mental life, but by living with them in the context of events, actions and personal destinies. Even when we do on occasion give consideration to mental experience as such, we do this only in a context of causes and effects as understood by us, or else we make a practice of classifying personalities into categories, etc. We never feel prompted to consider a mental phenomenon in isolation, e.g. a perception or a feeling *per se,* and to describe it in terms of its appearance and essence.

*****

Isolating the Phenomena

Now this attitude, which is not satisfied with understanding as mere experience but wishes to promote it to the level of knowledge that can be communicated, investigated and argued about, finds itself faced with an infinity of many-sided psychic phenomena, which are governed by correlations which are still far from clear and whose relations of dependence and consequence have yet to be elucidated. Without doubt, the first step towards a scientific comprehension must be the sorting out, defining, differentiating and describing of specific psychic phenomena, which are thereby actualized and are regularly described in specific terms.

We must begin with a clear representation of what is actually going on in the patient, what he is really experiencing, how things arise in his consciousness, what are his own feelings, and so forth; and at this stage we must put aside altogether such considerations as the relationships between experiences, or their summation as a whole, and more especially must we avoid trying to supply any basic constructs or frames of reference. We should picture only what is really present in the patient's consciousness; anything that has not really presented itself to his consciousness is outside our consideration. We must set aside all outmoded theories, psychological constructs or materialist mythologies of cerebral processes; we must turn our attention only to that which we can understand as having real existence, and which we can differentiate and describe. This, as experience has shown, is in itself a very difficult task. This particular freedom from preconception which phenomenology

demands is not something one possesses from the beginning, but something that is laboriously acquired after prolonged critical work and much effort – often fruitless – in framing constructs and mythologies. When we were children, we first drew things as we imagined them, not as we saw them; so as psychologists and psychopathologists we go through a stage where we form our own ideas, in one way or another, of psychic events, and only later acquire an unprejudiced direct grasp of these events as they really are. And so this phenomenological attitude is to be acquired only by ever-repeated effort and by the ever-renewed overcoming of prejudice.

How then do we proceed when we isolate, characterize and give conceptual form to these psychic phenomena? We cannot portray them, or bring them before our eyes in any way that can be perceived by the senses. We can only guide ourselves and others by a multiple approach. We have to be led, starting from the outside, to a real appreciation of a particular psychic phenomenon by looking at its genesis, the conditions for its appearance, its configurations, its context and possible concrete contents; also by making use of intuitive comparison and symbolization, by directing our observations in whatever ways may suggest themselves (as artists do so penetratingly) and by demonstrating already known phenomena which appear to play some part in the formation of the phenomenon studied. All this constitutes an incentive, reinforced by these indirect hints, for others to actualize these phenomena for themselves, while we too are encouraged to make use of our findings in later studies. The more numerous and specific these indirect hints become, the more well-defined and characteristic do the phenomena studied appear. Indeed, this personal effort to represent psychic phenomena to oneself under the guidance of these purely external hints is the condition under which alone we can speak of any kind of psychological work at all.

A histologist will provide an exhaustive description of particular morphological elements, but he will do it in such a way as to make it easier for others to see these elements for themselves, and he has to presume, or else induce, this "seeing for oneself" in those who really want to understand him. In the same way the phenomenologist can indicate features and characteristics, and show how they can be distinguished and confusion avoided, all with a view to describing the qualitatively separate psychic data.

But he must make sure that those to whom he addresses himself do not simply *think* along with him, but that they *see* along with him in contact and conversation with patients and through their own observations. This "seeing" is not done through the senses, but through the understanding. This is something quite special, irreducible and ultimate; and if we are to take even one single step forward in phenomenology we have to train ourselves in it and master it – including such things as "representing data to oneself", "understanding", "grasping" or "actualizing". Only so do we acquire a fruitful critical faculty which will set itself against the framing of theoretical constructions as much as against the barren deadly denial of any possibility of progress. Whoever has no eyes to see cannot practise histology; whoever is unwilling or incapable of actualizing psychic events and representing them vividly cannot acquire an understanding of phenomenology.

The Search for Irreducible Phenomena

This ultimate irreducible quality of psychic phenomena, which can only acquire identical meaning for numbers of people through the incentive and the multiple clues and leads mentioned previously, may already be found in the case of the simplest sensory qualities, such as red, blue, colour, tone; it comes into play also with spatial awareness, object awareness, perception, imagery, thought, etc. In psychopathology we have examples in pseudo-hallucination, the *déjàvu* phenomenon, derealization, heautoscopy, experience of the "double" and so on; though all these terms merely describe groups of psychic phenomena which are in themselves still more subtly differentiated from each other.

For the actualization to ourselves of all these phenomenologically ultimate characteristics, we have such expressions as "seeing", "viewing", "feeling oneself into", "empathy", "understanding" and so on. These expressions always denote the kind of ultimate concept-fitting experience which plays the same role in psychology as sensory perception plays in the natural sciences. Just as sense-perceptions are evoked by the demonstration of an object, so this meaningful empathic actualization will be evoked in us by the above-mentioned hints and indications, by our immediate grasp of expressive phenomena and our self-immersion in other people's self-description. From this terminology it follows that empathy and

understanding are by no means simple ultimate phenomena in themselves, but probably contain a whole series of elements yet to be defined. In the same way as perception, empathy has its tasks to set: first for phenomenology itself; of which it is the very foundation, and next for the investigation of psychogenesis. At this point we are not concerned with either of these; we need only to note the contribution made to our knowledge by this empathic, understanding experience, and to raise the question of the reliability of this way of gaining access to the facts. If, on the analogy of perceptual experience, we recognize empathic experience as ultimate, the question can be answered on these lines: in the field of empathic experience the technical means of retaining what has been seen but once, for later comparison and other purposes, are so inadequate that far more difficulties are encountered than in the case of sensory perception. But in principle reliability is established in the same way, i.e. by comparison, repetition and verification of such empathic experiences as reach actualization. In both fields there is much uncertainty; one cannot deny that in the psychological field it is greater than in the natural sciences, but this is only a difference of degree.

Whether we are representing our own past psychic experiences or those of other people is immaterial. The only important difference seems to be between observations which are systematic, experimental self-observations of persisting experiences, and those which are ordinary empathic representations. In the investigation of psychopathological phenomena, only the latter can really be considered, since patients can rarely be induced to carry out self-observation in the former sense, and then only in very favourable conditions, in regard to simple disturbances such as agnosias or hallucinations in clear consciousness. However, such empathic representations of phenomena among the mentally ill may well be furthered by concepts that have been won from the more elaborate phenomenological investigations of the former kind.

Methods of Phenomenological Analysis

The methods by which we carry out a phenomenological analysis and determine what patients really experience are of three kinds: 1. one immerses oneself, so to speak, in their gestures, behaviour, expressive movements; 2. exploration, by direct questioning of the patients and by means of accounts which they themselves, under our guidance, give of their own experiences; 3. written self-descriptions seldom really good, but then all the more valuable; they can, in fact, be made use of even if one has not known the writer personally. In all these instances we are pursuing phenomenology in so far as we are orientated towards subjective psychic experience and not towards object-ive manifestations, which in this context are only stages in our journey – the means, not the object, of our investigation. Of all these sources of information, good self-descriptions have the highest value.[2]

When, using these methods, we try to come closer to the patient's psychic life, our first impression is of an unsurveyable chaos of constantly changing phe-nomena. Our first aim must be to capture and delimit some particular item and by depicting it to form a conception of it, of which we and others can make permanent use; and we must supply it with a name by which we can always identify it. Psychopathological phenomena seem to call for just such an approach, one which will isolate, will make abstractions from related observations, will present as realities only the data themselves without attempting to understand how they have arisen; an approach which only wants to see, not to explain. Under pathological con-ditions, numerous psychic phenomena make their appearance without meaningful antecedents; psycho-logically speaking they emerge from nothing; seen causally they are occasioned by a disease process. Vivid memories of things never experienced; ideas held with a conviction of their truth without any intelligible basis for such conviction; moods and emo-tions appearing spontaneously and not based on any relevant experiences or ideas; all these, and many others, are common examples. These are the objects

of phenomenological investigation, which determines and represents them as they actually are.

Three groups of phenomena can be ascertained in this manner. The first consists of phenomena known to us all from our own experience. They come into existence in the same way as the corresponding psychic processes which in normal conditions arise out of others in an intelligible way; they differ only in their mode of origin from phenomena, otherwise quite similar, occurring in the mentally ill, e.g. many falsifications of memory. Next, there are phenomena which are to be understood as exaggerations, diminu-tions or combinations of phenomena which we ourselves experience, e.g. the ecstasies of some acute psychoses, pseudo-hallucinations, perverted impulses. How far our "understanding" can go in such cases, when we cannot base it on any conscious experiences of a similar kind, is a question that cannot be con-clusively answered. Sometimes it seems as if our understanding can go far beyond the possibilities afforded by experiences, even if similar ones, of our own.

The third group of pathological phenomena are distinguished from the two previous groups by their complete inaccessibility to any empathic understand-ing. We can only get closer to them by means of analogies and metaphors. We perceive them individu-ally, not through any positive understanding of them, but through the shock which the course of our comprehension receives in the face of the incom-prehensible. In this group we may perhaps include those "fabricated" thoughts and moods which many patients report as undoubted experiences (passivity experience), but which we can never identify except by using such terms as these, and by a series of observations designed to ascertain what these phe-nomena are not. Some patients who, notwithstanding their psychosis, have retained the awareness of their normal mental life readily admit the impossibility of describing their experiences in ordinary language. One patient explained: "Partly one has to do with things which simply cannot be expressed in human language. If I am to be understood, even to some extent, I shall have to use figures of speech and analo-gies which can do no more than get somewhere near the truth; the only way is to make some comparison with well-known facts of human experience . . . " In another context: "One has also to consider that it is mostly a matter of visions; I have the images in my head, but it is uncommonly difficult to describe them

---

2 For those interested, I list a few of the best self-descriptions so far published:

Schreber, *Memoirs of a Neurotic*, Leipzig, 1903.
Thomas de Quincey, *Confessions of an Opium Eater*.
Gerard de Nerval – *Aurilie*.
J. J. David – "Hallucinations." *Neue Rundschau*, No. 17, 874.
Kandinsky – "On the study of hallucination." *Archly. f. Psych. ix*, 453.
Klinke – *Jahr. f. Psych.*, 9.
Kieser – *Allgemeine Zeitschr. f. Psych.*, 10, 423.
Engeiken – Ibid., 6, 586.
Meinert – *An Alcoholic Madman*. Dresden, 1907.
[Original note]

in words, in part frankly impossible." Some – though not many – of the neologisms coined by patients are based on similar efforts to give a name to their own experiences; one patient sought to describe a sensation he felt in his hip more precisely in this way: When asked whether what he felt was a "twitching", he said: "No, it isn't a twitching, it's a 'plotching'."

From its beginnings, psychiatry has had to concern itself with delimiting and naming these different forms of experience; there could, of course, have been no advance at all without such phenomenological definitions. Delusions, sense-deceptions, depressive and expansive mood changes and much else have thus been described. All of this will remain the foundation for further phenomenological research. Often, however, we have first to clear away a ballast of theories concerning the supposed physical basis or psychological framework of these phenomena. Numerous phenomenological approaches have been smothered almost at once by such theoretical endeavours. We cannot now be satisfied with just a few meagre categories, but will devote ourselves without any preconceptions to the phenomena themselves, and whenever we can identify one we will seek to realize and describe it as completely as possible, without claiming to know in advance what the phenomenon is by virtue of our knowledge of psychology. The current classification of symptoms of insanity into sense-deceptions and delusions may be useful in a rough and ready way, but these terms conceal a hitherto unexplored multitude of diverse phenomena.

A few examples will illustrate the sort of phenomena that can be delimited. Kandinsky gave a description of pseudo-hallucinations, a particular kind of pathological imagery. They differ from normal images in their greater sensory concreteness, clarity and detail, their appearance independently of, and even against, the subject's will, and by the accompanying experience of passivity and receptiveness. On the other hand, they differ both from true hallucination and from normal perception in that they do not appear in external space as perceptions do, but in the internal space in which images also are experienced. This conception of pseudo-hallucinations has been attacked on the grounds of theoretical considerations. However, the problem is purely a phenomenological and descriptive one. It might be possible to represent the reported cases in some other more convincing way; one could adduce other cases (self-descriptions, the results of other investigations); but it is only through clearly realized

representations of this kind that Kandinsky's views could be refuted, never by mere theoretical considerations. The task of phenomenology is an independent one, and awareness of this will guard against criticism based on misunderstanding and hence unproductive.

Again, it is not uncommon for patients to report an experience, of which they are acutely aware, of there being somebody just behind or above them. When they look around, this somebody turns round, too; they "feel" it, there really is somebody there. But they have no sensation of actual contact, or indeed any sensation, nor can they ever come face to face with the supposed person. Some of these patients come to the conclusion that there is nobody there, others remain convinced of the existence of this someone whose presence they feel so vividly. Here it is obviously not a matter of sense-deception, since the sense-element is lacking; nor of a delusional idea, since there is an actual experience which is subjected to an act of judgment, and this judgment may be either correct or delusional. A third example, taken from the emotional sphere, will show how, simply by "sinking" oneself in the individual phenomena without the aid of any theory or system, one can arrive at a representation and delimitation of such phenomena. For instance, one hears of "feelings of ecstasy": among these one can readily distinguish if not different phenomena at least different shades of feeling. We are not here concerned with whether we are right or wrong in any particular instance. One can distinguish in the first place a general enthusiasm, emotion or rapture, embracing everything conceivable; secondly, a deep inner happiness out of which some joy-bringing image will occasionally arise; thirdly, a feeling of exaltation and grace, of holiness and high significance. In order to be of lasting value, such rapidly made differentiations should then be subjected to further phenomenological elaboration.

The methods of psychopathological phenomenology have now been discussed (grasp of expressive movements, exploration of patients' experience, and self-descriptions); also the indirect leads by which we are guided towards our own representation of the phenomena (noting their genesis, the conditions and circumstances under which they appear, their content, any already well-known elements they may contain, the symbolic indications, etc.); and the only question that remains is how we can provide an incentive for others to form their own representations of the phenomena in the light of all that has been brought forward. In a work on phenomenology, therefore, individual cases will be presented, general descriptions will be derived from them, and a terminology will be established. That phenomenology deals only with immediately presented data is no reproach to it, merely the statement of a fact. But it will always be difficult to find how one can lead from the individual case to a more general understanding and a more complete delimitation. It must be borne in mind that the experiences of individual patients are infinitely manifold; that phenomenology only extracts from them some general feature which can be found equally in some other case and therefore can be called the same feature, whereas the infinity of individual experience continues to change. We therefore have the position that on the one hand phenomenology abstracts from an infinity of constantly changing constituents, and on the other hand is definitely orientated towards the perceptible and the concrete, not the abstract. Only where something can be reduced to "reality" and becomes an immediate datum, i.e. becomes concrete, can it form the subject for phenomenology.

Classifying Groups of Phenomena

Let us assume that, in the ways described above, a number of phenomena can be delineated and clarified. We now seem to find ourselves once more in the presence of a fresh chaos of innumerable phenomena which have been described and defined, but still cannot satisfy our scientific needs. Delimitation must be followed by the bringing of phenomena into some kind of order, so that we can become aware of the diversity of psychic life in a systematic way, and make it possible to survey them up to the limits we have progressively reached. Phenomena can be arranged in quite different ways according to the purpose one has in view. For example, they can be arranged according to their origin, their physical determinants, their contents, their significance from some particular point of view, such as the logical, ethical or aesthetic. All these principles of classification should be made use of in their rightful place; but for phenomenology itself they are not very satisfactory. We seek a classification which will arrange psychic phenomena according to their phenomenological affinities with each other, somewhat in the way that infinite numbers of colours are arranged in the spectrum in a manner which is phenomenologically satisfying. Now in the present state of phenomenology, it would seem that there exist numerous groups of phenomena between which no relationship can be perceived. Sense-perceptions and ideas, hallucinations and delusions, seem to be phenomena separated by a gulf rather than united by transitions. Such totally unrelated phenomena can only be placed under separate headings and cannot be organized into any particular pattern within the psychic life.

But there are other groups of phenomena which can be related and arranged systematically. Between these, transitions can usually be made out (as between colours). An example of such a systematic arrangement of related phenomena can be given in the case of pseudo-hallucinations. On close consideration of individual cases, it appears that transitions exist between normal imagery and the completely developed pseudo-hallucination (which never becomes substantial but always remains in the internal psychic space, that occupied by imagery). Surveying these phenomena, it is possible to find four main points of contrast, between which they can oscillate through a whole series of transitions. If, then, we can describe each phenomenon in terms of where it can be approximately located in the series, we shall have satisfactorily characterized in phenomenological terms that particular phenomenon, lying as it does somewhere between an image and a pseudo-hallucination. These four points of contrast are as follows:

Fully formed pseudo-hallucination

1. Clear-cut, complete in detail.
2. The sensory elements are each adequately perceived, as in normal perception.
3. There is consistency and easy retention.
4. It is involuntary; nothing can be called forth or changed by choice. Associated with feelings of passivity and receptivity.

Normal imagery

1. Vague, incomplete and in detail
2. A *few* sensory elements are adequately perceived, or none, e.g. an imagined face is neutral in tone.
3. The images dissolve, disperse, have constantly to be recreated.
4. It is volitional; it can be changed by choice. Feelings are those of activity.

This example, which will not be discussed further here, shows how we set about grouping related phenomena on a purely phenomenological basis, using only those aspects of the phenomena which are really experienced as the points of difference, and excluding any added notions or theories. Further, it shows how vital it is to distinguish between phenomenological transitions and phenomenological gaps. Transitions will allow us to place phenomena in their order, but where there are gaps we can only enumerate or contrast opposites. It is at the same time evident that to recognize a group of phenomena as a phenomenologically new one, separated by a gap from those already recognized, is something only to be decided after careful consideration of clear evidence. At present, however, when so many people seek to reduce psychic data to the narrowest and simplest terms possible, it is preferable to accept rather too many phenomena – they can be organized later – than to lapse into some shallow psychological system made up of just a few elements.

For while the ideal of phenomenology is an infinity of irreducible psychic qualities, classified and ordered to permit of their survey, there exists another, opposite ideal, that of the fewest possible ultimate elements, as in chemistry. According to this school, all complex psychic phenomena could be derived from such elements, and all psychic phenomena could be satisfactorily presented by breaking them down into those elements. To be consistent, such an attitude must envisage the possibility of making do with a single ultimate psychic atom, everything psychic being built up from varying configurations of this particle. This ideal takes its cue from the natural sciences, and certainly has a meaning in relation to the origins of psychic qualities. Just as the infinite variety of colours can be traced to purely quantitative differences in wave-length, so one could wish to explain the origins of psychic qualities and perhaps establish different classifications on this basis. For phenomenology itself, however, such requirements seem quite pointless. The aim of phenomenological analysis is to increase its awareness of psychic phenomena by clearly delimiting them. As one procedure among others, phenomenology brings to light psychic qualities that appear as constituents of what is being studied. This breaking down of complex structures into constituents is only one way of proceeding; but those who adopt the point of view already described, which is valid only in relation to the origination of psychic phenomena, speak as if it were the only way. They would, for example, explain perception by analysing it into the elements of sensation, spatial

perception and intentional act, whereas true phenomenology would first compare perception with imagery, which is composed of the same elements, and come to the conclusion that perception must be characterized as an irreducible psychic quality. Even when occasionally the conception of "analysis into ultimate elements" does, like that of "analysis as a delimitation of ultimate qualities", appear to present itself as purely phenomenological and uninfluenced by the genetic point of view, it still tends to relapse at every opportunity into confusion with genetic considerations: once again complex psychic structures are said to arise from combinations of elements. Phenomenology, on the other hand, rejects the ideal of the fewest possible elements; on the contrary it has no wish to restrict the infinite variety of psychic phenomena, only, as far as possible (for the task is, of course, boundless), to try to make them more lucid, precise and individually recognizable at any time.

The Boundaries of Phenomenology

In the foregoing we have presented, if only in broad outline, the aims and methods of phenomenology, which has, of course, been practiced since psychiatry began, but has never yet been given its opportunity for unfettered development. Since it has suffered most harm from being confused with other lines of research, we will briefly restate what it is that phenomenology does *not* intend to pursue, and with what phenomenology should *not* be confused.

Phenomenology concerns itself only with actual experiences, only with the perceptible and concrete, not with any factors that may be thought to underlie psychic events and are the subject of theoretical constructs. For every one of its findings phenomenology must ask: has this actually been experienced? Does this really present itself to the subject's consciousness? Phenomenological findings derive their validity from the fact that the various elements of the psychic reality can be evoked repeatedly. Its findings can thus only be refuted if the facts of a case have previously been wrongly represented or are not represented correctly; they can never be refuted by demonstrating their impossibility or error on the basis of some theoretical proposition. Phenomenology can gain nothing from theory: it can only lose. The accuracy of a particular representation cannot be checked by its conformity to general criteria; phenomenology must always find its standards within itself.

Phenomenology, then, deals with what is actually experienced. It views psychic events "as from within", and brings them into immediate realization. It therefore does not concern itself with external manifestations, with motor phenomena, expressive movements as such, nor with any kind of objective performance. We have already explained to what extent expressive movements and self-descriptions can be used as the means, but not as the subject, of phenomenology.

Further, phenomenology has nothing to do with the genesis of psychic phenomena. Though its practice is a prerequisite for any causal investigation it leaves genetic issues aside, and they can neither refute nor further its findings. Causal studies relating to colour, perception, etc. are alien to it; yet such factual investigations have been less of a danger than those cerebral mythologies which have sought to interpret phenomenology and replace it by theoretical constructions of physiological and pathological cerebral processes. Thus Wernicke, who in fact did make important phenomenological discoveries, distorted them by interpretations in terms of "connective fibres", "sejunctions" and the like. These sort of constructs constantly prevent phenomenological investigations from reaching their proper goal. At first the originators of such constructs must necessarily practise phenomenology, but having reached this theory they feel on safer ground, and with a remarkable failure to recognize their own sources they declare all phenomenological conclusions to be "highly subjective".

Lastly, phenomenology must be kept separate from what we call the "genetic understanding" of psychic events, i.e. the comprehension of their meaningful relationships. This is a unique form of understanding which only applies to psychic events; it grasps as self-evident how one psychic event emerges from another; how a man attacked should be angry, a betrayed lover jealous. We have made use of the word "understanding" both for the "representations" of phenomenology and for this "grasp" of the psychic connections. To avoid confusion the former is termed "static understanding"; it is the basis on which their definition must rest, and comprehends only data, experiences, modes of consciousness and delimitation. The latter we call "genetic understanding" – the understanding of the meaningful connections between one psychic experience and another, the "emergence of the psychic from the psychic". Now

phenomenology itself has nothing to do with this "genetic understanding" and must be treated as something entirely separate; yet, where required, it may legitimately study regular sequences of psychic events, if these are actually experienced and as such together form a phenomenological unit *sui generis*. An example, perhaps, is the experience of the Will. But such a phenomenological sequence is quite a different thing from a meaningful flow of psychic events emerging one from the other. We restrict phenomenology to whatever can be understood "statically".

If we look at psychopathology as a whole, obviously our most essential interest lies in what is "genetically understandable", in extra-conscious causal connections, and in the ascertainment of the physical basis of psychic processes – in other words, in the way things are *related*. Phenomenology only makes known to us the different *forms* in which all our experiences, all psychic reality, take place; it does not teach us anything about the contents of the personal experience of the individual, nor anything about the extra-conscious basis on which psychic events seem to float like a thin layer of foam on the surface of the sea. Penetrating these extra-conscious depths will always be more attractive than merely demonstrating phenomenological findings, yet the completion of this latter task is an essential prerequisite for all further investigation. It is only in the setting of these phenomenologically established forms that actual life, accessible to our immediate understanding, unfolds itself; and it is, after all, in order to arrive at a better comprehension of this psychic life that we are prompted to investigate its extra-conscious relationships.

Future Tasks for Phenomenology

In conclusion we will indicate a few specific tasks for phenomenology. Not one field of psychopathological phenomenology can as yet be regarded as fully worked over. Even where the nature of a phenomenon is apparently clear-cut, as with some kinds of hallucinations, really good case-material that can serve to enlarge and verify one's experience is so scanty that careful and detailed case-descriptions are still of great value. Much work still needs to be done on the different types of hallucination, especially those of the higher senses, which ought be thoroughly investigated. An obvious instance is the problem of visual hallucinations occurring simultaneously with real perceptions in objective space. The phenomenology of delusional experiences has hardly been treated it all; all that exists so far on this subject is to be found in publications on emotional changes as the first symptom in paranoia. The phenomenology of pathological emotions is unbelievably scanty. The best is contained in the excellent work of Janet, in which, however, little value is placed on careful delimitation or classification. The subjective experience of one's own personality has been treated systematically by Oesterreich. For all these problems phenomenological descriptions by psychiatrists with material to hand, as well as self-descriptions more penetrating than those so far available, would be of the greatest value.

In histology, when examining the cerebral cortex, one is required to account for every fibre, every nucleus. In the same way phenomenology demands that we should account for every psychic phenomenon and every experience that comes to light in the investigation of our patients or in their own self-descriptions. We should in no circumstances be content with a general impression extracted from the total picture, but should get to know, as regards each detail, how it is to be viewed and assessed. Then, if we practise this method for some time, much will appear less startling to us because it has been frequently observed; whereas those who only go on "general impressions" will not have made themselves aware of the phenomena in question, and so, every time these do come to their notice through the momentary direction of their "impressionability", they will appear as novel and surprising. But the practised phenomenologist will pay attention to what is really new and unknown, and may then be justifiably surprised; one need not be afraid that surprises will ever cease! Needless to say, many psychiatrists already make it their practice to act on these lines and would rightly think it an impertinence if we claimed to be telling them something new. But the phenomenological approach is not yet so widespread as not to require repeated efforts to promote it. One may hope that its application will further enrich our knowledge of what the psychiatric patient really experiences.

Chapter

11

Jaspers' approach 2: Genetic understanding – 'Verstehen'

Jaspers, K. (1913–59), 'Meaningful psychic connections'

From (1962) *General Psychopathology*, Part 2, *Meaningful Psychic Connections (Verstehende Psychologie),* 7th edn. Translated by J. Hoenig and M. W. Hamilton. Manchester: Manchester University Press. Originally published as (1959) *Allgemeine Psychopathologie,* 7th edn. Berlin: Springer.

"We will assume the same theoretical distinction as has been made between subjective psychopathology (phenomenology) and objective psychopathology. 1. We sink ourselves into the psychic situation and *understand genetically by empathy* how one event emerges from another. 2. We find by repeated experience that a number of phenomena are regularly linked together, and on this basis *we explain causally.* Understanding the emergence of psychic events from each other has also been termed '*psychological explanation*', but this term is justifiably disliked by scientifically minded investigators … Meaningful psychic connections have also been called '*internal causality*', indicating the unbridgeable gulf between genuine connections of external causality and psychic connections which can only be called causal by analogy … Understanding is a fundamental human activity that from time immemorial has proceeded on its own methodical, conscious and scholarly way" (p. 301).

"In the natural sciences we find causal connections only but in psychology our bent for knowledge is satisfied with the comprehension of quite different sort of connection. Psychic events 'emerge' out of each other in a way which we understand. Attacked people become angry and spring to the defense, cheated persons grow suspicious. The way in which such an emergence takes place is understood by us, *our understanding is genetic.* Thus we understand psychic reactions to experience, we understand the development of passion, the growth of an error, the content of delusion and dream; we understand the effects of suggestion, and abnormal personality in its own context or the inner necessities of someone's life. Finally we understand how the patient sees himself and how this mode of self-understanding becomes a factor in his psychic development" (pp. 302–3).

"We can have no psychological understanding without empathy into the *content* (symbols, forms, images, ideas) and without seeing the *expression* and sharing the *experienced phenomena.* All these spheres of meaningful objective and subjective experience form the matter for understanding. Only in so far as they exist can understanding take place. They come into a context through the comprehension of our genetic understanding" (p. 311).

"In the psychology of meaningful phenomena, the application of directly perceived, understandable connections to an individual case never leads to deductive proof but only to probabilities. Psychological understanding cannot be used mechanically as a sort of generalised knowledge but a fresh, personal intuition is needed on every occasion. 'interpretation is a science only in principle, in its application it is always an art' (Bleuler)" (p. 313).

Minkowski's structural approach

Minkowski, E. (1933), 'The notion of a generating disorder and the structural analysis of mental disorders'

From (1970) *Lived Time: Phenomenological and Psychopathological Studies.* Translated by N. Metzel. Evanston, IL: Northwestern University Press: 220–71. Originally published as (1933) *Le temps vécu: Etudes phénoménologiques et psychopathologiques,* in the series *Collection de l'évolution psychiatrique.* Paris: D'Artrey.

From the Symptom to the Generating Disorder

Psychiatry, like all empirical science, endeavors first of all to set out the elementary notions assigned to the study of the group of phenomena which constitute the object of research of that field. Thus, at the beginning of every textbook of psychiatric medicine we find a chapter entitled "General Psychiatry," which contains a description of syndromes.

Psychopathology, the younger sister of psychology and physiology, as people like to call it, makes these symptoms precise from the angle that is imposed on it by its two older sisters. It takes its point of departure from notions which are elaborated by them, such as perception, memory, ideation, judgment, affectivity, and so forth, and attempts to determine the pathological modifications which these different functions can undergo. Consequently, psychopathology will talk of hallucinations (considering them as perceptual disorders), amnesia, dissociation, flight of ideas, delirious ideas (considering them to be judgmental disorders), morbid depression or euphoria, and indifference, and so forth.

The aspect adopted is evidently far from being an inconsequential factor; it automatically implies a certain grouping and a certain interpretation of symptoms. Thus, hallucinations arising from different senses are described as varieties of the same group, which is tantamount to saying that they are considered at once, and perhaps conclusively, as phenomena of the same nature which must therefore be referred to similar causes, such as, for example, the excitation of the corresponding nervous centers. The possibility of a fundamental divergence, of a psychological nature, between these various kinds of hallucinatory phenomena, for example, between visual and auditory hallucinations, is not even envisaged. In the same way, delusions are all considered to be the expression of judgmental disorder and are then subdivided, according to their content, into delusions of grandeur, persecution, guilt, negation, and so forth.

Defined and grouped according to current psychophysiological notions, symptoms will be considered to be on the more or less artificial frontiers of these notions. They will be aligned on the same level; each will primitively represent a particular fault of the psyche. In these conditions, it seems that psychiatry as a specialty can consist only in a description of the different combinations of symptoms learned through clinical experience. In any event, we would be forced to look for initial and essential disorders among the symptoms presented.

In reality, however, the case is otherwise.

Clinical psychiatry establishes the frequency and the regularity of certain associations and symptoms. In this way it substantiates syndromes. This process is common to all branches of medicine and should not surprise us. But in psychiatry we are dealing with mental disorders, that is, with phenomena belonging to psychic reality, and we ought to inquire whether special problems do not arise from this fact.

In somatic medicine we look for the anatomical and functional basis of the syndrome. Thus the Brown-Séquard syndrome came to stand for a unilateral lesion of the marrow, and it is thus that we are led to establish the syndrome of hepatic or renal insufficiency. The character of the symptoms is not changed in any way. Symptom – syndrome – anatomophysiological basis: this is the direction of our thought.

Things look different, at least in part, when we are concerned with mental medicine. To be sure, we can look for or, what is simpler, grant straight off an organic basis of a more or less hypothetical nature for the syndrome studied. But even these organicist tendencies in the long run will not be able to ignore an important step that comes to be interpolated between the mental syndrome and the organic disorder because of the very fact that we are dealing with psychic phenomena. This step will modify the whole problem noticeably.

In psychiatry, behind the symptom and, even more, behind the syndrome there is a whole *living personality*. And the need to penetrate through the symptoms to this living personality, to achieve an understanding of his whole being in one effort of mind, is so imperative that we could rid ourselves of it as little in the domain of the pathological as in the domain of the normal.

*****

Behind confusion always lies the confused person, behind melancholy, the depressed, behind the syndrome of influence, the influenced. The symptoms thus closely interpenetrate one another, and the syndrome is no longer based on a purely empirical or more or less contingent coexistence of isolated symptoms. It tends to be transformed into an organized and vital unity, in the psychological meaning of the term. The clinical syndrome tends to become a true psychological syndrome.

[I]t is precisely in this way that we come to distinguish "pure" cases in psychiatry and to establish the fundamental mechanisms which constitute them.

*****

Despite their relative rarity, the pure cases remain pure cases for us, which we recognize as such and which permit us to analyze related cases. Fundamentally, this "purity" is nothing other than the expression of the feeling we have in the presence of certain patients when we attempt to grasp their living personality, to which all the symptoms they present are related in that they all rest upon an initial disorder, are an organized unity, and represent a true psychological syndrome.

This need to unify each mental syndrome with the help of an act of penetration is so profoundly anchored in us that we could not renounce it even in the presence of a syndrome as paradoxical at first

sight as Cotard's syndrome, in which contradictory ideas, ideas of negation, ideas of enormity, of immortality, exist side by side. We will discuss it presently.

It is thus that the idea of *generating disorders* arises in psychopathology. The mental syndrome is for us no longer a simple association of symptoms but the *expression of a profound and characteristic modification of the whole human personality*. We must now study these different modifications – a task which has only scarcely been initiated.

The generating disorder essentially corresponds, on the psychological level, to the anatomophysiological basis of somatic syndromes. However, we will not be concerned with either organs or functions but with the one and indivisible living personality. Our scientific thought ought to be entirely preoccupied with this domain. The interpretation of symptoms and of all mental disorders in general will undergo a resultant change.

Thus the hypochondriacal preoccupations of a neurotic and the hypochondriacal ideas of a schizophrenic appear as completely dissimilar manifestations because the mental basis is completely different in the two cases. Their personalities are so different that we would not even dare to say that they both are overly concerned about their health. We are led to believe that there is only a superficial similarity in the ideational and verbal expression of two generating disorders that have nothing in common with each other at any time. The same applies to the delusions of grandeur of a schizophrenic or a general paretic and to the true obsessions and the pseudo-obsessions of a schizophrenic nature. This similarity in the expression of entirely different disorders ought not to be surprising. The number of concepts which sick people have at their disposal to express their states of mind is necessarily limited. And it is easier for them to have recourse to the same ideas in order to fill the void which develops in them than to draw from the restricted quantity of concepts formed for better or worse, they are forced to express their disorders by using the same ideas for disorders of different kinds. This does not prevent them from believing that they are correct, but we ourselves must take care not to interpret their statements literally.

The grouping of symptoms established by general psychiatry can no longer be considered as definitive and sacrosanct. In each case, we will no longer feel bound by the structure imposed by these groupings nor will we hesitate to disjoin the phenomena that they unite if the psychological analysis of syndromes demands it in any way. We have already said that we could not consider the delusions of grandeur of a schizophrenic and a general paretic as identical manifestations, nor will we be content with the simplistic formula which relegates the two cases to a judgmental disorder of the same kind. Examples of this kind can be multiplied indefinitely. In the same way, clinical experience tells us that auditory hallucinations occupy, as much from the diagnostic point of view as from the prognostic, a different place from that of visual hallucinations. The first are primarily characteristic of schizophrenic states, while the second, on the contrary, characterize confusional syndromes. I doubt that even the most fervent organicists would be led, on the strength of this conclusion, to reduce the differences between mental confusion and schizophrenia to the differences of nervous and cerebral localization of the two processes. In any case, as psychologists confronted by these facts, we will search to discover what in the living personality makes the difference between "hearing voices" and "seeing images," and we will attempt to see whether this difference is related to the dissociative character of the schizophrenic process, on the one hand, and to the global character of mental confusion, on the other. This study will easily lead us, beyond the frontiers of pathology, to a deeper examination of the place that visual and auditory phenomena occupy in the general contexture of the world.

A more detailed analysis of the intimate structure of syndromes will also be prompted by the same directives. In melancholic delirium, depression seems to constitute the link which unites all the elements of which the syndrome is composed into a synthetic whole; delusions of ruin, guilt, indignity, and imminent torture fit perfectly with this emotional foundation. One is tempted to believe that these represent only an attempt on the part of the patient *to explain* the depression that inexplicably overcomes him. We are familiar, however, as we said above, with states of profound depression without delusion, and nothing allows us to grant that in these cases the causal need is less developed than in the preceding ones. And, on the other hand, ideas just as depressing as these exist which rarely if ever develop into states of melancholic depression. Thus it seems difficult to accept the claim that the genesis of melancholic ideas is due simply to a judgmental disorder. The regularity with which the choice of these ideas occurs alone forces us to think that the choice obeys a precise law preformed in the normal personality, and we must attempt to discover whether or not, beyond their apparent ideational content, these ideas present, in terms of their inner structure, some details which would allow them, more than some others, to constitute a true psychological syndrome and to come to be superadded as a whole to the state of depression. We see a new problem dawning on the horizon: *the need to penetrate beyond the ideational elements and even the emotional factors of a syndrome to the inner structure of the morbid personality which serves as their framework and unites them.* The deviations observed, as a result of comparison with the structure of the normal personality, will allow us finally to establish the modalities of the generating disorders which are found at the base of the various psychopathological pictures.

A number of psychiatrists believe they ought to confine themselves to syndromes; others, on the contrary, attempt to go further and to specify true nosological entities, that is, true mental diseases. We have not taken a side in this debate. What interests us, above all, is that the nosological point of view projects a new light on the classification and the importance of symptoms and that it does so in the same sense as the syndromic point of view.

We can place the notion of dementia praecox at the center of the contemporary nosological efforts. Kraepelin's clinical synthesis necessarily led to the differentiation between primary and secondary symptoms and Bleuler's conception of schizophrenia.[1] This represents the first two stages in the evolution of the modern conception of dementia praecox.

Sooner or later, however – and here begins the third stage, which we are actually experiencing – we ought to feel the need of unifying the conception of schizophrenia even more by reducing the primary symptoms to one, and only one, generating disorder. Bleuler himself saw the problem very clearly. But faithful to traditional psychology, he chose the generating disorder from among the elementary symptoms imposed by this psychology and built his theory of schizophrenia upon a weakening of associations. He did so even though it was he who had introduced into the symptomatology of schizophrenia a new notion

---

[1] On this subject see E. Minkowski, "La Genèse de la notion de schizophrénie et ses charactères essentiels," *Evolution psychiatrique,* Vol. I (Paris: Payot, 1925). [**Original note**]

which could not be reduced to the traditional triad of psychology – intelligence, affectivity, and will – but which referred, rather, to a manner of being of the whole personality. We are speaking here of *autism*. Thus, Bleuler gave us an inkling of the existence of a particular form of the psychic life of schizophrenics, a form which serves as a framework for, and leaves its impression upon, intelligence, affectivity, and activity and determines the characteristic manner of being of the schizophrenic. But Bleuler considered autism as only one of the consequences of the weakening of associations.

It is this that has inspired recent efforts to complete the schizophrenic synthesis from the psychopathological point of view. The particular form of the schizophrenic personality, and not some one of its functions, will now be seen as the central problem. It is thus that, inspired by Bergsonian ideas, I have spoken of the *loss of vital contact with reality*.

We have learned to project our nosographic frameworks onto the classification of psychopathological constitutions and, even beyond that, onto the classification of normal constitutions. The psychological constitution not only determines in this way the behavior of the individual in life but determines his specific vulnerability as well as the character of the psychopathic reactions that could occur in him.

We have not touched on the clinical applications of the notion of constitution. What is important is that this notion, in establishing a relation of (qualitative) identity between certain clinical pictures and pre-existent constitutions, obliges us to abstract from the striking symptoms of mental illness in order to search behind them for several characteristic traits which are capable of being put in direct relation with one aspect of the behavior of the human personality. The opposition between the manic-depressive disease and schizophrenia is thus reduced finally to a difference of attitude of the mentally ill in relation to the environment, and this opposition leads us to the notions of syntony and schizoidism, which, far from being equivalent to current notions of intelligence, affectivity, or will, constitute two important "vital principles" (Bleuler) capable of conferring a particular tone on all the manifestations of the individual. Our efforts in psychopathology are more and more oriented toward the search for elementary disorders relating to the whole personality and not to some one of its functions. In this sense we speak of *generating disorders*.

Our knowledge here is still fragmentary. Only in the future will we succeed in making it more precise. In the meantime it seems useful to say something, even if it concerns only a general program, while reserving the right to rectify later the errors which are unavoidable in a provisional survey.

Among the generating disorders, we will primarily study the psychopathological processes. We are especially familiar with two processes of this order: intellectual impairment and schizophrenic processes. The first, characterized by a progressive debility of the intellectual faculties, is clearly distinguished from the second, which produces a decrease of the dynamic factors of life and causes a particular pragmatic deficiency.

But whatever our understanding of the psychopathological processes may be, they alone cannot exhaust the field of generating disorders. In penetrating in a more or less slow and insidious way into the human personality, they determine, each in its own way, a particular deficiency of that personality, but they stop there and are incapable of accounting for the appearance of more complex symptoms, such as hallucinations or delusions. Besides, before attempting the analysis of these symptoms, we ought, instead of examining each one of them separately, to ask whether they cannot be grouped in a natural way so that they can be then reduced by groups to particular generating disorders, more or less distinct from the psychopathological processes with which we were concerned. But it must be kept in mind that our analysis must not progress from the periphery to the center, as in the past, but from the center to the periphery: hallucination cannot be for us a simple perceptual disorder, nor can a delusion be a simple judgmental disorder; both must now be treated as phenomena which materialize in the morbid personality under certain conditions, and sometimes in different ways.

We are thus led to the conclusion that, in addition to the psychopathological processes, there are generating disorders of another order; these, intervening in a much more brutal fashion than the former, modify directly and radically – in the course of the psychopathological processes or quite independently of them – the very form of mental life.

Without dwelling on the form of mental life here, it will suffice to say at this point that it is conditioned in normal life by the faculty of affirming the ego, affirming it in relation to space as well as time. We thus ought to search for the particular generating disorders of which we have spoken in the domain of the affirmation of the ego. In so doing, it would seem obvious that we should compare Clérambault syndrome to melancholic delirium, as we have done above. In both cases the normal affirmation of the ego is disturbed, but each in a different way.

Speaking in a schematic manner, we can say that in the first case there is a complete damage of spatial orientation, in the second a damage of temporal orientation. And we now see how, in going beyond the ideo-affective content of mental disorder, we can penetrate as far as its intimate structure, as far as the particular form of mental life that they express. This ought to lead us to the question as to why Clérambault's syndrome has a neutral character, at least as long as other secondary elements are not joined to it, whereas melancholic delirium is intimately related to the state of depression and sadness. We cannot answer this question at this point, but what probably is of primary importance is the manner in which the human personality is situated with the aid of feelings and emotions in relation to time and to space.

We see now in which direction we are to search in psychopathology for the generating disorders which are of another order than those of psychopathological processes.

As for the name we will give to these disorders, I am willing to use the term "morbid mental subduction," which was introduced by my deceased colleague and friend Mignard.[2] This term appears appropriate because the generating disorders of which we have spoken seem truly to modify the very form of mental life in a radical fashion in reducing it, so to speak, to an inferior level and submitting it to a real mental subduction. We will speak in this sense, in referring to melancholic delirium, of a *mental subduction of time* and, in referring to Clérambault's syndrome, of a *mental subduction of space*. I add as well, in order not to be misunderstood, that in limiting the term "mental subduction" to generating disorders of the second order I am using the term in a more restrictive sense than Mignard used it. He extended it to nearly all the manifestations of mental illness, and it played an integral part in his conception of organopsychic

influence, of which we have already had occasion to speak. In sum, we can draw up the following outline for the study of generating disorders:

Psychopathological processes

a) Intellectual impairment
b) Schizophrenic processes
c) Epileptic processes

Morbid mental subduction

a) In time (melancholic delirium and probably the whole manic-depressive psychosis)
b) In space (Clérambault's syndrome)

This is merely a schema which is by no means complete. But it will do for now, to indicate the direction that we want to pursue.

Finally, I will put forth one more suggestion on the subject of morbid mental subduction. Perhaps we ought to distinguish different levels of it. These are the facts that suggest this to me. The intimate structure of melancholic delirium is reminiscent of the situation that the idea of death creates in normal life. This idea, when it surges forth or when it dominates the spirit, appears as an insuperable barrier before us, makes us anxious, brings forth a feeling of impotence, hinders all affirmation of the ego, stops all *élan*. But sometimes we descend even one level further in the negation of life. This negation no longer has the phenomenon of death for its basis, with all that is still vital in it; it becomes more abstract, more theoretical, and rests on the idea of the limitation, the smallness, of the ego in relation to the infinity and eternity of the world. It is expressed by the formula "What's the use?" – which some people think they can embrace. It is an open question whether this antithesis of the infinitely small and the infinitely large, in the presence of which our reason sometimes places us, constitutes the psychological basis of Cotard's syndrome. In any case, it would explain the origin of the structure of this syndrome, or rather the origin of the contradictory ideas of which it is composed, and it would allow us to consider it, in relation to simple melancholic delirium, as a more advanced level of morbid mental subduction. Certainly, at first sight, Cotard's syndrome has nothing in common with the philosophic attitude that some believe[3] they

---

[2] Maurice Mignard, "La Subduction mentale morbide," *L'Année psychologique*, XXV (May, 1924); *L'Unité psychique et les troubles mentaux* (Paris: Alcan, 5928). [**Original note**]

---

[3] We say they "believe" because in reality they can never carry this attitude through to the end. [**Original note**]

can adopt as a result of the antithesis of which we are speaking; but perhaps it does rest on that antithesis, with the sole difference that when it occurs in a morbid consciousness it penetrates into everyday life and, because of this, is expressed in a delirious manner.

Generating Disorder and Organopsychic Relations

The new orientation in psychopathology cannot help but have repercussions on all the problems with which the psychiatrist is concerned. We cannot list all of these problems; we will be content to examine the main ones.

Insofar as organopsychic relations are particularly concerned, the psychiatrist is at present content to search for an anatomophysiological explanation of isolated symptoms, primarily for those among them, such as hallucinations, which seem to be found on the periphery of the psyche; or, having established certain nosological entities, he tries to reduce them to anatomopathological or functional modifications which he would like to be able to consider as pathognomonic for them.

We obviously have no intention of doubting the utility of this research. On the contrary, we would not know how to do without it. However, even where we know the characteristic anatomopathological modifications of a mental disease, we are unable to establish a plausible relation between these modifications and all the psychopathic manifestations of which the given psychosis is composed.

The notion of generating disorders seems destined in time to bring a little more clarity into this domain. The various generating disorders representing, so to speak, the primitive lesions of the psyche now ought to serve as a point of departure for our organopsychic hypotheses. The latter will necessarily be inspired by the new notions that they imply.

We cite as an example Mignard's theory of organopsychic influence.[4] This theory attempts – and this is completely in accord with what was said above – to preserve the notion of mental unity as the primary psychic fact. "If the organism is normal," Mignard

writes, "it will be in control of thought, while, on the contrary, the diseased organism causes a morbid influence, which is expressed on the psychological level by feelings or delusions of influence, so frequent with the mentally ill." In other words, the well individual feels himself to be master of his thought, the normal functioning of his organism is related to a feeling of ease, which accompanies all of his acts and which is so habitual that we do not even notice it; but the disorder of this functioning involves a particular disturbance which gives rise to delusions of influence. Here it is a question of "an excessive preponderance which attacks certain particular neurocerebral functions normally subdued by the actions of properly so-called mental functions" (Mignard).

I cite Mignard's theory here simply as an example of the direction our organopsychic hypotheses are now taking under the influence of the notion "generating disorder." As for the theory itself, the very fact that it attempts to reduce all mental disorders to a single organopsychic disorder (attack and feeling of influence) obliges us to consider it (after what we said awhile back concerning the various kinds of generating disorders) as too general and, in consequence, as insufficient. It has the merit, however, of having been one of the first of the attempts in this area which conform to the tendencies of contemporary psychopathology.

The Double Aspect of Mental Disorders

Our conception of mental disorder, and especially of delirium, will also be inspired by the ideas which were discussed in the preceding pages. These ideas lead to what we can call the *double aspect* of psychopathic phenomena.

To describe delusions as judgmental disorders really tells us very little, after all. This is because the capacity for judgment in daily life has nothing to do with the nature of delusions. Certainly, we can, for our purposes, call "judgment" whatever it is that keeps us from having delusions; but this will be a purely verbal formula, incapable of telling us anything about either the nature of judgment or the genesis of delirious ideas. On the contrary, we believe that we have made an advance in the understanding of these ideas in assuming that behind them is found a phenomenon of normal life, distorted only in the place that it occupies in the psyche and in the manner in which it is expressed.

---

4 Mignard, "L'Emprise organo-psychique et les états d'aliénation mentale," *Encephale* (May, 1922). [**Original note**] This may be seen as an early example of 'neurophenomenology'. [**Editors' note**]

We said above that melancholic delirium is not, as far as we are concerned, solely the association of a depressive foundation and depressive ideas but that, in order to comprehend this syndrome, it appears possible and even necessary to assume that there is a particular structure behind the idea-emotional content that we term "morbid subduction in time." This structure appears to determine the choice of delusions and, in uniting them into one psychological syndrome, produces the most adequate means of expressing itself in an intelligible manner. Thus, from the psychological point of view, we have differentiated two separate aspects of the syndrome in question: first, the *idea-emotional* aspect – or, better, in certain cases, the *ideo-affective* aspect – which allows us to understand the patient, to establish an ideational rapport as well as a sympathetic relation with him; and second, the *structural aspect*, which constitutes the inner framework of the syndrome, which conditions the arrangement of these elements, and which explains why our reasoning has no grasp of the delusions of the patient. These delusions are nothing but the *secondary expression* of a particular form of mental life, different from our own and resulting from the morbid subduction of the personality in time.

We can generalize this perspective. In the presence of a hypochondriac we automatically feel that we are faced with an individual who is morbidly preoccupied with his state of being. We transpose his statements literally onto a normal psyche. Then, if we are organicists, we will search for the reason for these hypochondrial preoccupations in a problematic coenesthesis, or, if we are psychoanalysts, we will be led to consider hypochondria as deriving from narcissistic interest in the subject's organism, an interest born of autoeroticism. Perhaps, however, we should not abandon this point of departure too readily. Do the hypochondrial preoccupations of the patient always express the same thing? We have already spoken of the difference that exists between the hypochondrial preoccupations of anxious depressives and the hypochondrial ideas of a schizophrenic. While in the first case the preoccupations are closer to real preoccupations, in the second they seem to be only a secondary attitude for the purpose of filling the void made by the schizophrenic processes. But this is not all. Certain hypochondriacs confuse themselves with their morbid preoccupations; others, on the contrary, consider them to be foreign to their person. To cite only one example, one of my male

patients, of whom I will speak later, after having expressed a series of coenesthopathic and hypochondrial complaints, said to us:

> My obsession is to remain as I am, to bore everyone with my complaints. This is completely contrary to my nature. It irritates me to be concerned with things that I don't care a damn about. However, I am not a hypochondriac. This isn't the reason that I am so concerned about everything I don't want to attach so much importance to my movements, but I am only grub and defecation. I am only a sort of animal function, and one that injures himself. I have the feeling of being nothing but living tripe. I have neither sensations nor precise ideas. I have the feeling of being nothing but vegetative functions, of being nothing but a mass.

It seems that here the phenomenon of organopsychic solidarity and the feeling of ease and quietude which are an integral part of this phenomenon have been attacked; the result is a feeling of *increased materiality*, which, by infiltrating the personality of the patient and in then attempting to express itself, can do so only with the aid of multiple and varied complaints of a coenesthopathic and hypochondrial order. Other traits of the patient's behavior confirm this interpretation. We will return to them later. What is important at this point is that a different structure may be hidden behind the same facade, behind the same hypochondrial preoccupation; and if in certain cases this preoccupation is exactly what, according to its ideo-emotional content, it should be, namely, a "hypochondrial preoccupation," in other cases it is only the secondary expression of a particular dislocation of the innermost structure of the personality (increased materiality) and is in complete accord with the other symptoms with which it unites to form a particular psychological syndrome.

*****

This whole discussion concerning the relation between the first personality (the one before the illness) and the second personality (created by the patient) rests, I believe, on a misunderstanding of the double aspect of mental disorders, of the ideo-affective aspect, on the one hand, and of the structural aspect, on the other. The first aspect – more human, more comprehensive, at first sight – ought not to allow us to neglect the study of the problems posed by the second.

In quite a few cases, as Clérambault maintains,

> I do not deny all affective support to the group of ideas that have been observed; I only deny that the appearance of this group of ideas, its intensity and form, can, as a

whole, be explicable in terms of affective causes. If affectivity really evoked it, at least the general process has amplified and deformed it, and the evocation itself is most frequently the result of this general process.

*****

Phenomenological Compensation

The idea of compensation will now be given an additional significance. Psychiatry has been concerned with compensation for a long time. For example, this is the way the fabulations of demented seniles, which come to fill the gap left by the deficiency of the memory, have been interpreted. In these cases it is a matter of a completely *mechanical compensation*. Presented as such, it does not pose any new problem for us. For the time being, it is sufficient to make note of this. We will come back to it later, when we will have occasion to show that this compensation is more complex than it may have appeared to be.

Important progress has already been made with the introduction into psychiatry of the idea of affective compensation, primarily under the influence of Freud's work. In his view of delirium, as in his view of dreams, the individual achieves what he has been denied or what he has repressed in a more or less conscious manner.

*****

[The double aspect of mental disorders] leads us more particularly to a new form of compensation which, found by means of the extension of the structural analysis of mental disorders, limits the importance of the affective compensation. I propose to call this sort of compensation "phenomenological compensation," since it refers to the essential characteristics of the phenomena of which life is composed and grants only a secondary role to their affective content, which is always more or less contingent and which varies from individual to individual. I have studied this compensation especially in schizophrenia. Here is how I have considered it.[5]

The essential disorder in schizophrenia resides in a loss of vital contact with reality. This loss conditions the autistic manifestations of the patient. With this understood, it becomes possible to order the phenomena of normal life from this point of view. Certain of them appear immediately as *retreat reactions* in relation to reality; examples are reverie, daydreaming,[6] or regrets. In the same way, in the intellectual domain, interrogation engages the activity of the subject much less than affirmation. Since the goal of interrogation is the response that ought to follow it, it has an unfinished character. Isolated artificially from its natural end, it seems destined to play – compared to normal contact with reality – a role of strategic retreat. An individual who adopts an interrogative attitude and who passes his time asking questions (regardless of whether he asks them of himself or of others) without concern for the responses that could be made to these questions is a schizophrenic. Because of the aspect of retreat contained in them, these diverse phenomena are in harmony with the essential feature of the mental life of schizophrenics, constituted as it is by loss of contact with reality. We find this to be completely natural, since the schizophrenic stops with the predilection for these phenomena in order to fill up the void that opens up in him because of the schizophrenic process, and as a result of a compensationary tendency he attempts to add vivid color to the arid countryside of the autistic life. For me, this is the prototype of a phenomenological compensation, modeling itself on the particular structure of the morbid consciousness. I have grouped these various modalities of the phenomenological compensation of the schizophrenic under the rubric "schizophrenic attitudes."

Certainly, in reverie the mentally ill person is able to achieve his desires, just as his regrets can color events with a high degree of affectivity; but what seems to be of as much, if not more, significance than the ideo-affective content of this reverie or these regrets is the fact that, independently of their content, these phenomena effect a form of psychic activity which accords perfectly with the fundamental nature of the schizophrenic mind. Thus the schizophrenic clings to it quite naturally. He dreams; he simply dreams before dreaming of anything in particular. It is better to give oneself up to sterile reverie or adopt an attitude of regret or an interrogative attitude than to fall into the void. Moreover, the content sometimes fades away; the patient daydreams without being able to describe what he is dreaming about, or else he poses

---

[5] Please refer to p. 241. [**Editors' note**]

[6] Morbid daydreaming was described by A. Borel, "Rêveurs et boudeurs morbides," *Journal de psychologie*, XXII (1925). [**Original note**]

questions in an incoherent manner without concern for the subject of all the objects which occur to him, without the least concern for the pragmatic importance of these questions or the responses which could be given to them. It seems much more a question of a phenomenological compensation than an affective compensation. This appears all the more plausible since these mechanisms participate in the mental foundation from which they develop and become recognizable in schizophrenics by their rigidity and their unpragmatic nature, so that, basically, on the psychological level, these schizophrenic attitudes strongly resemble psychomotor stereotypes. In time, however, they follow the same course as the schizophrenic process; their content becomes weakened, and they crumble away and disintegrate to the same extent that the schizophrenic personality does.

In order to clarify these relations, we appeal to the following schema, which represents a progressive degradation of our activity. Confronted by a deception, we can try to achieve our desires in our dreams. However, sooner or later, it is better to discover some compensation in real life by putting forth a new effort. The situation will be even more compromised if, following a failure of vital contact with reality, regardless of the cause, the individual becomes immobilized, even without previous deception, in an attitude of reverie, and will no longer search for any outlet in the world around him. This reverie thus becomes an end in itself; and even if in certain cases it has an affective tone, it will be entirely lost, along with the others, in vagueness. But even in these latter cases it will appear more preferable than the absolute void.

In this way we are led to assert that phenomenological compensation plays an important role in psychopathology. To be sure, in a number of cases it superimposes itself upon affective compensation, as, for example, with schizophrenic dreamers. In the last analysis, however, it seems to be not only a distinct entity, but even assumes an enormous importance.

The very fact that in schizophrenia various mechanisms, diverse attitudes – reverie, daydreaming, the attitude of regret, the interrogative attitude, etc. – can fill the same role confirms this kind of analysis, just as the fact that the same complexes can be found at the source of dissimilar symptoms greatly limits the role of the former in the pathogenesis of the latter.

The Problem of Primary and Secondary Symptoms – The Tendency for Ideo-Affective Expression

The problem of primary and secondary symptoms in psychiatry offers us the occasion to insist once again upon the double aspect of mental disorders ...

For Bleuler, schizophrenia is an organic illness. It is from this angle that he approaches the problem of primary and secondary symptoms. He considers the morbid manifestations which seem to depend directly upon the subjacent organic process as primary symptoms. We will not enumerate all of these manifestations here; this could be of little interest to us. What is important is to point out that, on the psychological level, he considers the initial disorder to be that which can be linked with the subjacent organic process in the most plausible way; he sees it; as we know, in a particular disorder of associations. He tries then to deduce from it the other fundamental symptoms of schizophrenia, such as logical deficiency, affective disorders, autism, ambivalence, etc. He arrives then at the superstructure determined by the ideo-affective content of complexes. Even though Bleuler considers schizophrenia to be an organic disease more than anything else, he still accords a very large place in his conception to the affective factors, understood as secondary mechanisms. And it is in this way that he comes to envisage the pathogenesis of certain accessory symptoms, such as delirium and certain hallucinations, almost uniquely from the point of view of their content, sometimes without taking sufficient account of the fact that from the psychological point of view a complex by itself, whatever its content is, is incapable of providing an explanation of the genesis of particular phenomena, such as delusions and hallucinations.

A reaction to this conception was inevitable ...

*****

It always seems unproductive to me, when confronted by a work of great breadth, to search for its weak points. It is much more fruitful to emphasize its essential points so that a broad perspective may be opened for further efforts. We must avoid destroying what is positive in a work, but it would also be useless to consider it as definitive and untouchable. Our task is to attempt to build further while dutifully rendering it homage.

Two points are essential for Bleuler's theory: first, the initial disorder is related to a subdivided function – more precisely, to the associative function;

second, the whole conception is placed under the rubric of "disease," which means that the mental life of the schizophrenic is represented as a *pathological* modification of the normal psyche. For these reasons I will speak readily of an *anatomomedical* theory; the word "anatomical" designates not so much Bleuler's organicist point of departure as the fact that the human spirit is here dissected into isolated functions, of which one becomes, on the psychological level, the seat of the initial disorder. For Bleuler the word "medical" indicates that the whole situation is seen from the point of view of a person who is sick rather than a being who is "different" with respect to normal life.

It is now clear that we will change nothing essential in the general orientation of this conception if we replace the associative function with another function, such as affectivity or volition, in the current sense of these terms, and then try to deduce the other "pathological" manifestations of a schizophrenic nature.

But we can take a completely different attitude toward the so-called psychopathological phenomena.

Whenever we are faced with psychic manifestations, we have a tendency to conceive of them as a *whole*. This is a general principle that has no exception. It is the same whether we have a schizophrenic or any other mentally ill person before us. Here we are dealing not so much with a psyche that has been dissociated and disfigured by a morbid process as with a *sui generis* psychic life, forming a whole which we wish to penetrate.

Indeed, it is a psychic life which is different from our own, but we ought now to make this difference precise in a completely different way. We will no longer be concerned with a disorder which is related to a function of some kind; rather, we will be concerned with a *general* modification of the *structure* of the psychic life, insofar as it is an indivisible whole. In the foreground we will not find a "diseased person" but a "person who is different," who obviously, as a consequence, but only as a consequence, can be interpreted for medical purposes as an expression of a pathological modification. As Gruhle says, we replace the 'lack' by a "difference." This attitude will be the *phenomenopsychopathological* attitude.

Among our Bleulerian notions there is one which agrees indisputably with this attitude much more than with association-ism. This is autism. We can speak of an autistic form of mental life and attempt to create a living picture of it in ourselves. Certainly, from the pragmatic point of view, the autistic life is in discord with the exigencies of ambient reality. But

so is non-Euclidean geometry if we compare it, from this point of view, with Euclidean geometry. It still constitutes an edifice whose parts agree perfectly with one another; the discord with ambient reality is not a criterion of dislocation or intrinsic contradiction. Will not autistic life, viewed from within, be completely uniform, even though, viewed from without, it would have one "axiom" less than normal life?

Thus the idea of autism seems the indicated starting point for the new efforts which are destined to allow us to deepen our understanding of the schizophrenic form of psychic life. It is scarcely necessary to recall that autism cannot be reduced to a deposit of complexes, or even less to narcissism or to autoeroticism. Autism simply refers to a particular form of mental life.

The problem of primary and secondary symptoms or, now more preferably, primary and secondary manifestations observed in the course of a given mental affliction, appears now under another aspect. Thus the psychic stereotypes in schizophrenia, particularly insofar as they are general attitudes, seem to serve to effectuate a kind of phenomenological filling-in of the void that was hollowed out in the psychic life by the initial disorder. The ideo-affective content intervenes in this case only in the second or, more precisely, the third place (the first level being constituted by the generating disorder) ...

Certainly, it would be premature to attempt to explicate all the psychic manifestations we have observed in schizophrenics in this fashion. To mention only one group of them, the hallucinatory phenomena, particularly, do not lend themselves to interpretations of this order. Be that as it may, we have the impression of being confronted with a new method, capable of accounting for the linking-up of diverse phenomena in the morbid consciousness.

*****

But does anything remain of the psyche if we take away, one after another, the ideas, the feelings, the volitions – and isn't the structure of which we are speaking simply a myth? Yes, something remains – something essential remains. What remains is the way in which the *living ego situates itself in relation to space and time*, not, obviously, in relation to measurable time and geometrical space, but to time and to space which, even deprived of their concrete and material content, are not simply dead forms but appear, on the contrary, as we know, full of life.

We ought to search for the basis of the structural aspect of mental disorders through a phenomenological analysis of these spatiotemporal relations of the living ego.

*****

Example: Analysis of a Case of Pathological Jealousy based on Mental Automatism

We choose the following case history to demonstrate how, in a given case, the various factors – clinical, [ideo-]affective, and structural – in becoming entangled are related to one another.

Mme. L., 35 years old, comes to consult us at the Dispensaire de Prophylaxie Mentale. She is a worker who has been employed for some years in a factory; her husband is a foreman there. At the first examination the patient complains that she has the impression that people are making fun of her, of not being like others, of having her head caught in a vise; but the purpose of her visit is mainly a feeling of jealousy with regard to her husband. Around two years ago her husband brought one of his friends to the house. Without knowing why she felt so, she became jealous of this man; the idea that her husband could have relations with him arose in her mind; from that day forward she had not ceased to be jealous of her husband, "of everything and everyone"; she was thus driven to create "hideous scenes" with him, especially at the time of her period; discouraged, she had a few days ago gone to drown herself.

Her husband supplied the following information:

They had been married since June, 1914. Several months later the husband was inducted, wounded, and made a prisoner. He did not return home until December, 1918.

Up until the appearance of the existing disorder, he noticed nothing particularly abnormal about his wife. He remembered, however, that she had made a small scene the day after their marriage, declaring that he had had to marry her against his will. Also, she had a fairly jealous character; she was jealous of her sister, who was in a better situation than she. After her husband's return home, from 1918 to 1925, she was nervous from time to time but did not present any bizarre ideas.

The actual disorder appeared suddenly two years ago. One day he went out for an hour; when he returned, she accused him of unnatural activities. Since then, scenes of this sort had occurred fairly frequently over nothing – because he was five minutes late, for example. The husband went to a doctor; the latter, after administering a sedative, drew up a commitment

certificate, but the husband hesitated to put his wife in an asylum.

The father of the patient was an alcoholic. A cousin was mentally ill.

The patient is an excellent worker. She is a good housekeeper and is very affectionate with her children, and, except for the scenes of jealousy, she takes good care of her husband, too. He is perfectly aware of the morbid character of these scenes.

We also had the occasion to see the patient's children, who, as far as manners were concerned, showed particular care on the part of the mother.

At her next visit the patient tells us the following:

At the age of 19 she had the measles; following this illness she was bothered for several months by the idea that people were making fun of her, that people looked at her sideways, that her feet perspired in an abnormal manner and emitted a nauseous odor which others could not help but notice. Around the same time, someone at the workroom caused a "row," accusing her of intimate relations with another young girl. She was furious. At this time she was in love with a young man, but he preferred one of her friends. This made her jealous.

At the age of 23 she had made a sensible marriage. Her husband was from the beginning indifferent with regard to her; she herself had gained little pleasure from him.

As a child she was very happy; then, as a young girl, she had attacks of despair following her first unhappy love affair and at the time of her wedding.

During the war she had an affair; after the war she had one other. She believed herself to be influenced by this man and felt incapable of resisting him.

Two years ago her husband evinced suspicions concerning her fidelity. Then she in turn begins to accuse him and becomes jealous of him; discouraged, she thinks of suicide.

She remembers very well the circumstances where she felt this jealousy for the first time; her jealousy was directed at an old friend of her husband's; one day, seeing them return together, she was convinced that they had done horrible things. Since then she has remained jealous of her husband. She is jealous of men and women in the same way.

In the past she has often had indefinable illnesses. These illnesses disappeared as soon as she got these jealous ideas. She remarks also that these attacks of jealousy had resulted the next day in intimate relations with her husband.

One is thus led to believe that, in this case, it is mainly a question of manifestations of jealousy of a pathological nature in a person who has always had a certain tendency to be jealous. The patient spontaneously gave us the details of her intimate life which were capable of playing the role of affective complexes and established a direct relation between these passionate manifestations and her instinctive life. Thus it seemed legitimate to assume that it was primarily affective factors that were the basis for the mental disorders that she exhibited.

However, a more careful examination disclosed symptoms of a completely different order. The presence of these symptoms, as well as the way in which these various disorders are arranged in the morbid consciousness of Mme. L., leads us to submit this conception that we have just formulated to a more extensive analysis. They orient our pathogenetic research in another direction.

We saw our patient regularly every eight days for many months. Let us see what she said.

May 11, 1927. She has been calmer this week, has not felt jealous of her husband.

When she is better, she wonders what caused her to be that way. There is something strange, mysterious, bizarre in her. She doesn't recognize herself at all in these ideas of jealousy; she would never have experienced such ideas by herself; these are not her ideas; she wonders whether she did not experience these ideas under the influence of a third person.

When she is jealous of a woman, she often recognizes in this woman her own gestures, recognizes something of herself; at the same time, she "cannot find herself anymore."

She is convinced, and it is a conviction that she holds to, despite everything, that the woman of whom she is jealous knows everything that she thinks, in sum, that she has taken her place. "However, I tell myself that no one can change places with another person"; she also finds that she is different from other people.

When she thinks, it is as if she were having a conversation with someone. When she works, it is as if someone commands her, says to her, for example, "Go to the rest room"; she then argues with this someone. She does not know whether these are her own thoughts or not.

She believes that someone is doing something to her, transforming her; if she knew who it was, she would be better able to defend herself.

During her second affair she felt that her lover and even his wife enticed her to their house despite herself. Her lover influenced her, suggested all her ideas to her. He was a vicious man. She had never loved him, but something pushed her toward that man despite herself.

At the age of 19 she often changed jobs because she thought people were making fun of her, that she smelled bad. She held onto these ideas for a long time, until just after her marriage – in reality until her first affair; she was attached to that man.

Here, too, the patient establishes a direct connection between the affective factors and the genesis of her disorder. But at the same time, even if we do not take the crisis of jealousy into consideration, we see a group of signs clearly forming that are all relevant to Clérambault's syndrome: flight of ideas, interior dialogues, enunciation of acts, ideas of influence. Further, we see mechanisms of identification and projection (recognition of her own gestures in the woman of whom she is jealous), which, as we know, constitute an integral part of thought interference. These same symptoms are recognizable in the patient's accounts of her past. Thus, according to her, she had to submit to a foreign influence in the same way at the time of her affair after the war.

In the course of our successive examinations the details that we have just enumerated tended to occupy a more and more important place in the clinical picture.

May 18. Sunday she found her husband completely changed. He had a headache, he was in a bad mood. She wondered whether it was really he who had changed her like that.

One day in October, last year, her child was sleeping in her arms; she had the idea that her husband had put them both to sleep. From that time she found her child completely changed; the lover that she had during the war coughed; she recognized that same cough in the youngster. She now suspects that someone is inflicting the same things on another woman.

What seems strange to her is that her husband changes so often, that he is not always the same. When she feels well, her husband is sick. She wonders sometimes if someone has not done something to both of them (she cries). She also sometimes wonders if her husband does not have the key to the mystery, but that he does not want to disclose it to her. Her mother-in-law, who lives with them, also has been completely changed for a month; she is always thinking, whereas, before, she used to speak more often.

*****

We can add some further details to the picture sketched above. The patient often had the impression that mysterious changes were occurring, either in her or around her. Sometimes it was she who was completely changed; sometimes it was one of her relatives who had changed. At the same time, banal and natural events, such as the fact of seeing her child sleeping in her arms, became problematic for her, obliging her to seek a special reason for them. We had the impression of being confronted by a particular disorder relating to the sensation of *the natural flux of life*. Events which usually pass unnoticed or which are considered to be completely natural easily become separated from this flux, emerge as independent facts.

In a secondary manner, these events, once separated from the *natural flux*, often become the starting point of morbid identifications, of which we have spoken above. In this way she recognized her lover's cough in her child's cough or came to believe that someone inflicted upon another woman what she herself experienced.

Certain of our patient's words could make us believe that she was conscious, at least in part, of her condition. In reality, she always held to the morbid conviction that something bizarre and mysterious happened around her. At best, she admitted the idea of illness as one of the manifestations of the maleficent actions which she suffered, and wanted very much to have a doctor cure her of this.

All of these facts are found again and again during the course of subsequent examinations.

June 1. She feels better; has had no more jealous ideas; this makes her very happy. Has had instead ideas that someone has accused her of having had unnatural relations with her sister. For a moment such ideas take her in, but then they make her laugh; she tells herself that someone has done it on purpose, to make fun of her.

*****

June 8. She has had no unhealthy ideas this week; feels the taste of life return; has taken pleasure in putting up new wallpaper in her apartment. She is aware that she has tortured her husband for nothing.

Before, she often felt that she was the person with whom she spoke; this exasperated her, and she wondered if she were destined to live all her life like that, in someone's else's tow. Today again, at noon, has asked her husband if she could not possibly be he.

June 15. For three days she has had to think of a dog, has seen everyone with heads of dogs; the scenes of her childhood, of which she spoke the other day, came back to mind. It is as if someone were sending her ideas directly. Then she believed that she was elsewhere, that there must be two of her for her to be just like that. Each time she saw someone, she thought that that person knew her thoughts, knew that she thought of a dog; she got it into her head that someone had watched those childhood scenes and was now using them against her.

*****

Our patient sometimes suggested delusions of persecution. She believed, for example, that someone had been watching at the time of the scene with the dog and was now using it against her. These ideas, however, had a completely episodic character; they were not crystallized or systematized at any moment. This fits well with the patient's general attitude; easily approachable and often confident, she did not behave at all like a paranoiac.

But what interested us primarily was the way in which the past intervened in her morbid consciousness. First of all, it could be said that she searched for a stable point in the past to counteract the perpetual changes which she felt she experienced, changes which we have connected to a disorder in the feeling of the natural flux of becoming, changes which give, among other things, the impression of a particular splitting-up of the ego in time. This is why she tells us that she "finds herself" again when she thinks of her parents, and then she feels good. This is a mechanism which is easy to understand; the past, with all its affective attachments, was, in her daily life, one of the foundations of self-identity and the stability of the ego.

*****

The patient constantly attached present events to past events. It is interesting to note that for her it was not a question of simple remembrances which were evoked but rather a true identification, a reliving of the past, with all of the characteristics of the present. It was thus that, at the time of her natural brother's visit, she saw herself as she was at the age of 18; or when she broke down and cried, she saw herself as a little girl. This was also probably one of the effects of the splitting-up of the ego and of becoming in time, about which we were concerned above. The living perspective which allows us to envisage the past from the point of view of the present is missing, and because of this the slices of the past become identified with the present. We have spoken of this phenomenon in an earlier work.[7] It is perhaps useful to recall here, as well, that, even if it is not a question of facts which are entirely identical to those which we are here studying, the impression of *déjà vu* does not rest, according to the ingenious conception of Pierre Janet, on the presence of a false memory but rather on a disorder in the function of presentification. The failure of this function, which is of a complex and synthetic nature, will result in a projection of a present impression onto the past.

We only mention these facts here in passing, since it is time to outline a total view.

If we open the classical psychiatry textbooks, such as Chaslin's work,[8] we will find there, in addition to the delusions of jealousy which occur in alcoholics, a description of two kinds of cases of pathological jealousy: 1) pathological jealousy as a variety of abnormal passions occurring in maladjusted and sometimes mentally deficient subjects and 2) systematized jealous madness, where there is a modality of systematized chronic insanity based uniquely upon delirious interpretations.

Our case does not fit into either one of the two categories. The feeling of jealousy appeared in our patient in a paroxysmal manner and occurred on a particular mental basis. This basis was constituted by Clérambault's syndrome, to which the relevant symptoms of identity and projection mechanisms (transference) are added.

The coexistence of these diverse symptoms is not made artificially, for they are related to one another through a feeling of depersonalization or, as is perhaps a preferable way of saying it, they express a disorder of the affirmation of the ego in relation to space. In Clérambault's syndrome, it is the inner life of the ego which finds itself reflected outside. In transference it is the whole ego which is projected elsewhere in space and attributed to other persons. Here we have a kind of repetition, that is, a kind of echo of the ego, as if there was an echo of thoughts somewhere else.

In order to complete our picture, we ought to add to this the phenomenon of a particular splitting of the notion of duration, which is expressed by the fact

that the events stand out more than is necessary from the natural flux of becoming and, once separated from it, are either experienced as uninterrupted and extraordinary changes occurring around the patient or in him, or are projected on the foundation of mystery which seems to float around him.

The problem which ought to occupy us now is the way in which the feeling of jealousy becomes attached to the mental basis from which it originates.

From this point of view, let us first of all establish one fact. We observed our patient for more than a year, and during this time we witnessed oscillations in her condition. These oscillations allowed us to see how the various disorders which we have described were arranged, so to speak, in the patient's consciousness. On the whole, jealousy was the least constant symptom; she appeared to overcome it again and again, so that it did not return for many months. But its absence did not indicate a return to normalcy. Behind it existed the mental basis which we have clarified above.

*****

Clérambault has shown in his studies of psychoses based on mental automatism how the constitutional factors can come to be added to the central nucleus of the psychoses.

Shouldn't this be the place to search for an analogous origin of our patient's delusions of jealousy? Certain facts argue in favor of this conception: her husband brought out a certain jealous tendency in her. However, in pushing our study of our patient further, we see that she not only did not establish a true delusion of jealousy around the syndrome of mental automatism, as paranoiacs do, for example, by adding a delusion of persecution, but that, properly speaking, she did not have an umbrageous and jealous character. Quite confident, she manifested her jealousy only in an episodic way and in a particular form.

This obliges us to search for another explanation. We have already seen that affective factors constantly intervened in our patient's statements. There is a connecting thread which we can follow from the first childhood conflicts through the first romantic disappointment, the marriage out of vexation, the later affairs, up to the feeling of jealousy and the content of certain symptoms of the present psychosis. A question arises as to whether it is not justifiable to see in this an argument for a purely affective

---

[7] E. Minkowski, "Les Regrets morbides," *Annales medico-psychologiques* (November, 1925). [**Original note**]

[8] Ph. Chaslin, *Elements de sémiologie et clinique mentales* (1912). [**Original note**]

interpretation of the symptoms. Here again, certain details argue in favor of this hypothesis. Thus our patient attributed the affair she had after the war, which left a particularly painful memory in her, to a foreign influence. She told us also that something bad happened in her against her husband and that she told herself that that did not come from her; or, expressing herself more clearly concerning one of her ideas, she said, "This idea did not come from me because I never thought of such horrible things." On the other hand, sexual details, such as the characteristic admission of her frigidity in the marriage – frigidity which was replaced by a feeling of pleasure when she became jealous of her husband – tended to establish a direct connection, not only with the affective life in the narrow sense of the term, but also with the instinctive life of the subject.

We do not wish to discuss these hypotheses in detail here. We recall only that, in searching for the affective genesis of disorders, we find that they immediately establish too great an analogy, if not an absolute identity, between the ideo-affective manifestations of the normal consciousness and the ideo-affective manifestations of the morbid consciousness.

*****

Whenever the patient tried to animate this mental base to some degree by the introduction of affective factors, she seemed inevitably led to the feeling of jealousy. This feeling fitted perfectly, in effect, with the essential traits which ruled over her mental activity; for if, in transference, she identified with another – put herself in *her place*, said she was just like her – in her jealousy she *desired to be in her place*, desired to have what the other possessed and what she herself did not have. The frame remains fundamentally the same; the difference consists simply in the presence, in the second case, of an affective or, if you prefer, passionate factor. In jealousy the ego no longer affirms itself; it is a feeling which depersonalizes, and this is perhaps what primarily distinguishes it from vanity and pride. A man's vanity is affected when he discovers he is second and not first; this is a painful situation he must settle with himself – his rival plays, basically, only a secondary role. In jealousy it is the inverse that occurs: we suffer because the other is first and we ourselves occupy only a second place; the accent falls on the person of the "other," whose place we want to occupy. Consequently, vanity is born out of the desire to conquer; jealousy, on the contrary, provokes one to vengeance and destruction. Because it is negative in relation to affirmation of the ego, jealousy is in perfect accord with the principles which characterized the mental basis of our patient. Dominated by the principles of similitude and identity, the psyche studied found jealousy on its route when it appealed to the affective sphere. All the same, this is a desire, a suffering, but one which always rests upon a partial identification with the other, in the sense of coveting what the other has. Jealousy is thus a defense reaction, tending to fill with affective factors the form of mental life determined by the generating disorder of the affection. Thus it is, as we have seen – and this confirms our way of seeing the matter – a jealousy which in no way has the same tonality as habitual jealousy; it is a bizarre jealousy, a jealousy without love.

*****

We are too often inclined to consider the delusions of our patients as real beliefs, exactly comparable to our own, while in reality their beliefs are an ideational or ideo-affective expression of the profound modification which the very form of their mental life has undergone. This is the form which we should investigate.

*****

Chapter 13

Binswanger's existential approach

Binswanger, L. (1946), 'The existential analysis school of thought'

From (1958) *Existence: A New Dimension in Psychiatry and Psychology*. Edited by R. May, E. Angel and H. Ellenberger and translated by E. Angel. New York: Basic Books: 191–213. Originally published as (1946) Über die Daseinsanalytische Forschungsrichtung in der Psychiatrie. *Schweizer Archiv für Neurologie und Psychiatrie* 57: 209–25.

Existential Analysis – Its Nature and Goals

By existential analysis we understand an anthropological[1] type of scientific investigation – that is, one which is aimed at the essence of being human. Its name as well as its philosophical foundation are derived from Heidegger's Analysis of Being, *"Daseins Analytics."* It is his – not yet properly recognized – merit to have uncovered a fundamental structure of existence and to have described it in its essential parts, that is, the structure of being-in-the-world. By identifying the basic condition or structure of existence with being-in-the-world, Heidegger intends to say something about the condition of the possibility for existence. The formulation "being-in-the-world" as used by Heidegger is, therefore, in the nature of an ontological thesis, a statement about an essential condition that determines existence in general. From the discovery and presentation of this essential condition, existential analysis received its decisive stimulation, its philosophical foundation and justification, as well as its methodological directives. However, existential

analysis itself is neither an ontology nor a philosophy and therefore must refuse to be termed a *philosophical anthropology*; as the reader will soon realize, only the designation of *phenomenological anthropology* meets the facts of the situation.

Existential analysis does not propose an ontological thesis about an essential condition determining existence, but makes *ontic statements* – that is, statements of factual findings about actually appearing forms and configurations of existence. In this sense, existential analysis is an empirical science, with its own method and particular ideal of exactness, namely with method and the ideal of exactness of the *phenomenological* empirical sciences.

Today we can no longer evade recognition of the fact that there are two types of empirical scientific knowledge. One is the *discursive inductive* knowledge in the sense of describing, explaining, and controlling "natural events," whereas the second is the *phenomenological empirical* knowledge in the sense of a methodical, critical exploitation or interpretation of phenomenal contents. It is the old disagreement between Goethe and Newton which today – far from disturbing us – has changed by virtue of our deepened insight into the nature of experience from an "either/or" into an "as well." The same phenomenological empirical knowledge is used regardless of whether we deal with the interpretation of the aesthetic content of an artistic style-period, with the literary content of a poem or a drama, or with the self-and-world content of a Rorschach response or of a psychotic form of existence. In phenomenological experience; the discursive taking apart of natural objects into characteristics or qualities and their inductive elaboration into types, concepts, judgments, conclusions, and theories is replaced by giving expression to the content of what is purely phenomenally given and therefore is not part of "nature as such" in any way. But the phenomenal content can find expression and, in being expressed, can unfold itself only if we approach and question it by the phenomenological method – or else we shall receive not a scientifically founded and

---

[1] Binswanger uses this word not in its usual American meaning, which is cultural anthropology, the comparative study of races, mores, etc., but rather in its more strictly etymological sense, that is, anthropology as the study of man (*"anthropos"*) and specifically, as he goes on to say above, the study of the essential meaning and characteristics of being human. [**Translator's note**]

verifiable answer but just an accidental *aperçu*. In this, as in every science, everything depends upon the method of approach and inquiry – i.e., on the ways and means of phenomenological method of experience.

Over the last few decades the concept of phenomenology has changed in some respects. Today, we must strictly differentiate between Husserl's pure or eidetic phenomenology as a transcendental discipline, and the phenemonenological interpretation of human forms of existence as an empirical discipline. But understanding the latter is not possible without knowledge of the former.

In this we should be guided, to mention only one factor, by abstinence from what Flaubert calls *la rage de vouloir conclure*, that is, by overcoming our passionate need to draw conclusions, to form an opinion, or to pass judgment – a task which in the light of our one-sided natural-scientific intellectual training cannot be considered an easy one. In short, instead of reflecting on something we should let the something speak for itself or, to quote Flaubert again, "express the thing as it is." However, the "as it is" contains one more fundamental ontological and phenomenological problem; for we finite human beings can acquire information on the "how" of a thing only according to the "world-design" which guides our understanding of things. Therefore, I have to return once more to Heidegger's thesis of existence as "being-in-the-world."

The ontological thesis that the basic constitution or structure of existence is being-in-the-world is not a philosophical *aperçu* but rather represents an extremely consistent development and extension of fundamental philosophical theories, namely of Kant's theory about the conditions of the possibility of experience (in the natural-scientific sense) on the one hand, and of Husserl's theory of transcendental phenomenology on the other. I shall not elaborate on these connections and developments. What I want to emphasize here is only the identification of being-in-the-world and transcendence; for it is through this that we can understand what "being-in-the-world" and "world" signify in their anthropological application. The German word for transcendence or transcending is *Ueberstieg* (climbing over or above, mounting). An *Ueberstieg* requires, first, that toward which the *Ueberstieg* is directed and, secondly, that which is *ueberstiegen* or transcended; the first, then, toward which the transcendence occurs, we call "world," whereas the second, which is transcended, is the being itself (*das Seiende selbst*) and especially that in the form

of which a human existence itself "exists." In other words, not only "world" constitutes itself in the act of transcending – be it as a mere dawn of world or as objectifying knowledge – but the self also does so.

Why do I have to mention these seemingly complicated matters?

Only because through the concept of being-in-the-world as transcendence has the fatal defect of all psychology been overcome and the road cleared for anthropology, the fatal defect being the theory of a dichotomy of world into subject and object. On the basis of that theory, human existence has been reduced to a mere subject, to a worldless rump subject in which all sorts of happenings, events, functions occur, which has all sorts of traits and performs all sorts of acts, without anybody, however, being able to say (notwithstanding theoretical constructs) how the subject can ever meet an "object" and can communicate and arrive at an understanding with other subjects. In contrast, being-in-the-world implies always being in the world with beings such as I, with coexistents. Heidegger, in his concept of being-in-the-world as transcendence, has not only returned to a point prior to the subject–object dichotomy of knowledge and eliminated the gap between self and world, but has also elucidated the structure of subjectivity as transcendence. Thus he has opened a new horizon of understanding for, and given a new impulse to, the scientific exploration of human existence and its specific modes of being. The split of Being into subject (man, person) and object (thing, environment) is now replaced by the unity of existence and "world," secured by transcendence?[2]

---

[2] Where we speak of "world" in terms of existential analysis, there world always means that toward which the existence has climbed and according to which it has designed itself: or, in other words, the manner and mode in which that which is (*Seiende*) becomes accessible to the existence. However, we use the expression "world" not only in its transcendental but also in its "objective" sense, as, *e.g.*, when we speak of the "dull resistance of the world," of the "temptations of the world," "retiring from the world," etc., whereby we have primarily the world of our fellow men in mind. Similarly, we speak of a person's environment and of his "own world" as of particular regions of that which exists in the objective world, and not as of transcendental world designs. This is terminologically troublesome, but not open to change any more. Hence, where the meaning is not self-evident, we have to place "world" always in quotation marks, or use the term "world design." [**Original note**]

Transcending, therefore, implies far more, and something much more original, than knowing, even more than "intentionality" in Husserl's sense, since "world" becomes accessible to us first and foremost already through our "key" (*Stimmung*). If for a moment we remember the definition of being-in-the-world as transcendence and view from this point our psychiatric analysis of existence, we realize that by investigating the structure of being-in-the-world we can also approach and explore psychoses; and realize furthermore that we have to understand them as specific modes of transcending. In this context we do not say: mental illnesses are diseases of the brain (which, of course, they remain from a medical–clinical viewpoint). But we say: in the mental diseases we face modifications of the fundamental or essential structure and of the structural links of being-in-the-world as transcendence. It is one of the tasks of psychiatry to investigate and establish these variations in a scientifically exact way.

As can be seen from all our analyses published so far, spatialization and temporalization of existence play an important part in existential analysis. I shall confine myself here to the still more central problem of time. What makes this problem so central is the fact that transcendence is rooted in the very nature of time, ill its unfolding into future, "having been" (*Gewesenheit*), and present. This will help to explain why, in our anthropological analyses of psychotic forms of being-human, we are not satisfied with our investigation unless we gain at least some insight into the respective variations of the structure of our patients' time . . . .

All this takes us only to the outermost gate of Heidegger's fundamental ontology or *Daseins* Analytics" and just to the gates of anthropological or existential analysis which has been inspired by and founded on the former. But I hasten to outline the method of existential analysis and the area of its scientific function. At this point, I have to mention that my positive criticism of Heidegger's theory has led me to its extension: being-in-the-world as being of the existence for the sake of *myself* (designated by Heidegger as "care") has been juxtaposed with "being-beyond-the-world" as being of the existence for the sake of *ourselves* (designated by me as "love"). This transformation of Heidegger's system has to be considered especially in the analysis of psychotic forms of existence where we frequently observe modifications of transcendence in the sense of the "overswing" of love, rather than in the sense of the "overclimb" of care. Let us only remember the enormously complex shrinkage of the existential structure which we so summarily call "autism."

The Differentiation Between Human Existence and Animal Being

"World" in Its Existential Analytical, and "World Around" (Umwelt) in Its Biological Meaning

However sketchy and incomplete my statements have been so far, I hope they have indicated why in our analyses, the concept of "world" – in the sense of world-formation or of "world-design" (Husserl's "mundanization" [*Mundanisierung*]) – represents one of the most important basic concepts and is even used as a methodological clue. For the *what* of the respective world-design always furnishes information about the *how* of the being-in-the-world and the *how* of being oneself. In order to clarify the nature of the world-design, I shall now confront it with some world-concepts of a biological nature. First comes to mind Von Uexküll's biological world-concept, particularly because it shows, in spite of its differences, a certain similarity in its methodological application. I shall start with the methodological agreement.

Von Uexküll distinguishes a perception world (*Merkwelt*), an inner world, action world of the animal and combines perception world an inner world under the name environment (*Umwelt* or "world-around"). The "circular interaction" occurring between these worlds he designates as *function-circle*. And just as we would say that it is not possible to describe the psychosis of a person without having fully encompassed (*umschritten*) his "worlds," so Von Uexküll states: "It is not possible to describe the biology of an animal unless one has fully encompassed its function-circles."[3] And as we would continue by saying: "Therefore, we are fully justified in as the existence of as many worlds as there are psychotics," so Von Uexküll continues: "Therefore, one is fully justified in assuming the existence of as many environments (*Umwelten*) as there are animals."[4] He comes similarly close to our viewpoint when he says: "Also, to understand each person's actions, we have to visit his 'special stage.'"[5]

Von Uexküll's concept of environment however is much too narrow to be applied to man, because he understands by this term merely the "island of the

---

[3] *Theoretische Biologie*, 2 Aufl., 1928, S. 100. [Original note]
[4] *Ibid.*, S. 144. [Original note]
[5] *Nie geschaute Welten. Die Umwelten meiner Freunde*, S. 20. [Original note]

senses" – i.e., of sensory perceptions which "surround man like a garment." Hence it does not surprise us that in his brilliant descriptions of his friends' environments he continuously transgresses that narrow concept and demonstrates throughout how these friends are really "in-the-world" as *human beings*.

We further agree, for the present, with Von Uexküll's statement: "It is nothing but mental inertness to assume the existence of a single objective world [we psychiatrists naïvely call it reality] which one tailors as closely as possible to one's own environment, and which one has extended in all directions in space and time."[6]

However, Von Uexküll overlooks the fact that man, in contrast to animal, has his own world as well as an objective one which is common to all. This was known already to Heraclitus, who said that in the state of wakefulness we all have a common world, while in our sleep, as in passion, emotional states, sensuous lust, and drunkenness, each of us turns away from the common world toward his own. That common world – and Heraclitus recognized this, too – is one of phronesis, or rational deliberation and thinking. We psychiatrists have paid far too much attention to the deviations of our patients from life in the world which is common to all, instead of focusing primarily upon the patients' own or private world, as was first systematically done by Freud.

There is, however, one factor which not only differentiates our existential analytical concept of world from Von Uexküll's biological concept but places it even in diametrical opposition. It is true that, in Von Uexküll's theory, the animal and its environment form at times a genuine structure within the function-circle and that they appear there as "made to order for each other." However, Von Uexküll still considers the animal as subject and its environment as an object separated from it. Unity of animal and

environment, of subject and object, is, according to Von Uexküll, guaranteed by the respective "blueprints" (action-plans, but also perception-plans) of the animal which, in turn, are part of an "overwhelmingly vast planful system." It now becomes clear that in order to proceed from Von Uexküll's theory to existential analysis, one must perform the Kantian–Copernican turn; instead of starting with nature and its planful system and dealing in natural science, one has to start at transcendental subjectivity and to proceed to existence as transcendence. Von Uexküll still throws both into one pot, as one deduces from the following ideas (which are quite impressive in themselves):

> Let us take as an example a certain oak tree and then ask ourselves what kind of of environmental object will that oak tree be, in the environment of an owl that perches in its hollow trunk; in the environment of a singing bird that nests in its branches; of a fox which has its hole under its roots; of a woodpecker which goes after wood-fretters in its bark; in the environment of such a wood-fretter itself; of an ant which runs along its trunk, etc. And, eventually, we ask ourselves what the role of the oak tree is in the environment of a hunter, of a romantic young girl, and of a prosaic wood-merchant. The oak, being a closed planful system itself, is woven into ever new plans on numerous environment stages, the tracing of which is a genuine task for the science of nature.

Von Uexküll is a natural scientist and not a philosopher. So it should not be held against him that he, like most natural scientists, makes light of the essential difference between animal and man and does not "keep sacred" (Spemann) the division between them. And yet, just at this point, this division becomes almost tangible. In the first place, the animal is tied to its "blueprint." It cannot go beyond it, whereas human existence not only contains numerous possibilities of modes of being but is precisely rooted in this multifold potentiality of being. Human existence affords the possibility of being a hunter; of being romantic of being in business, and thus is free to design itself toward the most different potentialities of being; in other words, existence can "transcend" the being – in this case the being which is called "oak" – or make it accessible to itself, through the most diverse world-designs.

Secondly, we remember – now departing completely from the biological point of view – that transcendence implies not only world-design bin, at the same time, self-design, potential modes of being for the self. Human existence is a very different being for the self, according to whether it designs its world as a

---

[6] See *Umwelt und Innenwelt der Tiere*, 2 Aufl., 1921, S. 4: "Only to the superficial observer it seems as if all sea-animals were living in a homogeneous world, common to all of them. Closer study teaches us that each of those thousands of forms of life possesses an environment peculiar to itself which is conditioned by and, in turn, conditions the 'building plans' of the animal." Also, viz., *Theoretische Biologie*, S. 232: "We now know that there is not one space and one time only, but that there are as many spaces and times as there are subjects, as each subject is contained by its own environment which possesses its own space and time. Each of these thousandfold worlds offers to the sensory perceptions a new potentiality to unfold themselves." [**Original note**]

hunter and *is* a hunter or, as a young girl, is a romantic self, or as a wood-trader is a prosaic-calculating self. All these are different ways of being in the world and of potential modes of the self which are joined by numerous others, particularly that of the genuine potentiality of being oneself, and of the potentiality of being *we* in the sense of love.[7]

The animal, not being able to be an *I-you-we*-self (since it is kept from even saying "*I-you-we*") does not have any world. For self and world are, indeed, reciprocal concepts. When we speak of the environment (*Umwelt*) the paramecium, the earthworm, the cephalopod, the horse, and even man *has*, this "*has*" possesses a very different meaning from the one we use when saying that man "*has*" a world. In the first case; the "*has*" signifies the establishment of a "blueprint," especially of the perception-and-action-organization, limited by nature to quite definite possibilities of stimulation and reaction. The animal has its environment by the grace of nature, not by the grace of freedom to transcend the situation. That means; it can neither design world nor open up world nor decide independently in and for a situation. It is, and always has been, in a once and for all determined "situational circle."[8] On the other hand, the "having" of a "world" on the part of man implies that man, although he has not laid his own foundation himself but was thrown into being and, insofar as that, has an environment like the animal, still has the possibility of transcending this being of his, namely, of climbing above it in care and of swinging beyond it in love.

Somewhat closer to our viewpoint than Von Uexküll's theory is Von Weizsaecker's concept of the "gestalt-circle"

as a self-contained biological act. "In so far as a living being through its movement and perception integrates itself into an environment, these movements and perceptions form a unit – a biological act."[9]

*****

All these theories are not only of the greatest interest to psychology and psychopathology but in addition bring clearly into focus the fact that only the concept of being-in-the-world as transcendence is genuinely consistent and penetrating; at the same time, they demonstrate that this concept can be applied consistently only to *human* existence.

Finally, I would like to remind the reader of Goldstein's world-concept, which proves so fruitful for the understanding of organic disturbances of the brain. Even where he uses the expression "milieu" in place of "world," we are still dealing with a genuine biological world-concept. As we know, it is one of his fundamental propositions that "a defective organism . . . can produce organized behavior only by such limitation of its milieu as corresponds to its defect."[10] At other times he speaks of a "loss of freedom" and of a "tightening of the tie to the environment" on account of a defect. We remember the fact that certain organic patients are no longer able to orient and conduct themselves in the world of "ideas," while being perfectly able to do so in the world of action or of practice where, as Goldstein put it more recently, "effects can come about through concrete acts in handling material presently at hand." In speaking, like Head, of a "disturbance of the symbolic expression" or, jointly with Gelb, of a "disturbance of categorical behavior," Goldstein in both instances formulates only a modification of "being-in-the-world" as transcending.[11]

This chapter has tried to demonstrate the degree to which biological thinking today endeavors to view and investigate organism and world as a unity in a unitary gestalt, symbolized by the circle. What prevails is the insight that everything here is connected with everything, that no partial change within the circle can occur without a change of the whole and that, in general, no isolated facts exist any more. This, however, carries with it a change in the concept of *fact*, of the fact itself, and of the methods in studying

---

[7] We therefore differentiate in the structure of the existence as being-in-the-world: (a) the ways in which it designs world and builds world – in short, the ways of world-design and world images; (b) the ways in which it, accordingly, exists as a self – i.e., establishes itself or does not establish itself; (c) but also the ways of transcendence as such, that is, the ways in which the existence is in the world (*e.g.*, acting, thinking, creating, fancying). Thus, doing existential analysis in the area of psychiatry means to examine and describe how the various forms of the mentally ill, and each one for himself, design world, establish their self and – in the widest sense – act and love. [Original note]

[8] This was already emphasized by Herder in his essay, "On the Origin of Language": Each animal has its circle within which it belongs from its birth, in which it remains for its life time, and in which it dies. (*Ausgew. Werke* [Reclam.] Ili, S. 621.) [Original note]

[9] "Der Gestaltkreis," *Theorie der Einheit vom Wahrnehmen und Bewegen*, 1940, S. 177. [Original note]
[10] *Der Aufbau des Organismus*, 1934, p. 32. [Original note]
[11] Please refer to p. 132 for an example of Goldstein's approach. [Editors' note]

facts. For the goal is now no longer to arrive at conclusions by induction through mere accumulation of facts but to delve lovingly into the nature and content of the single phenomenon. Goldstein is well aware of this when he says: "In the formation of biological knowledge, the single links that are integrated into the whole cannot simply be evaluated quantitatively, as though the insight became the more certain the more links we establish. Rather, all the single facts are of a greater or, lesser qualitative value." And he continues: "If in biology we see a science dealing with phenomena that can be established by analytical natural-scientific methods alone, we have to forego all insight which grasps the organism as a whole, and with it actually any insight into the life processes at all."[12]

This already carries us close to a phenomenological view of life in the widest sense, a view, that is, which aims at the grasping of the life-content of phenomena and not at their factual meaning within a precisely circumscribed object-area.[13]

The Existential-Analytical School of Thought in Psychiatry

As compared with biological research, which exhausts or interprets the life-content of the phenomena, existential-analytical research has a double advantage. Firstly, it does not have to deal with so vague a "concept" as that of life, but with the widely and completely uncovered *structure of existence* as "being-in-the-world" and "beyond-the-world." Secondly, it can let existence actually speak up about itself – let it have its say. In other words, the phenomena to be interpreted are largely language phenomena. We know that the content of existence can nowhere be more clearly seen or more securely than through language; because it is in language that our world-designs actually ensconce and articulate themselves and where, therefore, they can be ascertained and communicated.

As to the first advantage, knowledge of the structure or basic constitution or existence provides us with a systematic clue for the practical existential-analytical investigation at hand. We know, now, what

to focus on in the exploration of a psychosis, and how to proceed. We know that we have to ascertain the kind of spatialization and temporalization, of lighting and coloring; the texture, or materiality and motility, of the world-design toward which the given form of existence or its individual configuration casts itself. Such a methodical clue can be furnished only by the structure of being-in-the-world because that structure places a norm at our disposal and so enables us to determine deviations from this norm in the manner of the exact sciences. Much to our surprise it has turned out that, in the psychoses which were so far investigated, such deviations could not be understood merely negatively as abnormalities, but that they, in turn, represent a new norm, a new *form* of being-in-the-world. If, for example, we can speak of a manic form of life or, rather, of existence, it means that we could establish a norm which embraces and governs all modes of expression and behavior designated as "manic" by us. It is this *norm* which we call the "world" of the manic. The same holds true for the far more complicated, hitherto incalculably manifold world-designs of the schizophrenic. To explore and ascertain the world of these patients means, here as everywhere, to explore and ascertain in what way everything that is – men as well as things – is accessible to these forms of existence. For we know well enough that that-which is as such never becomes accessible to man, except in and through a certain world-design.

As to the second advantage, the possibility of exploring language phenomena, it is the essence of speech and speaking that they express and communicate a *certain content of meaning*. This content of meaning is, as we know, an infinitely manifold one. Everything, therefore, depends upon the precise criteria by which we explore the language manifestations of our patients. We do not – as the psychoanalyst systematically does – focus merely upon the historical content, upon references to an experienced or conjectured pattern of the inner life-history. And we do not at all watch the content for all possible references to facts pertaining to life function, as does the psychopathologist in focusing on disturbances of speech or thinking functions. What attracts our attention in existential analysis is rather the content of language expressions and manifestations insofar as they point to the world-design or designs in which the speaker lives or has lived or, in one word, their world-content. By world-content, then, we mean the content of facts

---

[12] *Ibid.*, S. 255 f. [**Original note**]

[13] *Viz.*, again Goldstein, *Der Aufbau des Organismus*, S. 242: "Biological insight is the virtuous process through which we experience increasingly the idea of the organism, curing of a 'ken' which is always based on the grounds of very empirical facts." [**Original note**]

pertaining to worlds; that is, of references to the way in which the given form or configuration of existence discovers world designs and opens up world – and is, or exists, in the respective world. There are, furthermore, indications of the way in which the existence is *beyond-the-world*; that is, how it *is*, or *is not*, at home in the eternity *(Ewigkeit)* and haven *(Heimat)* of love.

In "The Case of Ellen West," my first study planned as an example of existential analysis as applied to psychiatry, conditions were particularly favorable for existential analysis. In this case I had at my disposal an unusual abundance of spontaneous and immediately comprehensible verbal manifestations such as self-descriptions, dream accounts, diary entries, poems, letters, autobiographical drafts, whereas usually, and especially in cases of deteriorated schizophrenics, we have to obtain the material for existential analysis by persistent and systematic exploration of our patients over months and years. First and foremost it is our task to assure ourselves, over and over again, of what our patients really mean by their verbal expressions. Only then can we dare to approach the scientific task of discerning the "worlds" in which the patients are or, in other words, to understand how all partial links of the existential structure become comprehensible through to the total structure, just as the total structure constitutes itself, without incongruity, from the partial links. In this, as in any other scientific investigation, there do occur errors, dead ends, premature interpretations; but, also as in any other, there are ways and means of correcting and rectifying these errors. It is one of the most impressive achievements of existential analysis to have shown that even in the realm of subjectivity "nothing is left to chance," but that a certain organized structure can be recognized from which each word, each idea, drawing, action, or gesture receives its peculiar imprint – an insight of which we make continuous use in existential-analytical interpretations of the Rorschach test and recently also in the Word Association Test. It is always the same world-design which confronts us in a patient's spontaneous verbal manifestations, in the systematic exploration of his Rorschach and Word Association responses, in his drawings; and also, frequently, in his dreams. And only after having encompassed *(umschritten)* these worlds – to speak in Von Uexküll's words – and brought them together can we understand the form of our patient's existence in the sense of what call "neurosis" or "psychosis." Only then may we dare to attempt to understand single, partial links of those forms of world and existence (clinically evaluated as symptoms) from the modes and ways of the patient's total being-in-the-world.

Naturally, the connections of the life-history, too, here play an important part but, as we shall soon realize, by no means in the same way as in psychoanalysis. Whereas for the latter they are the goal of the investigation, for existential analysis they merely provide material for that investigation.

The following examples will illustrate the kind of world-designs with which we have to deal in psychopathology; but the number of such deviations is infinite. We are still at the beginning of describing and investigating them.

For my first clinical illustration I shall report the case of a young girl who at the age of five experienced a puzzling attack of anxiety and fainting when her heel got stuck in her skate and separated from her shoe.[14] Ever since, the girl – now twenty-one years of age – suffered spells of irresistible anxiety whenever a heel of one of her shoes appeard [sic] to loosen or when someone touched the heel or only spoke of heels. (Her own had to be nailed to her soles.) On such occasions, if she could not get away in time, she would faint.

Psychoanalysis proved clearly and convincingly that hidden behind the fear of loose or separating heels were birth phantasies, both about being born herself and therefore separated from mother and about giving birth to a child of her own. Of the various disruptions of continuity which psychoanalysis revealed as being frightening to the girl, the one between mother and child was fundamental and most feared. (I am omitting completely, in this context, the masculine component.) Before the period of Freud, one would have stated that the skating accident, harmless as it was per se, had "caused" the "heel phobia." Freud demonstrated subsequently that the pathogenic effect is produced by phantasies connected with and preceding such an accident. Yet in both periods still another explanation would be drawn upon to account for the fact that a specific event or phantasy had such a far-reaching effect precisely upon this person – namely, the explanation of "constitution" or "predisposition." For each of us has experienced the

---

[14] *Viz.*, "Analyse einer hysterischen Phobie," *Jahrbuch Bleuler und Freud*, III. [**Original note**]

"birth trauma," but some lose their heels without developing a hysterical phobia.

We do not, of course, propose to unfold, let alone solve, the problem of "predisposition" in all its aspects; but I dare say that we can throw some more light on it when we view it from an "anthropological" angle. In later studies we were able to demonstrate that we could reach even *behind* the phantasies insofar as we could trace and investigate the world-design which made possible those phantasies and phobias in the first place.

What serves as a clue to the world-design of our little patient is the category of *continuity*, of continuous connection and containment. This entails a tremendous constriction, simplification, and depletion of the "world content," of the extremely complex totality of the patient's contexts of reference. Everything that makes the world significant is submitted to the rule of that *one* category which alone supports her "world" and being. This is what causes the great anxiety about any disruption of continuity, any gap, tearing or separating, being separated or torn. This is why separation from the mother, experienced by everyone as the arch-separation in human life, had to become so prevalent that any event of separation served to symbolize the fear of separation from the mother and to invite and activate those phantasies and daydreams.

We should, therefore, not explain the emergence of the phobia by an overly strong "pre-oedipal" tie to the mother, but rather realize that such overly strong filial tie is only possible on the premise of a world-design exclusively based on connectedness, cohesiveness, continuity. Such a way of experiencing "world" – which always implies such a "key" [15] – does not have to be "conscious"; but neither must we call it "unconscious" in the psychoanalytical sense, since it is outside the contrast of these opposites. Indeed, it does not refer to anything psychological but to something which only makes possible the psychic fact. At this point we face what is actually "abnormal" in this existence – but we must not forget that where the world-design is narrowed and constricted to such a degree, the self, too, is constricted and prevented from maturing. Everything is supposed to stay as it was before. If, however, something new does happen and continuity is disrupted, it can only result in catastrophe, panic,

anxiety attack. For then the world actually collapses, and nothing is left to hold it up. The inner or existential maturation and the genuine time-orientation toward the future are replaced by a preponderance of the past, of "already having-been-in." The world must stop here, nothing must happen, nothing must change. The context must be preserved as it has always been. It is this type of temporal orientation that permits the element of *suddenness* to assume such enormous significance; because suddenness is the time quality that explodes continuity, hacks it and chops it to pieces, throws the earlier existence out of its course, and exposes it to the Dreadful, to the naked horror. This is what in psychopathology we term, in a most simplifying and summarizing manner, anxiety attack.

Neither the loss of the heel nor the womb and birth phantasies are "explanations" of the emergence of the phobia. Rather, they became so significant because holding on to mother meant to this child's existence – as is natural for the small child – having a hold on the world. By the same token, the skating incident assumed its traumatic significance because, in it, the world suddenly changed its face, disclosed itself from the angle of suddenness, of something totally different, new, and unexpected. For that there was no place in this child's world; it could not enter into her world-design; it stayed, as it were, always outside; it could not be mastered. In other words, instead of being accepted by the inner life so that its meaning and content could be absorbed, it appeared and reappeared over and over again without having any meaning for the existence, in an ever-recurring invasion by the Sudden into the motionlessness of the world-clock. This world-design did not manifest itself before the traumatic event occurred; it did only on the *occasion* of that event. Just as the a priori or transcendental forms of the human mind make experience only into what experience is, so the form of that world-design had first to produce the condition of the possibility for the ice-skating incident in order for it to be experienced as traumatic.

It should be mentioned that this case is not at all an isolated one. We know that anxiety can be tied to various types of disruption of continuity; *e.g.*, it may appear as horror at the sight of a loose button hanging on a thread or of a break in the thread of saliva. Whatever the life-historical events are to which these anxieties refer, we are always dealing here with the same depletion of being-in-the-world, narrowed down to include only the category of continuity. In

---

[15] Or attunement (*Gestimmheit*). [**Translator's note**]

this peculiar world-design with its peculiar being-in-the-world and its peculiar self, we see in existential terms the real key to the understanding of what is taking place. Like the biologist and neuropathologist, we do not stop at the single fact, the single disturbance, the single symptom, but we keep searching for an embracing whole within which the fact can be understood as a partial phenomenon. But this whole is neither a functional whole – a "Gestalt-circle" – nor a whole in the sense of a complex. Indeed, it is no objective whole at all but a whole in the sense of the unity of a world-design.

We have seen that we cannot progress far enough in our understanding of anxiety if we consider it only as a psychopathological symptom per se. In short, we must never separate "anxiety" from "world," and we should keep in mind that anxiety always emerges when the world becomes shaky or threatens to vanish. The emptier, more simplified, and more constricted the world-design to which an existence has committed itself, the sooner will anxiety appear and the more severe will it be. The "world" of the healthy with its tremendously varied contexture of references and compounds of circumstance can never become entirely shaky or sink. If it is threatened in one region, other regions will emerge and offer a foothold. But where the "world," as in the present case and in numerous others, is so greatly dominated by one or a few categories, naturally the threat to the preservation of that one or those few categories must result in a more intensified anxiety.

Phobia is always an attempt at safeguarding a restricted, impoverished "world," whereas anxiety expresses the loss of such a safeguard, the collapse of the "world," and thus the delivery of the existence to nothingness – the intolerable, dreadful, "naked horror." We then must strictly differentiate between the historically and situationally conditioned *point of breakthrough* of anxiety and the existential *source* of anxiety. Freud made a similar distinction when he differentiated between phobia as a symptom and the patient's own libido as the real object of anxiety.[16] However, in our concept the theoretical construct of libido is replaced by the phenomenological–ontological structure of existence as being-in-the-world. We do not hold that man is afraid of his own

libido, but we state that existence as being-in-the-world is, as such, determined by uncanniness and nothingness. The source of anxiety is existence itself.[17]

Whereas in the preceding instance we had to, deal with a static "world," as it were, a world in which nothing was supposed to "come to pass" or happen, in which everything had to remain unchanged and no separating agent was to interfere with its unity, we shall in the following example meet a torturously heterogeneous, disharmonious "world," again dating from early childhood. The patient, displaying a pseudo-neurotic syndrome of polymorphous schizophrenia, suffered from all sorts of somata-, auto-, and allopsychic phobias.[18] The "world" in which that which is – everything-that-is (*alles Seiende*) – was accessible to him was a world of push and pressure, loaded with energy to the point of bursting. In that world no step could be made without running the danger of being knocked against or knocking against something, whether in real life or in phantasy. The temporality of this world was one of *urgency* (René Le Senne), its spatiality therefore one of horribly crowded narrowness and closeness, pressing upon "body and soul" of the existence. This came clearly to light in the Rorschach test. At one point the patient saw pieces of furniture "on which one might knock one's shin"; at another, "a drum that strikes one's leg"; at a third, "lobsters which squeeze you," "something you get scratched with"; and finally, "centrifugal balls of a flywheel which hit me in the face, me of all people, although for decades they had stayed fixed with the machine; only when I get there something happens."

As the world of things behaves, so does the world of one's fellow men; everywhere lurk danger and disrespect, mobs or jeering watchers. All this, of course, points to the borderline of delusions of "reference" or "encroachment."

It is very instructive to observe the patient's desperate attempts to control this disharmonious, energy-crammed, threatening world, to harmonize it artificially, and to belittle it in order to avoid the constantly imminent catastrophe. He does this by keeping himself at the greatest possible distance from the world, rationalizing this distance completely – a

---

16 "Neue Folge der Vorlesungen zur Einführung in die Psychoanalyse," S. 117 (*Ges. Schr., XII*, 238 f.) [**Original note**]

17 *Viz., Sein und Zeit*, 40, S. 184 ff. [**Original note**]

18 A reference to concepts by Wernicke, meaning simply phobias relative to the patient's own body, to his own psyche, and to the external world. [**Translator's note**]

process which, here as everywhere, is accompanied by the devaluation and depletion of the world's abundance of life, love, and beauty. This is particularly demonstrated in his Word Association Test. His Rorschach responses, too, bear witness to the artificial rationalization of his world, to its symmetrization and mechanization. Whereas in our first case everything-that-is (alles Seiende) was only accessible in a world reduced to the category of continuity, in this case it is a world reduced to the mechanical category of push and pressure. We are therefore not surprised to see that in this existence and its world there is no steadiness, that its stream of life does not flow quietly along, but that everything occurs by jerks and starts, from the simplest gestures and movements to the formulation of lingual expression and the performance of thinking and volitional decisions. Everything about the patient is jagged and occurs abruptly, while between the single jerks and pushes emptiness prevails. (The reader will notice that we are describing in existential–analytical terms what would clinically be called schizoid and autistic.) Again, very typical is the patient's behavior in the Rorschach test. He feels a desire to "fold up the cards and file them away with a final effort," just as he would like to fold up and file away the world as such with a final effort, or else he would not be able to control it any more.

But these final efforts exhaust him to such a degree that he becomes increasingly inactive and dull. If in the first case it was continuity of existence that had to be preserved at all costs, in the present case it is its dynamic *balance*. Here, too, a heavy phobic armor is employed in the interest of that preservation. Where it fails, even if only in phantasy, anxiety attacks and complete desperation take over. This case, whose existential and world-structure could be only very roughly suggested here, was published as the second study on schizophrenia under the title of "Juerg Zuend."

Whereas the above case permitted us a view of the kind of world in which "delusions of reference and encroachment"[19] become possible, a third case, that of Lola Voss, gave us some insight into the world-structure which makes possible delusions of persecutions. It offered us the rare opportunity to watch

the appearance of severe hallucinatory delusions of persecutions, preceded by a pronounced phobic phase. This expressed itself in a highly complicated superstitious system of consulting an oracle of words and syllables, whose positive or negative dicta guided the patient in the commission or omission of certain acts. She would feel compelled to break up the names of things into syllables, to recombine these syllables in accordance with her system and, depending on the results of these combinations, to make contact with the persons or things in question or to avoid them like the plague. Again, all this served as a safeguarding for the existence and its worlds against catastrophe. But in this case, catastrophe was not felt to be in the disruption of the world's continuity nor in the disturbance of its dynamic balance, but in the invasion by the unspeakably Uncanny and Horrid. This patient's "world" was not dynamically loaded with conflicting forces which had to be artificially harmonized; hers was not a world-design reduced to push and pressure but one reduced to the categories of familiarity and strangeness – or uncanniness (*Vertrautheit* and *Unvertrautheit – oder Unheimlichheit*). The existence was constantly threatened by a prowling, as yet impersonal, hostile power. The incredibly thin and flimsy net of artificial, syllable-combinations served as a safeguard against the danger of being overwhelmed by that power and against the unbearable threat of being delivered to it.

It was very informative to observe how, simultaneously with the disappearance of these safeguards, a new, quite different, because now quite unintended, safeguard made its appearance, namely the actual delusions of persecution.

The place of the impersonal power of the bottomless Uncanny (*Unheimlichen*) was now taken by the secret (*heimliche*) conspiracy of personalized enemies. Against these the patient could now consciously defend herself – with accusations, counterattacks, attempts at escape – all of which seemed like child's play compared with the constantly helpless state of being threatened by the horrible power of the incomprehensible Uncanny. But such gain in the security of existence was accompanied by the patient's complete loss of existential freedom, her complete yielding to the idea of hostility on the part of her fellow men, or, in psychopathological terms, by delusions of persecution.

I am reporting this case in order to demonstrate that we cannot understand these delusions if we begin

---

[19] The Swiss School differentiates between delusions characterized by ideas of reference and being encroached upon (*Beeintraechtigung*), on the one hand, and of persecutions on the other. [**Original note**]

our investigation with a study of the delusions themselves. Rather should we pay close attention to what *precedes* the delusions – be it for months, weeks, days, or only hours. We would then surely find that the delusions of persecution, similarly to the phobias, represent a protection of the existence against the invasion of something inconceivably Frightful, compared with which even the secret conspiracies of enemies are more tolerable; because the enemies, unlike the incomprehensible Frightful, can be "taken at something"[20] – by perceiving, anticipating, repelling, battling them.

In addition, the case of Lola Voss can show that we are no longer constrained by the bothersome contrast of psychic life with which we can empathize and that with which we cannot, but that we have at our disposal a method, a scientific tool, with which we can bring closer to a systematic scientific understanding even the so-called incomprehensible life of the psyche.

Of course, it still depends upon the imagination of single researcher and physician how truly he is able to reexperience and resuffer, by virtue of his own experiential abilities, all the potential experience which existential–analytical research methodically and planfully opens to his insight.

In many cases, however, it does not suffice to consider only *one* world-design, as we have done so far for the sake of simplicity of presentation. Whereas this serves our purpose in the morbid depressions, as in mania and melancholia, in our investigations of what is clinically known as schizophrenic processes we cannot neglect the bringing into focus and the describing of the various worlds in which our patients live in order to show the changes in their "being-in-the-world" and "beyond-the-world." In the case of Ellen West, for instance, we saw the existence in the shape of a jubilant bird soaring into the sky – a flight in a world of light and infinite space. We saw the existence as a standing and walking on the ground in the world of resolute action. And, finally, we saw it in the form of a blind worm crawling in muddy earth, in the moldering grave, the narrow hole. Above all, we saw that "mental illness" really means for the "mind," how the human mind really reacts under such conditions, how its forms actually change. In this case it was a change to a precisely traceable

narrowing-down, to a depletion or excavation of existence, world, and beyond-world to the point where, finally, of all the spiritual riches of the patient's world, of its abundance in love, beauty, truth, kindness, in variety, growth, and blossoming, "nothing was left except the big unfilled hole." What did remain was the animalistic compulsion to cram down food, the irresistible instinctual urge to fill the belly to the brim. All this could be demonstrated not only in the modes and changes of spatiality, of the hue, materiality, and dynamics of the various worlds, but also in the modes and changes of temporality, up to the state of the "eternal emptiness" of so-called autism.

As to manic-depressive insanity, I refer to my studies on *The Flight of Ideas*[21] and to the investigations of the manifold forms of depressive states by E. Minkowski, Erwin Straus, and Von Gebsattel, all of which, although not existential–analytical in the full sense of the word, were definitely conducted in an empirical–phenomenological fashion. In mentioning E. Minkowski we must gratefully acknowledge that he was the first to introduce phenomenology into psychiatry for practical purposes, particularly in the area of schizophrenia where he immediately put it to fruitful use. I wish to mention further the work of Erwin Straus and Von Gebsattel on compulsion and phobias, and of the late Franz Fischer on *Space and Time Structure in the Existence of the Schizophrenic*. Applications of existential–analytical thinking can be found in Von Gebsattel's excellent study, *The World of the Compulsive*, and in Roland Kuhn's study, *Interpretations of Masks in the Rorschach Test* (1945).

Apart from the deepening of our understanding of psychoses and neuroses, existential analysis is indispensable to psychology and characterology. As to characterology, I shall confine myself here to the analysis of miserliness. It has been said that miserliness consists in persisting in the state of potentiality, in "a fight against realization," and that only from this angle can the bondage to money be understood (Erwin Straus). But this is still too rationalistic an interpretation. One has rather to analyze the miser's world-design and existence; in short, to explore what world-design and what world-interpretation lie at the root of miserliness, or in what way that-which-is (*Seiende*) is accessible to the stingy.

---

[20] A Heideggerian concept which, in this context, serves to emphasize that these enemies can be "handled" by the patient. [**Translator's note**]

[21] L. Binswanger, *Über Ideenflucht* (Zurich: 1933). [**Original note**]

Viewing the behavior of the miser and his description in literature (as by Molière and Balzac) we find that he is primarily interested in *filling*, namely the filling of cases and boxes, stockings and bags with "gold," and only consequently in refusing to spend and in retaining. "Filling" is the a priori or transcendental tie that allows us to combine faeces and money through a common denominator. It is only this that provides psychoanalysis with the empirical possibility of considering money-addiction as "originating" from the retention of faeces. But by no means is the retaining of faeces the "cause" of stinginess.

The above-mentioned empty spaces, however, are designed not only to be filled but, in addition, to hide their content from the eyes and hands of fellow men. The miser "sits" or "squats" on his money "like the hen on her egg." (We can learn a great deal from such phrases of idiomatic language since language has always proceeded, to a high degree, phenomenologically rather than discursively.) The pleasure of spending money, of giving it out – possible only in sympathetic contact with one's fellow men – is replaced by the pleasure of secret viewing, rummaging, touching and mental touching, and counting the gold. Such are the secret orgies of the miser, to which may be added the lust for the glittering, sparkling gold as such as the only spark of life and love which is left to the miser. The prevalence of filling-up and its worldly correlate, the cavity, points to something "Moloch-like"[22] in such a world and existence. This, naturally, carries with it (according to the unitary structure of being-in-the-world) also a certain Moloch-like form of the self-world, and in this case particularly of the body-world and of body-consciousness, as rightly emphasized by psychoanalysis. As to temporality, the very saying that one can be "stingy with one's time" proves that the miser's time is here spatialized in a Moloch-like sense, insofar as small portions of time are eagerly and constantly being saved, accumulated, and jealously guarded. From this follows the inability to give "of one's time." Of course all this implies at the same time the loss of the possibility of true or existential temporalization, of maturation of personality. The miser's relation to death which here, as in all existential–analytical investigations, is of the greatest importance, can in this context not be discussed. It is closely linked to his relations to his fellow men and linked also to his profound lack of love.[23]

In the same way in which we investigate and understand a characterological trait, we investigate and understand what in psychiatry and psychopathology is so summarily termed feelings and moods. A feeling or a mood is not properly described as long as one does not describe how the human existence that has it, or is in it, is in-the-world, "has" world and exists. (See in my studies on *The Flight of Ideas* the description of the optimistic moods and the feelings of exhilarant gaiety.) What has to be considered here is, in addition to temporality and spatiality, the shade, the lighting, the materiality and, above all, the dynamics of the given world-design. All this can be examined again through the medium of individual verbal manifestations as well as through metaphors, proverbs, idiomatic phrases in general, and through the language of writers and poets. Indeed, idiomatic language and poetry are inexhaustible sources for existential analysis.

The peculiar dynamics of the world of feelings and moods, their ascending and descending motion, their Upward and Downward, I have pointed out in my essay on "Dream and Existence."[24] Evidence for this kind of motion can be found in waking states as well as in dreams, introspective descriptions, and Rorschach responses. Gaston Bachelard, in his *"L'Air et les Songes,"* gives a brilliant, comprehensive presentation of the verticality of existence, *de la vie ascensionnelle* on the one hand and *de la chute* on the other.[25]

He impressively and beautifully demonstrates the existential–analytical significance of the fundamental metaphors *de la hauteur, de l'élevation, de la profondeur, de l'abaissement, de la chute* (earlier referred to by E. Minkowski in his *Vers une cosmologie).* Bachelard quite correctly speaks of a psychology– we would call it an anthropology – *ascensionnelle.*

---

22 The author here refers not to the cruel aspects of Moloch-worship but to the hollowness of the idol which had to be filled. [**Translator's note**]

23 L. Binswanger, "Geschehnis und Erlebnis," *Monatsschrift f. Psychiatrie,* S. 267 ff. [**Original note**]

24 *Neue Schweizerische Rundschau,* 1930, IX, S. 678. [**Original note**]

25 But we also know of a horizontality of existence, particularly from Rorschach responses. This horizontality is characterized by the road, the river, the plain. It does not reveal the "key" of the existence, but the ways of its "life-itinerary," that is, the way in which it is able or unable to stay, or not stay, in life. [**Original note**]

Without this background, neither feelings nor "keys" (*Stimmung*) nor "keyed" (*gestimmte*) Rorschach responses can be scientifically understood and described. Bachelard, too, has realized what impressed itself so urgently upon us in the case of Ellen West – that the imagination obeys the "law of the four elements" and that each element is imagined according to its special dynamism, We are particularly happy to find in Bachelard insight into the fact that those forms of being which are characterized by dropping and falling, those of a descending life in general, invariably lead to an *imagination terrestre*, a turning into earth, or a bogging down of the existence. This, in turn, is of the greatest importance for the understanding of Rorschach results.

This *matérialité* of the world-design, originating from the "key" (*Gestimmtheit*) of the existence is by no means confined to the environment, to the world of things, or to the universe in general, but refers equally to the world of one's fellow men (*Mitwelt*) and to the self-world (*Eigenwelt*) (as demonstrated in the cases of Ellen West and Juerg Zuend). For them, self-world and environment were only accessible in the form of the hard, energy-loaded material, while the world of their fellow men was only accessible by way of an equally energy-loaded, hard, and impenetrable resistance. When the poet speaks of the "dull resistance of the world" he demonstrates that the world of one's fellow men can be experienced in the form not just of a metaphor but of an actually and bitterly felt hard and resistant matter. The same is expressed in sayings such as "a tough guy" and "a roughneck."

Finally, what part is existential analysis equipped to play in the total picture of psychiatric investigation and research?

Existential analysis is not a psychopathology, nor is it clinical research nor any kind of objectifying research. Its results have first to be recast by psychopathology into forms that are peculiar to it, such as that of a psychic organism, or even of a psychic apparatus, in order to be projected onto the physical organism.[26] This cannot be achieved without a greatly simplifying reduction whereby the observed existential–analytical phenomena are largely divested of their phenomenal contents and reinterpreted into functions of the psychic organism, psychic "mechanisms," etc. However, psychopathology would be digging its own grave were it not always striving test its concepts of functions against the phenomenal contents to which these concepts are applied and to enrich and deepen them through the latter. Additionally, existential analysis satisfies the demands for a deeper insight into the nature and origin of psychopathological symptoms. If in these symptoms we recognize "facts of communication" – namely, disturbances and difficulties in communication – we should do our utmost to retrace their causes – retrace them, that is, to the fact that the mentally ill live in "worlds" different from ours. Therefore, knowledge and scientific description of those "worlds" become the main goal of psychopathology, a task which it can perform only with the help of existential analysis. The much-discussed gap that separates our "world" from the "world" of the mentally ill and makes communication between the two so difficult is not only scientifically explained but also scientifically bridged by existential analysis. We are now no longer stopped at the so-called borderline between that psychic life with which we can, and that with which we cannot, empathize. Quite a number of case reports show that our method has succeeded beyond earlier hopes in communicating with patients, in penetrating their life-history, and in understanding and describing their world-designs even in cases where all this seemed impossible before. This applies, in my experience, particularly to cases of hypochondriacal paranoids who are otherwise hardly accessible. Thus we also comply here with a *therapeutic* demand.

This insight – that the world-designs as such distinguish the mentally ill from the healthy and hamper communication with the former – also throws new light on the problem of the projection[27] of psychopathological symptoms onto specific brain

---

26 We are speaking here of the role of psychopathology within the total frame of psychiatric medical research. We do not neglect the fact that in the psychoanalytical investigation, as well as in every purely "understanding" psychopathology, germs of existential–analytical views can always be found. But they indicate neither a

methodical scientific procedure nor a knowledge of why and in what way existential analysis differs from the investigation of life-historical connections and from an "empathic" or "intuitive" entering into the patient's psychic life. [**Original note**]

27 The German term "projection" used here in the sense of localizing or assigning. [**Translator's note**]

processes. Now it cannot be so important to localize single psychic symptoms in the brain but rather, primarily, to ask where and how to localize the fundamental psychic disturbance which is recognizable by the change of "being-in-the-world" as such. For indeed, the "symptom" (e.g., of flight of ideas, of psychomotor inhibition, neologism, stereotypy, etc.) proves to be the expression of a spreading change of the soul, a change of the total form of existence and the total style of life.

Chapter

14

Introduction

The texts presented in this section are on clinical questions, but are deeply rooted in the philosophical work outlined in Parts I and II. We have selected texts which address issues of psychiatric practice, such as what influences the doctor–patient relationship and how to retain a whole-person level approach to the patient. We have made an effort to include texts that deal with common clinical problems. For this purpose, we have translated for the first time into English early key work on phenomena such as the beginning of schizophrenia and affective disorder. All texts have been significantly shortened by the editors and are introduced by short paragraphs that aim to stimulate a sympathetic but critical reading.

Brain injury

Goldstein, K. (1940), 'Pathology and the nature of man: the abstract attitude in patients with lesions of the brain cortex'

From (1940) *Human Nature in the Light of Psychopathology.* Cambridge, MA: Harvard University Press.

Editors' commentary

In this text Goldstein examines the effect of brain injury upon the whole behaviour and mental state of the affected person. Goldstein thinks that in order to see the full effects of brain injury, the frame of observation needs to be wide. He is guided by a philosophical distinction between a symbolic, or conceptual, ability which is able to abstract away from individual instances in an environment (he calls this the 'abstract' attitude) and an ability to respond directly to cues in an environment (he calls this the 'concrete' attitude). In drawing this distinction he owes a lot to the neo-Kantian philosopher Ernst Cassirer (please see p. 89, footnote 3). Frontal brain injury, Goldstein argues, can show us what the unique symbolic capacities of the human being are in a negative sense, i.e. they give us instances of behaviour and mental state where these capacities are absent. Although neuropsychology has moved on since Goldstein, and the philosophical weight he places on the 'abstract' attitude may be excessive, we think this text demonstrates a descriptive, philosophically sensitive approach to the phenomena of brain injury which is needed when assessing a person's global functioning, or their decision-making capacity.

Before considering the phenomena observable in patients with mental diseases we must answer two questions: 1. Is it not dangerous to use pathological phenomena for formulating ideas about normal human nature? 2. Why do we use observations of pathologically changed human beings? What is the advantage of that procedure as compared with the use of the observation of normal persons?

In regard to the danger involved in using pathological phenomena, if one considers pathological facts – as has very often been done – as curiosities caused by illness and therefore not intelligible in the same way as the behavior of normal individuals, opposition to the use of pathological findings for the understanding of normal behavior is justified. There is no doubt, however, that such an assumption is false. If it were correct, we should not have the systematic statements about pathological facts that we do have; we should not even be able to describe them satisfactorily. Pathological phenomena are of a kind accessible to the understanding of the normal person. They are performances which have been modified according to definite laws, and they become intelligible if one takes into consideration the characteristic alterations which illness produces. To be sure, we are not able at present to understand all pathological phenomena from such a point of view, and those which are not understandable should not occupy the psychologist.

Here we shall deal only with phenomena of the understandable type. For this reason we shall choose a special kind of patient as a basis for our discussion. It is quite usual, particularly in textbooks of psychopathology, to start from observations of mentally ill persons, of psychotics and neurotics. We shall not omit evidence which can be gained from such cases, but this material will not constitute our main source. It is too complicated, and it still resists unambiguous analysis ... Another type of patient provides better material, allows of better observation and much better understanding and explanation of modifications in behavior – the patient with an organic defect of the brain caused by injury or disease.

We shall first take into consideration patients with circumscribed lesions of the brain cortex, in whom the damaged brain process has healed but with some irreparable defect. We begin with these cases instead of with patients who have acute illnesses, because in acute stages of illness (stages in which the struggle of the organism with the damage has not ended) the behavior picture is much more complicated, and it is much more difficult to analyze and to form an opinion of the changes that occur. We shall not overlook this acute condition, however, for we can also learn very much from it, particularly about the struggle of the organism against the damage done to it.

A great part of my own material has come from brain injuries incurred during the first World War. These injuries were very well suited for study, because they occurred in young people in good general physical condition. Furthermore, we had the unusual opportunity of being able to observe our patients for a very long period of time, some for more than eight years, in a relatively favorable environment. These circumstances gave us a much better insight into behavior than it is possible to obtain with patients who have brain lesions that are due to other causative factors, though the examination of the latter has not been omitted and has led us to the same conclusions.

For those phenomena with which we have to deal first the special localization of the lesion in the brain cortex is relatively unimportant. The phenomena are especially clear in lesions of the frontal lobe, and therefore we shall take our examples especially from patients with lesions of this part of the brain.

However, to come back to our two questions, why use pathological findings for understanding normal behavior? The answer is that we try to learn from the observation of sick people because we can acquire better information in this way, and acquire it more easily, than by observing normal individuals. Normal life is determined by so many factors, and these factors are interwoven in such various and complicated ways, that very often the reaction of a normal organism even to an apparently simple stimulation is exceedingly difficult, sometimes quite impossible, to analyze and to understand. Now the greater the defect of the organism, the simpler are its responses to stimuli, and therefore the easier to understand. Furthermore, pathological behavior is particularly revealing concerning the organization of behavior. The destruction of one or another substratum of the organism gives rise to various changes in behavior, showing how these substrata and forms of behavior are interrelated and giving an insight into the organization of the total organism. Just as it is easier to gain

an insight into the organization of performances in sick people, so it is easier to understand their ways of adjusting to changing conditions. For the sick organism, to find an adjustment to the abnormal condition produced by sickness is a question of being or not being. Thus we have an especially good opportunity of observing the forms and rules of adjustment, which are not always easily observed in normal persons.

The changes to be observed in patients with brain lesions are manifold, and concern both mental and bodily performances. Even if we restrict ourselves to mental performances we are faced with a very complex picture. Usually the disturbances have been described as separate changes in single fields of performance, as in perception, action, speech, emotions, memory, etc. Researches in the last few decades have shown more and more, however, that these complex pictures can be understood only if we regard them as expressions of a change in the total personality of the patient concerned.

We shall consider our findings in reference to two problems: first we shall concentrate on the change in personality; then on the adaptation of the patient to his defect. The study of the change of personality will give us some insight into the organization of the personality of the normal human being. The study of adaptation of the patient to his defect will inform us about the way the normal person comes to terms with the outer world. There would be no better way of getting to the heart of our problem than to give demonstrations with actual patients; I regret very much that this is impossible and that I must confine myself to a description of the behavior of certain patients.

The patient whom I have first in mind is a man thirty years of age, with a lesion of the frontal lobe. His customary way of living does not seem to be very much disturbed. He is a little slow; his face is rather immobile, rather rigid; his attention is directed very strictly to what he is doing at the moment – say, writing a letter or speaking to someone. Confronted with tasks in various fields, under certain conditions he gives seemingly normal responses, but under other conditions he fails completely in tasks that are apparently very similar to those he has performed quite well. These differences will be the starting point of our discussion. We shall ask: What is the reason for the failure in the one situation, the correct performances in the others?

Let us take as an example the behavior of this patient in a simple test. We place before him a small wooden stick in a definite position, pointing, for example, diagonally from left to right. He is asked to note the position of the stick carefully. After a half minute's exposure the stick is removed; then it is handed to the patient, and he is asked to put it back in the position in which it was before. He grasps the stick and tries to replace it, but he fumbles; he is all confusion; he looks at the examiner, shakes his head, tries this way and that, plainly uncertain. The upshot is that he cannot place the stick in the required position. He is likewise unable to imitate other simple figures built up of sticks. Next we show the patient a little house made of many sticks, a house with a roof, a door, a window, and a chimney. When he is asked to reproduce the model, he succeeds very well.

If we ask what the reason may be for the difference in the behavior of the patient in the two tasks, we can at once exclude defects in the fields of perception, action, and memory. For there is no doubt that copying the house with many details demands a greater capacity in all these faculties, especially in memory, than putting a single stick into a position seen shortly before.

At first sight the difference may seem inexplicable, but the following experiment clarifies the situation. We put before the patient two sticks placed together so as to form an angle with the opening pointing upward. The patient is unable to reproduce this model. Then we confront him with the same angle, the opening pointing down this time, and now he reproduces the figure very well at the first trial. When we ask the patient how it is that he can reproduce the second figure but not the first one, he says: "This one has nothing to do with the other one." Pointing to the second one, he says, "That is a roof"; to the first, "That is nothing."

These two replies lead us to an understanding of the patient's behavior. His first reply makes it clear that, to him, the two objects with which he has to deal are totally different from one another. The second answer shows that he apprehends the angle pointing downward as a concrete object out of his own experience, and he constructs a concrete thing with the two sticks. A concrete apprehension and concrete behavioral action are sufficient to meet the conditions of this test. In the former test the two sticks did not arouse an impression of a concrete thing. He had to conceive of the positions of two meaningless sticks in a meaningless connection with each other. He had to regard the sticks as mere representations indicating directions in abstract space. Furthermore, he had to

keep these directions in mind and rearrange the sticks from memory as representatives of these abstract directions.

In the second test the patient needs to deal simply with a known concrete object; in the first he must give an account to himself of relations in space, and act on the basis of abstract ideas. Thus we may conclude that the failure of the patient in the first test lies in the fact that he is unable to perform a task which can be executed only by means of a grasp of the abstract. The test in which the opening of the angle points down does not demand this, and the patient is able to execute it perfectly. It is for the same reason that he is able to copy the little house, which seems to us to be much more complicated.

Some examples of performances by another patient – a woman with a disease of the frontal lobe – may illustrate this defect still more clearly. This patient was also able to copy the angle pointing upward, and an analysis of her procedure revealed that this model was recognized by her as a concrete known object, namely, as a V. She was unable to copy a square, and it was obvious that this figure did not mean anything to her. However, she could copy the following model:

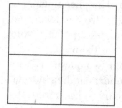

Asked what it was, she explained: it was a window. It could be demonstrated by many examples that if she recognized a model presented to her as a concrete object she could always copy it; if not, she failed. When she was unable to copy a model because it did not mean anything to her, she sometimes changed it so that it assumed for her the characteristics of a concrete object, and then she was able to copy it. Faced with a square

she produced the following picture:

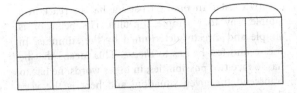

When asked what these figures meant, she answered, "The windows of a church." She drew not meaningless squares but three church windows in a position in which they might actually be found; apparently where we see an abstract geometrical figure, she had seen a concrete object.

This lack of an attitude toward the abstract is found not only in such tests as we have mentioned but also in the behavior of the patient in general. Thus, for instance, the patient is unable to execute everyday activities if the latter demand an attitude toward the imaginary. For example, he may be able to perform expressive movements (say, the act of threatening) in situations to which they belong but is unable to demonstrate them outside of the situation which demands them. He is unable simply to demonstrate. He may have no difficulty in using known objects in a situation that requires them, but he is totally at a loss if he is asked to demonstrate the use of such an object outside of the concrete situation, and still more so if he is asked to do it without the real object. For example, one of our patients was able to drink water normally out of a glass, but if he was given an empty glass and asked to demonstrate how one brings the glass to the mouth in drinking and to make the appropriate movements with his mouth, he was unable either to do so or to imitate the action after it had been demonstrated to him.

There is a real gradation of difficulty in these various procedures, depending on the degree of concreteness in the action. The easiest performance is to drink during dinner, if one is thirsty. Under these very concrete conditions only patients with the very greatest impairment of function fail; if the impairment is less marked, the patient may fail if he has to drink, let us say, not at mealtime or if he is not thirsty, but simply on demand. If he is asked to demonstrate how to drink with an empty glass or without a glass – that is, in a situation involving a very high degree of abstraction – he is unable to do it at all. The reason why the patient's capacity for performing these steps

corresponds somewhat to the degree of impairment of function is that his capacity for abstraction is disturbed by this to a greater or lesser degree.

Let us consider some other examples. The patient is asked to drive a nail with a hammer into a piece of wood. He takes the nail and drives it correctly by successive strokes of the hammer. Now the nail is taken away, and he is asked to imagine that there is a nail and that he is to drive it in. But this he is incapable of doing. He does not seem to know how to make the movement of driving it in either with the fist or with the hammer. Furthermore, even if he sees the nail and has the hammer in his hand, he is unable to make the movement of driving the nail in when he is not allowed to touch it.

The patient is asked to blow away a slip of paper. He does this very well. If the paper is taken away, and he is asked to think that there is a slip of paper and blow it away, he is unable to do so. Here again the situation is not realistically complete. In order to perform the task the patient would have to imagine the piece of paper there. He is not capable of this.

The patient is asked to throw a ball into boxes situated respectively at distances of three, nine, and fifteen feet. He does it quite well. When he is asked how far the several boxes are from him, he is not only unable to answer this question but unable even to say which box is nearer, which farther.

What is the difference between the two tasks? In the first, the patient has only to deal with objects in a behavioral fashion. It is unnecessary for him to be conscious of his act and of objects in a world separated from himself. In the second, however, he must separate himself from objects in the outer world and give himself an account of his actions and of the space relations in the world facing him. Therefore he fails.

That we do not have to deal here with a disturbance of space perception may be illustrated by another example which shows clearly that these patients are able to deal with complicated space relations when there is the possibility of doing it in a concrete way but fail as soon as an attitude toward the abstract is necessary.

In a conversation a patient was asked what she had been doing during the day. She answered, "I have been working." When asked where, she offered to lead the way to the workroom situated on an upper floor of the hospital. She went directly across the floor to the end of the ward, where there was a closed door, and glanced at the nurse, apparently realizing that the door was locked and desiring her to open it. The patient opened the door with a key given to her, locked it from the outside, returned the key to the nurse, went straight to the elevator situated on the other side of the corridor, rang correctly, and entered it on its arrival. On reaching the floor of the workroom she left the elevator at the direction of the operator, went directly to the door of the workroom, and immediately took her place at the table. She then asked the supervisor of the workroom for her needlework, prepared her material, and started to knit. All this was done without the least hesitation, even with alacrity. Later she was asked to go back to the ward. She arose and left, taking the correct route out and heading for the elevator. When she was stopped before reaching it, however, and was led into the corridor on the same floor (which was identical in structure with the floor on which her ward was located), she believed it to be the floor where her ward was. She then walked through the corridor as if she were on the ward floor and turned to the right at the end of the corridor as though she were about to enter her sleeping room. She was surprised to find herself in a room unknown to her. When told that she was on the wrong floor she became perplexed and looked around but was unable to find the correct way to the ward. She not only was ignorant of where she was but did not know how to return to the elevator. When, on another occasion, she was allowed to go straight to the ward, she did it in the same correct way as on her trip to the workroom. Plainly, she was able to take a complicated path in the same way as a normal person, but she failed immediately when the task demanded that she give herself an account of it – that is, of relations in space, the way from one place to another, etc. This may be deduced also from the fact that she could not describe the route, although she had followed it correctly.

*****

As a further example from another performance field we may choose a simple reaction test. The patient is instructed to execute a simple movement in response to an abruptly flashed light signal. After some practice he learns the situation. He reacts correctly in a relatively short time. We now flash a red light, then a blue light; and the patient is instructed to execute the movement on seeing the red light but to do nothing on seeing the blue. In this and similar selective reactions his performance is inadequate. He seems to become confused, and either does not react at all or makes many errors. What is the difference between the two tests? In one the patient has to react in a simple way to a simple stimulus. His behavior is simple and directly determined by the stimulus. In the second test he has to *choose*. This means that he has to face two possibilities; in other words, he has to transcend the given situation, and here is the very thing he cannot do.

These and similar examples show that the patient is unable to deal with any merely "possible" situation at all. Thus we may also describe the deficiency in these patients as a lack of capacity for approaching a "possible" situation.

Results with another task in quite a different field yield confirmation. A simple story is read to the patient. He seems unable to understand it. He may repeat some single words, but he does not understand their meaning and is unable to grasp the essential point. Now we read him another story, which would seem to a normal person to be no easier to understand. This time he understands the meaning very well and recounts the chief points. What was the difference between the two stories? The first one dealt with a simple situation, but a situation which had no connection with the actual environment of the patient. The second story had a direct bearing on his own situation. Again we observe that the failure is due to an incapacity to approach a situation presented only in imagination. Choosing stories with this point of view, we are able to predict beforehand which ones the patient will be able to understand.

The same difficulty is observable in tests with graphic representations. Pictures of single objects are almost always recognized. In pictures which contain a number of things and persons in contact with each other, the patient may pick out some details, but he is unable to understand the picture as a whole and is unable to react in response to the whole. A precise examination reveals that the patient's real understanding does not depend on the greater or smaller number of components in a picture but on whether the components, whatever their number, hang together concretely and in ways familiar to him, or whether an understanding of their connection requires a more abstract synthesis on his part. In the first case the patient may apprehend pictures with many details. In the second he may lack understanding even if there are only a few details. If the picture does not reveal its essence directly, by bringing the patient into the situation which it represents, he is not able to recognize it. Thus one may characterize the deficiency as an inability to discover the essence of a situation.

This change in behavior finds its expression in characteristic changes in memory and attention. Under certain circumstances the faculty for the reproduction of facts acquired long ago may be normal. For example, things learned in school may be recalled very well in some situations, but not in all. The situation must reawaken old impressions. The patient must be able to regard the present situation in such a way that facts from the past belong to it. If this is not the case, he is completely unable to recall facts which he has reproduced very well in another situation. Repeated observation in many different situations demonstrates clearly that such memory failures are not caused by an impairment of memory content but by a failure in the approach that is requisite for a specific test. The patient has the material in his memory, but he is unable to use it freely; he can use it only in connection with a definite concrete situation, to which it must seem to him to belong. Only in this way, too, is he able to learn new facts. He may be able to learn numbers, syllables, or movements by heart; he is able to hold in memory situations, facts connected with his environment, and so on, but he is able to do so only in a concrete situation, and he can reproduce them only in the situation in which he learned them.

That such patients keep in mind essentially those patterns which they are able to comprehend – that is, grasp in a concrete way – the following simple example may illustrate. We put before a patient a single vertical line, or a circle or a square alone. She is able to copy each figure. Now we present the vertical line, the circle, and the square together. When asked to reproduce the patterns a minute later, the patient draws only the square; the others she has not held in mind. She apparently remembers only the one among several patterns which is a *concrete* figure for her – that is, the square, which she interprets as a window of a church. Obviously, her memory of an object is determined by the concreteness or abstractness of the object in question. Her ability to copy pictures is not bad if the pictures are seen by her as concrete figures.

We arrive at the same result in testing attention. At one time the patient appears inattentive, at another attentive, even abnormally so. Attention is usually weak in special examinations, particularly at the

beginning, before the patient has gained the real approach to the whole situation. In such a situation he ordinarily seems much distracted. If he enters into the situation, however, his attention may be satisfactory, sometimes even abnormally keen. Under these circumstances he may be totally untouched by other stimuli from the environment to which normal persons will react unfailingly. His attitude, in short, depends upon whether he is equal to the task set him or not. In some tests he will always seem distracted – for example, in those which demand a change of approach (a choice reaction), because he is incapable of making a choice. Consequently, it is not correct to speak of a change of attention in these patients in terms of plus or minus. The state of the patient's attention is but a part of his total behavior and is to be understood only in connection with it.

The lack of an ability to grasp the abstract impairs all voluntary activities. Our patients have the greatest difficulty in starting any performance which is not determined directly by external stimuli. Thus, for example, they may be unable to recite the series of numbers on demand, although they are able to do it if the examiner begins the series. This difficulty finds its expression in a marked lack of initiative. They have great trouble in voluntary shifting, in switching over voluntarily from one topic to another, or from one part of a situation to another. Consequently they fail in performances in which such a shift is necessary. Since, as we have shown, they are hindered in the making of choices, they are unable to follow a conversation between various people, especially if the contents change, and they seem rigid and lifeless, mentally and bodily, in everything they do.

This difficulty in voluntary shifting can be explained in the following way. Shifting presupposes that I have in mind simultaneously the object to which I am reacting at the moment and the one to which I am going to react. One is in the foreground, the other in the background. But it is essential that the object in the background be there as a possible object for future reaction. Only then can I change from the one to the other. This presupposes the capacity for approaching things that are only imagined, "possible" things, things which are not given in the concrete situation. If, for example, we normal people do not understand a complicated picture immediately, we voluntarily look first at this and then at that part; we keep changing our attitude until we achieve success. This changing presupposes the capacity for freeing oneself from a concrete situation and turning to something that is already in mind. The mentally sick man is incapable of doing either because of his inability to grasp what is abstract.

To be sure, we normal people do not always shift in an arbitrary manner. Shifting may be directed by the changing significance of one part or another for the best and most adequate performance, and this happens somewhat passively. But if the situation itself does not bring about this change we can focus voluntarily upon one part or another. Normal performances usually demand both active and passive shifting. Among the abnormal, the incapacity for voluntary shifting makes the fulfillment of certain tasks impossible.

We have already mentioned the fact that our patients are unable to imitate or copy anything that is not a part of their immediate concrete experience. It is a very interesting expression of this incapacity that they have the greatest difficulty in repeating a sentence which is meaningless for them – that is, the contents of which do not correspond to the reality they are capable of grasping. Thus a patient of mine was unable to repeat such sentences as "The snow is black." I was able to induce him to repeat the individual words, isolated, and then to repeat the words one after the other in the correct succession, but he stopped before he spoke the word "black," looked startled, and said, "white," or, if he said the word "black," he did it very quickly and apparently with great uneasiness, and then said very quickly afterwards, "white." To say such things apparently requires the assumption of a very difficult attitude. It demands, so to speak, the ability to live in two spheres, the concrete sphere where "real" things take place and the non-concrete, the merely "possible" sphere, for in saying meaningless things we must shift from one to the other. This the patient is unable to do.

... He frequently exhibits a dulling of the emotions, but in other situations he does not appear to be without feeling; on the contrary, we observe in him a great excitability. If we analyze both situations carefully, we find that the presence or absence of emotional expression corresponds to his entire behavior in a given situation, and that his emotional behavior is best understood in terms of his attitude toward the situation. The fact seems to be this: If the patient does not seem to react emotionally in a satisfactory way, it is in situations in which he also fails to comprehend the essentials to which a definite feeling attaches. This frequently demands a grasp of the abstract. He may have grasped only a part of the situation because only that part could be grasped concretely. His reaction seems inappropriate to us because we regard the whole situation and not merely a part of it. If we consider his behavior from this point of view, we see that, in the situation as it is experienced by him, his feeling is not abnormal.

This also helps us to understand why it is that a patient who appears very dull may suddenly become excited in a situation which at first seems to contain no cause for irritation. For example, a patient of mine had a friend who was his close companion. One day the friend went to a cinema with another man. He did not take our patient because the latter had seen the picture before and would not go to see it a second time. When the friend came back our patient was in a state of great excitement and refused to speak to him. He was not to be quieted by any arguments. No explanation – that his friend did not want to offend him, that his friendship had not changed – made any impression. From that time on, our patient was his old friend's enemy.

This reaction, at first so unintelligible, can be understood if we remember that the patient was able to make only a direct concrete approach to any situation. This was the case in his approach to his friend. He saw only that his friend was the companion of another man, and he felt himself slighted. He was unable to understand that his friend's conduct in no way actually affected their relations. He could not understand why his friend went without him, and he could not perceive the situation as a whole. He saw only the concrete separation between himself and his friend, and his exaggeration is thoroughly understandable if we consider how difficult it is, in the case of such a change of attitude, to enter into the relation of friendship. The patient felt his loneliness, and sank into a "catastrophic situation" of confusion and anxiety. He regarded his friend as the cause of his bad condition and reacted to him in a way that is easily understandable in terms of his grasp of the situation.

It is in general very difficult for our patients to come into close contact with other people ... Only a concrete situation by which they are affected brings them into and keeps them in contact with others; then their feelings may correspond to normal feelings. Outside the actual situation, however, they may be without any inner contact with the members of their society. An example may make this clear. One of our patients never seemed to be concerned about his family. He never spoke of his wife or children, was unresponsive when we questioned him about them, and when it was suggested to him that he should write to his family was utterly indifferent. Thus he appeared to lack all feeling. Now it was an established practice that at times he should visit his home, which was situated in another town, and stay there several days. While at home he conducted himself, as we learned, like a normal man in the bosom of his family. He was kind and affectionate to his wife and children, and interested in their affairs in so far as his abilities would permit. Yet after his return to the hospital from such a visit, upon being asked about his people, he would smile in an embarrassed way and give evasive answers; he seemed utterly estranged from his home situation. Unquestionably what ailed this man was not really a deterioration of his character on the emotional and moral side. Rather, he could not represent the home situation to himself, and consequently the corresponding feelings did not arise. This lack of real contact with others, taken in connection with the impairment of a grasp of the abstract, will give us a basis for our discussion of the social relationship in normal persons.

We have characterized the patient's deficiency in different terms – as lack of a grasp of the abstract, lack of an approach to imagined things, inability to give himself an account of his own acting or thinking, inability to make a separation between the ego and the world, and lack of freedom. At bottom all these terms, and others which one may use to characterize the facts, mean basically the same thing. We speak, in brief, of the lack of an attitude toward the abstract.

To avoid misunderstanding, let me say here that the perception of concreteness by different patients need not be expressed in the same way in a given task. What is concrete for one individual can only be understood within the frame of reference for that particular patient, as it is related to his pre-morbid individuality and his changed capacity and the situation given. Therefore it may express itself in different ways in different patients with the same type of lesion.

I know that the designation of the two kinds of behavior as "abstract" and "concrete" is misunderstandable and has often been misunderstood. I am sorry that I do not know any more appropriate words with which to characterize the facts. Now I am very anxious not to be misunderstood at this point because what I am about to say concerns the most important problem in our attempt to characterize human nature on the basis of our findings.

Thus I should like to review briefly what has been said. In "concrete" performances a reaction is determined directly by a stimulus, is awakened by all that the individual perceives. The individual's procedure is somewhat passive, as if it were not he who had the initiative. In "abstract" performances an action is not determined directly and immediately by a stimulus configuration but by the account of the situation which the individual gives to himself. The performance is thus more a primary action than a mere reaction, and it is a totally different way of coming to terms with the outside world. The individual has to consider the situation from various aspects, pick out the aspect which is essential, and act in a way appropriate to the whole situation. True, this procedure may have various degrees of complexity. Sometimes the situation demands nothing more than a singling out of one property of an object, as, for instance, when we are asked to sort objects according to their colors. In the highest degree of complexity we have not only to apprehend objects by means of certain simple characteristics but to choose aspects for consideration in accordance with a certain task which demands a conceptual organization. Even in its simplest form, however, abstraction is separate in principle from concrete behavior. There is no gradual transition from the one to the other. The assumption of an attitude toward the abstract is not more complex merely through the addition of a new factor of determination; it is a totally different activity of the organism. Perhaps it would be better not to designate both conditions by the term "behavior," since behavior connotes real activity and is especially well suited to the concrete performance. Abstraction represents, rather, a preparation for activity; it involves an attitude, i.e., an inner approach, which leads to activity. Therefore it is better to speak of an attitude toward the abstract. Real action is never abstract; it is always concrete. The difference between the two conditions is shown in the difference between the processes which precede action. In the concrete situation action is set going directly by the stimuli; in the situation involving the abstract, action is begun after preparation which has to do with a consideration of the whole situation.

Yet these explanations are not entirely correct. From them it might seem as if concrete behavior could take place in complete independence of the abstract attitude, determined by the external situation alone. This, however, is not the case. The arousal and the normal course of an action presuppose in any case an abstract attitude. In normal life we are rarely forced into action by the stimulus situation itself. Usually we have to place ourselves – at least in imagination –in the appropriate situation. The outside world merely gives us the impulse to do this. Thus even the initiation of an action demands the abstract attitude. Nor is the latter entirely excluded during the performance of a concrete act. On the contrary, the concrete performance is always somewhat dependent upon the abstract attitude, which becomes effective in restoring order as soon as any disturbance in the normal course of concrete performances occurs. Thus concrete performances are grounded upon the abstract attitude in their initiation and receive its regulative control during their course.

This is very evident in our patients. Their concrete behavior can begin only if it is stimulated by the outer world, and it is to an abnormal degree dependent upon the outer world. It runs in an abnormal, compulsive way, and is disturbed very easily by changes in external events. It lacks spontaneity and, so to speak, an adequate context within the individual.

From what we have said it is clear that normally we do not distinguish sharply between performances carried out on the basis of the abstract attitude and those carried out in a concrete way. Normal performance demands both kinds of behavior. If I stress the importance of the abstract attitude for normal human beings, I do not mean that normal performances – or even the larger part of them – are carried out only in the abstract way. In ordinary life concrete behavior plays a very great role; most of our everyday performances are of this sort. Many performances consist of parts, some of which demand the one, others the other behavior.

Whether abstract attitude or concrete behavior plays a more prominent role depends upon various factors – first, on the situation. There are situations in which most normal persons react in a very concrete way without thinking about their behavior. A person enters his bedroom in the evening and puts on the light without realizing that he is doing so. Here and in similar cases our actions are determined directly by stimuli. But even here we do not act without employing an abstract attitude to a certain extent. We are acting somewhat passively, but we are not

forced to act in this way. Under certain conditions we can go to bed without putting on the light – if, for instance, we want to avoid disturbing someone else. This shows that, even where we react in a very concrete direct way, our actions are determined somewhat by our general mental set – that is, by some abstract attitude. Thus even in very familiar everyday actions we have to deal with a combination of abstract and concrete behavior.

The same is the case in activities of such high rank as scientific and artistic work. Perfection in any field demands the concrete execution of at least some parts of our actions without our thinking about them. Thinking itself is very often just such a concrete process; one thought involuntarily brings about another. The same is true in artistic expression. In all productivity concrete action plays a very great role. We must stress the point, however, that productive action is never possible unless it is embedded in an abstract set. The importance of concrete behavior in artistic creativeness has perhaps been overemphasized. Creative work can never be produced without an ideational basis – that is, without the abstract attitude. In this respect nothing in our patients is so impressive as their lack of productiveness.

*****

The role which this attitude plays in the life of an individual depends further upon the latter's individual organization, his constitutional and mental type. There are some persons who are more strongly directed toward the concrete than the abstract, and others who prefer by nature to assume an abstract attitude in all their doings. Thus one may easily arrive at a wrong judgment about the importance of the abstract attitude for human behavior by the observation that very intelligent people seem to behave very concretely. Behavior in performance tests provides a case in point. Take, for example, the following simple test, which I devised for this purpose with the material of the Kohs blocks.

The subject is faced with various simple designs and is asked to reproduce them with cubes, each cube having a different color on each side. The cubes are of the same size as the entire design. Thus the product built up from the blocks is four times as big as the model. On first looking at the models one is impressed by certain figures which stand out, and one may try to reproduce them. With this procedure, however, one can be at most only partially successful.

One has to abstract from the outstanding figures, divide the model in imagination into squares corresponding to the blocks, and copy the divided pictures. Our patients fail in various ways because of the impairment of their ability to abstract: they cannot abstract from the size or from the figures given, and they are not able to divide the model into squares in imagination. Now we sometimes observe in normal people behavior similar to that of our patients. Sometimes it takes a long time before a subject gets the idea of dividing the model in imagination, and sometimes the examiner has to demonstrate the successful procedure. This may suggest that intelligent normal persons, like our patients, are very concrete in their reactions and that the capacity for abstracting cannot be so essential as we have asserted. Yet there is one great difference between these normal persons and our patients which shows that such assumption is wrong. Immediately after a demonstration by the examiner the normal individual is able to continue in the correct way. This proves that he has grasped the abstract method and is following it. But a demonstration of the abstract method does not help our patients at all. They really lack the abstract attitude which normal persons possess. Although normal persons may have a tendency to behave primarily in the concrete manner and often begin in this way, they can shift very easily to the other mode of procedure and so gain the insight that is necessary for success.

Thus these and similar observations of normal people do not affect our conception of the significance of the abstract attitude; they show only that there are two types of normal persons – one that prefers the more concrete behavior, and another that prefers the abstract. This difference reveals a characteristic which has to be taken into consideration in any analysis of the structure of the personality, but it does not reveal any essential difference in the organization of various human beings ... Normal behavior is characterized by an alternation between an attitude involving abstract and one involving concrete behavior, and this alternation is appropriate to the situation and the individuality, to the task for which the organism is set. If either attitude becomes independent and governs the behavior of a normal person too completely, then we are faced with an anomalous form of behavior.

*****

To the characteristic deviation of behavior from the normal shown in the various examples I have given, there naturally corresponds a change in the world in which the patient lives. We may say that the patient has no world at all outside himself and opposed to him, in the sense that we do: he is impaired in his capacity for separating himself from the world which surrounds him; he is embedded in his own world. His inability to achieve performances which demand an abstract attitude means not only a shrinkage of his personality but also a shrinkage of the world in which he lives. In addition, not only are the contents of his environment diminished, and his own capacities shrunken, but there is a decrease in his freedom of action.

Perhaps we are now justified in drawing some conclusions as to the structure of the normal human being. We may start from this point: In the type of cases we have used as a basis for our discussion we never observe that an impairment of concrete behavior occurs while the attitude toward the abstract remains intact. The attitude toward the abstract is always impaired first, and to a higher degree. Now we may assume that those capacities which are first impaired by a brain lesion are those which demand the best functioning of the most complicated substratum of the brain. Thus it is not accidental that we find the loss of this capacity especially in lesions of the frontal lobe, which we consider to be the most complex part of the human brain. Further, we may assume that the performances corresponding to the best functioning of the most complex part of the brain are the most important – that is, represent the highest capacity of the organism in question. Thus we are led to the conclusion that we must distinguish in the human being two types of behavior, the concrete and the abstract, and that abstract behavior represents the highest capacity – in fact, the essential capacity – of the human being.

Chapter 16

Schizophrenia

Jaspers, K. (1913–59), 'The worlds of schizophrenic patients'

From (1962) *General Psychopathology*, 7th edn. Translated by J. Hoenig and M. W. Hamilton. Manchester: Manchester University Press: 283–4. Originally published as (1959) *Allgemeine Psychopathologie*, 7th edn. Berlin: Springer.

Editors' commentary

Jaspers is famous for characterizing core schizophrenic experience (e.g. primary delusions) as 'un-understandable'. Kurt Schneider's 'first rank symptoms' were an attempt at operationalizing these experiences. By 'un-understandable', Jaspers meant that the experiences resist attempts by another to understand them 'genetically' or in terms of meaningful connections (please refer to p. 101). However, the psychiatrist can delineate the experiences descriptively – attending to the form of the experiences (please refer to Chapter 10, pp. 91–100 and Chapter 11, p. 101) – and attempt to explain them using the principles of natural science. As well as this, Jaspers thought that some headway could be made toward understanding schizophrenic experience in terms of his philosophy of 'Existenz'. This kind of understanding for Jaspers is not scientific (either in the sense of causal explanation or in the sense of meaningful connection): it is quasi religious. Very tentatively, he attends to the content of core schizophrenic experiences and points, almost in a mood of fear and trembling, to their social and spiritual significance. This text illustrates that Jaspers must not be taken too literally when he refers to 'un-understandability' but it also shows that when Jaspers undertakes an existential analysis of core schizophrenic experience he is in some danger of constructing a stereotype.

Schizophrenic psychic life, particularly thinking and delusion, can be analysed as a particular phenomenon of experience (experience of primary delusion) and as a disturbance of the thought process (schizophrenic thinking). In both cases attention has to be given to the form of the disturbance. We may rightly feel that this is an advance on the old classification of delusion according to content, but we should be wrong to neglect the question of the possible components of the disturbance, the enquiry into the specific schizophrenic nature of the patient's world-formation. There is without doubt a typical and common connection between content and psychosis: delusions of catastrophe, cosmic delusions, delusions of reprieve ... von Bayer quite rightly says the schizophrenic world discloses itself in the delusion more tangibly, vividly and in greater detail than in any other of the psychopathological phenomena ... Rather it is an established fact that schizophrenia brings with it a transformation of the *content of experience*. It is not merely chance contents of a general human kind haphazardly interpreted into meaningless structures, but primary contents themselves that constitute the character of the disturbance.

Schizophenics, however, are not surrounded by a single schizophrenic world, but by a number of such worlds. If there were a single, uniform world-formation schizophrenics would understand each other and form their own community. But we find just the opposite. They hardly ever understand each other ... A community of schizophrenics is certainly almost an impossibility, since in every case it has to grow artificially and is not there naturally, as with all communities of healthy people.

*****

Why is schizophrenia in its initial stages so often (though not in the majority of cases) a process of cosmic, religious or metaphysical revelation? It is an extremely impressive fact: this exhibition of fine and subtle understanding, this impossible, shattering, piano-performance, this masterly creativity (van Gogh, Hölderlin), these peculiar experiences of the end of the world or the creation of fresh ones, the spiritual revelations and this grim daily struggle in the transitional periods between health and collapse. Such experiences cannot be grasped simply in terms of the psychosis which is sweeping the victim out of his familiar world, an objective symbol as it were of the radical, destructive event attacking him. Even if we speak of existence or the psyche as disintegrating, 'we are still only using analogies. We observe that a new world has come into being and so far that is the only fact we have.

Minkowski, E. (1927), 'The essential disorder underlying schizophrenia and schizophrenic thought'

From (1987) *The Clinical Roots of the Schizophrenia Concept*. Edited by John Cutting and Michael Shepherd, translated by J. Cutting. Cambridge: Cambridge University Press. Originally published as (1927) Chapter 2, Le trouble essentiel de la schizophrénie et la pensée schizophrénique. In *La schizophrénie*. Paris: Payot.

Editors' commentary

Minkowski's first research was on the psychopathology of schizophrenia. He was an experienced clinician and respected Kraepelin and Bleuler's schizophrenia concept. Yet he thought schizophrenia manifested in such psychologically diverse ways that it was not credible to locate the unity of the disorder in the psychological domain. He also thought that, phenomenologically, schizophrenia was most unlike organic dementias. This made him reticent about locating the unity of the disorder in the organic domain. Instead, he looked for the underlying unity of schizophrenia at the level of the whole person (please see p. 102) and inspired by Bergson's metaphysical contrasts: the intellect and intuition; the immobile and the flowing; the dead and the living; space and lived time (please see p. 10), he interpreted schizophrenia as a disturbance in the balance between these two principles as they manifest in the human being. The person with schizophrenia, he contended, was someone in whom there was an atrophy of the second principle across the whole gamut of psychological functions and a hypertrophy of the first. He summarized this as a 'loss of vital contact with reality' or a loss of the 'me-here-now' and contended that it resulted in a 'pragmatic dementia' quite different from what we see in organic dementias. In this text he puts forward a striking metaphor for schizophrenia
and compares it with the metaphors of Kraepelin, Bleuler and others.

Vital contact with reality

In forming the concept of dementia praecox Kraepelin fused several clinical conditions which hitherto had been regarded as more or less independent. These conditions included catatonia, hebephrenia and dementia paranoides. Later the condition known as simple dementia praecox was brought in to join them.

This synthesis posed a new problem. By becoming fused, the individual symptoms and even the syndromes lost their separate value. The symptoms, according to Kraepelin, were interchangeable, inconstant and all led to the same terminal state. There must, therefore, be some shared element. They could not merely be the accidental expression of an underlying morbid process. For this reason it became necessary to reduce the richness of the symptoms and the various clinical pictures to a single fundamental disorder and to clarify its nature.

This disorder could not be sought among the ordinary clinical symptoms, such as hallucinations, delusions, catatonic manifestations or states of excitement and depression. These symptoms have nothing constant or characteristic about them as we shall see. The disorder, therefore, had to be sought on another plane. The efforts to perfect the synthesis of dementia praecox and to make a true nosological entity of it required a new look at elementary psychic functions. It is here that one hopes to find the key to the particular behaviour which all patients with dementia praecox present, despite the infinite variations which distinguish them from one another symptomatically.

Contemporary psychological notions, however, rapidly proved inadequate for this purpose. Take, for example, the traditional triad – intelligence, feeling and will. It is obvious that the disorder in question is not related to any of these faculties. Neither lack of will, indifference, inability to show emotion or, even less, intellectual deterioration are characteristic of dementia praecox. It is more a question of the selective eclipse of each of these faculties, occurring in relation to certain situations, rather than their total abolition.

Psychopathological concepts are not static. They take on new meanings as ideas about normal psychic mechanisms change. Kraepelin himself, after having talked about a weakness in the emotional impulses of will and a loss of inner unity, reduced these two disorders to a weakening of ideas and feelings, and a tendency towards a disorganised mental life. He was speaking, in this sense, of a disorder of abstraction. Under these conditions, a subject would no longer be able to transform perceptions into abstract ideas, simple feelings into more organised ones, or isolated impulses into more constant inclinations. Kraepelin even sketched out a psychophysiological hypothesis of dementia praecox, by localising this faculty of abstraction in the higher layers of the cortex. Masselon placed primary emphasis on a disorder of attention and regarded an individual with dementia praecox as being in a state of perpetual distraction. Weygandt took over Wundt's ideas and talked about apperceptive dementia. None of these concepts, based on ideas about normal psychological functioning, persisted in the long run. As they were unable to express the essential disorder of dementia praecox they eventually gave way to notions of a different type.

Expressions such as 'discordance' (Chaslin), 'intrapsychic ataxia' (Stransky), 'intrapsychic dysharmony' (Urstein), 'loss of inner unity' (Kraepelin) or 'schizophrenia' (Bleuler) all imply that the disorder is not to be found in a particular function but rather in their total cohesion, in their harmonious interplay. To use a metaphor, the essential disorder does not affect one or more mental functions, whatever their place in the hierarchy, but is to be found among them all, in the 'interstitial space'. All these expressions constitute no more than an observation of fact, a description of the particular disturbance which occurs in dementia praecox or schizophrenia. This is already, however, an important statement, because the use of the term discordance neatly separates the condition from true dementia. But to a psychologist, and all psychiatrists should be that, this is inadequate. Chaslin's claim that hebephrenia consists of a discordance of psychic functions begs the question: what factors give rise to concordance of these same functions in normal people? This question remains for the moment unanswered. We have not yet achieved a clear idea of the fundamental disorder in dementia praecox, as we do not yet know to which factor in normal mental life it is linked.

For these reasons we have recourse to comparisons and metaphors. One might say that they suggest themselves in order to set the essentials of the condition in relief. Kraepelin talked of an 'orchestra without a conductor' and Chaslin of a 'machine without fuel' which, because it could be set in motion again, was entirely different from a broken-down machine. Anglade disliked using the term dementia praecox; he talked simply of 'dissociated patients'. To characterise their state, he compared them to a second-hand book: the pages might be out of place and the text partly illegible but none of the pages was actually missing. Compare this with a book whose pages have been irretrievably torn out. I myself, in thinking of the schizophrenic process, have been attracted by the following image: a building is made of bricks and cement; either the bricks *or* the cement can crumble; in either case the whole edifice can no longer hold up and it collapses; however, the ruins are not the same; they look different and have a different value; it is, moreover, easier to reconstruct a new house with intact bricks than with dust.

These metaphors express as well as possible the need to separate the schizophrenic process from intellectual impairment. But more than this, they seem to express the true nature of schizophrenia much better than any of the psychological definitions which we considered above.

Our sense of precision, however, is upset by these metaphors, which seem to be merely ingenious and pleasant methods of discourse. Scientific method and the search for truth should forbid such diversions. However, one should not forget that Henri Bergson, one of the most eminent of contemporary philosophers, believes that a whole side of our life, and not the least important, entirely escapes discursive thought. Things which impinge immediately on our consciousness, in some ways the most essential, belong to this category. They are irrational but are no less part of our life for that. There is no reason to sacrifice them to the spirit of precision. In fact, on the contrary, one should try and capture their true essence. The discipline of psychology has nothing to say on this matter as it is too constrained by the rules of scientific method. Were it to relax these rules it would be transformed from an arid subject to a fertile one, and would come to resemble life itself. How would we profit from this transformation in tackling the problem of schizophrenia?

It is at this point that the idea emerges of *vital contact with reality*.

Bleuler laid down what he saw as the cardinal symptoms of schizophrenia. They were all to do with the ideas, emotions and will of his patients. At the same time, however, his introduction of the concept of autism rendered environmental factors increasingly important. His emphasis on the lack of real goals and guiding ideas, and absence of emotional warmth, steered the concept of schizophrenia down a new path. All these disorders seem to converge on a single and unique notion, that of *loss of vital contact with reality*.

Vital contact with reality appears to be linked with the irrational factors in life. The ordinary concepts elaborated by physiology and psychology, such as excitation, sensation, reflexes and motor reactions, continue in parallel, largely unnoticed. The blind, the mutilated and the paralysed may be able to live in even more intimate contact with their environment than individuals whose sight is intact and whose limbs are whole; schizophrenics, on the other hand, can lose this contact even with an intact sensory-motor apparatus, memory or intelligence. The vital contact with reality is in touch with the depths, with the very essence of our personality, in which it links with the world around us. And this world is not just a collection of external stimuli, of atoms, forces and energy. It is a moving stream which envelops us at all points and constitutes the milieu without which we would not know how to live. 'Events' emerge from this like islets; they penetrate the personality by disturbing its most intimate parts. And then, by making these events part of its own make-up, our personality puts its own stamp on them, not by muscular contractions but through action, feelings, joy and tears. In this way there is established that marvellous harmony between ourselves and reality, a harmony that allows us to follow the progress of the world while at the same time safeguarding the notion of our own life.

These considerations lead one to conclude that vital contact with reality concerns the intimate dynamism of our life. We can never achieve this through the rigid concepts of spatial thought. Metaphors, not definitions, hold pride of place in this sphere of our life. Only they can impart some clarity to the notion of vital contact with reality.

This notion is not new. In his theory of psychasthenia Janet talks at length about the reality function. This idea, although not quite the same as ours, has many points in common with it. And the fact that two different paths lead in the same direction suggests that we are dealing with real and important matters which are currently 'in the air'.

The notion of a vital contact with reality, and the interpretation of schizophrenia in terms of a loss of this contact, is both simple and plausible. The newcomer to psychiatry can pick it up quickly and use it without difficulty. I am tempted to say that the notion follows on naturally from the evolution of the concept of dementia praecox.

But then, one might ask, has the considerable knowledge about clinical psychiatry merely led, in the end, to no more than a single psychological and psychopathological idea? I do not think so. As we shall see, the idea is capable of fostering further developments, and even if this were not so it is of some consequence in its own right, as is the case with many other clinical notions in psychiatry. The term 'mental confusion', for example, owes its origin to the need to tighten up the boundaries of dementia. It replaced the category of acute, curable dementia introduced by Pinel. Originally a French idea, promoted by Delasiauve, it was then exported to other countries. In the course of its evolution, having undergone many alterations in meaning, it is again being studied in its country of origin, particularly by Chaslin. Finally, through the efforts of Toulouse and Mignard, it has come to mean a general disorder of mental functions. This pattern in the evolution of our clinical notions in psychiatry should not surprise us. Does not any clinical term become clear and precise when we have succeeded in giving it a solid psychological foundation? Also we should appreciate that modern psychiatry strives to uncover the *causative disorder* underlying the clinical conditions which it studies.

I believe that I have staked a claim for the correct paternity of the idea of vital contact with reality in respect of its central role in schizophrenia. I have certainly not invented it, for ideas which have no link with past or present are usually of little value. On the one hand, the work of Bergson has influenced me greatly. On the other hand, Bleuler's book on schizophrenia contains the notion of a profound disturbance in the relationship with the outside world. Bleuler, however, laid most emphasis on the cardinal and elementary symptoms in this condition, symptoms which arise through the attrition of the ideas, emotions and will of the patient. Although he mentioned loss of contact with reality (autism), he did not regard this as the cause of these symptoms. A vital contact with reality, in his view, was not an essential regulatory factor in life to which other mental functions were subordinate. Faithful to associationism, he put forward, in his theory of schizophrenia, the opinion that a particular disorder in the association of ideas was at the root of this condition. He then looked for an underlying organic substrate.

In introducing French psychiatrists to the notion of schizophrenia, I cannot avoid a personal note. When one has genuinely tried to understand someone else's ideas, to live them rather than merely to adopt them, it is not always possible to be dispassionate. But this is of little significance. Science advances through the efforts of its practitioners, but we are merely agents and not part of the actual process.

In putting forward the idea that a vital contact with reality is central to the understanding of schizophrenia, I am aware that there is a certain conflict between Bleuler's work and my own analysis. The difference is well set out by Villey-Desmesaret, and the French psychiatrist Claude supports my point of view: 'We are struck by the fact that the profound disequilibrium in the contact with reality is not just a consequence of some other mental disorder, but is itself the underlying disturbance out of which emerge all the cardinal symptoms of this condition.'

The notion of a loss of vital contact with reality as the essential disorder in schizophrenia has led me to consider how this deficit could be formulated further. I shall try to present the evidence in the following pages.

Intellectual Dementia and Schizophrenic Dementia

It is now necessary to look at the consequences of the disorder which we have just outlined. Bergson, in particular, has influenced my thinking on these matters. As we saw in the previous section, my notion of vital conduct with reality is itself a point of contact between the Zurich school of psychiatry and Bergsonian ideas. I also believe that psychology and psychopathology benefit from having closer links with philosophy.

It is hardly necessary to set out Bergson's ideas in detail. The main thing to remember is his maxim that intelligence and instinct are in fundamental conflict. 'Instinct', says Bergson, 'is modelled along the same lines as life itself; intelligence, on the other hand, is characterised by a complete lack of understanding of life.'

Intelligence, although it is the product of nature, has as its principal object inorganic matter. It can only reflect things which are discontinuous and immobile. It only feels at home when dealing with dead things. It always acts as if it were fascinated by the contemplation of inert matter. Hence it is disturbed when faced with living things and finds itself face to face with organisation.

From the very fact that it is always striving to reconstruct what is there, intelligence cannot capture what is new at any moment in history. It has no room for the unpredictable. It rejects anything creative. Preoccupied only by repetition and similarity, intelligence cannot appreciate the changes produced by time. It ignores the fluidity inherent in things, and petrifies everything it touches. 'We may not think in real time, but we live in it' (Bergson).

Psychopathology cannot be expected to provide a complete answer as to whether Bergson's ideas shed any new light on problems which current psychological thinking has by-passed. They may do so, however, because morbid processes, by acting selectively, can 'dissect' the various psychological functions and reveal them in their naked state. Pathology sometimes succeeds where physiological methods fail to unravel the complexity of the factors involved.

Intelligence and instinct, i.e. the part of our mind dealing with solid inert and spatial aspects of reality on the one hand, and the part dealing with temporal and dynamic considerations on the other hand, are normally fused harmoniously. On its own neither can account for existence, but together they are complementary while at the same time limiting the other's sphere of influence in an entirely natural and appropriate way. But can this harmony be undermined by pathogenic influences? Cannot instinct, for example, be damaged on its own? Would not intelligence, in such circumstances, freed from its natural restraints, try to make up for the missing instinct and come up with bizarre ideas? Conversely, could not intelligence be the seat of a primary lesion with secondary involvement of other factors, depending on its chronicity? Questions of this type do not lead to abstract speculations. On the contrary, they lead, as we shall see shortly, to a series of facts which have been neglected by earlier investigators of psychopathology.

First, let us compare, in this respect, the two major mental processes which psychopathology has so far separated – schizophrenia and intellectual impairment. Most writers in recent times have insisted on a fundamental difference between these two. Nonetheless, it is not easy to say precisely in what this difference consists. We can say with some certainty that intellectual impairment affects judgement and memory. But there is no such certainty about the schizophrenic deficit. The term 'dementia' provides a very poor description of its essential nature.

To quote Bleuler: 'In schizophrenia, even when well-advanced, all the simple mental functions, as far as we know, are intact. In particular, memory, unlike the case in true dementia, is unaffected ... One may find surprisingly that under an apparent envelope of dementia the intelligence is much less affected than one might imagine, as if it were only asleep.' Or, as Chaslin noted: 'It is as if in discordant insanity (schizophrenia) the symptoms resemble those of true dementia. The cold delirious incoherence, the indifference, the bizarre acts, the complete cessation of intellectual activity and its substitution by behaviour of an inferior order, the stupor and bizarre postures, and the incoherent actions all suggest this. Despite the symptomatology, however, there is rarely any sign of true intellectual impairment, such as loss of memory or errors of judgement. In contrast to genuine organic dementia, where the intellectual functioning is actually worse than it appears at first sight, in the discordant form of insanity nothing seems to have been irretrievably lost and only a little effort seems to be required to revive the cerebral activity.'

What, then, is lacking in schizophrenia? And what is the key to the difference between it and true dementia? It is this very difference which we will try to uncover by making use of the opposition of intelligence and instinct which we discussed earlier. As well as noting the differences in psychological *deficits* between these two condition: we shall also draw attention to differences in *intact functioning* between them.

We will begin the study of the two processes by comparing the extreme degrees of deterioration which can occur in each.

We have chosen general paralysis of the insane as a good example of intellectual impairment. For our purpose this condition has the advantage that it usually affects individuals in the prime of life. The intellectual impairment is not then complicated by other factors, such as the physiological consequences of old age, which affects senile dementia. It exists, therefore, in a relatively pure state.

If I ask someone with general paralysis: 'Where are you?' he will reply: 'Here.' Lest he is only responding in a purely verbal and automatic way, I insist: 'But where is here?' The patient taps his foot to indicate the place where he is, or points to it with his finger, or even demonstrates the room with a gesture. 'But here,' he says to us, apparently surprised and annoyed by our insistence on the matter.

There is no question here of some simple semi-automatic response. This type of reply is found surprisingly often in these patients.

The schizophrenic, on the other hand, in reply to the same question, will give the name of the place quite correctly. But he will often say that, although he *knows* where he is, he does not *feel* as if he is in that place, or that he does not feel as if he is in his body. The term 'I exist' has no real meaning for him.

Two different types of factor are involved in our spatial orientation. There are those static factors concerned with the appreciation of how objects relate to one another in a geometrical space where everything is immobile, relative and reversible. But in fact we *live* in space, and we are always aware of the notion: 'I am here at this instant.' Under normal circumstances, therefore, our spatial concepts must accommodate this awareness. Our knowledge of things and our memory images come to be grouped around the notion of 'I am here at this instant.' This allows us to tell in any set of conditions where we are: in Paris, for example, or in Finland, or at our desk.

In patients with general paralysis, the static factors that I discussed earlier, the knowledge of things and memory, are impaired. Such patients are disorientated in space, in the usual sense of the word. Despite this, the structure of their notion of themselves as being 'me in this place' remains intact and active. Schizophrenics, by contrast, know where they are, but their notion of 'me in this place' has no longer its usual quality and finally breaks down.

At a less advanced stage of general paralysis we encounter reactions which are more complex, but whose general character is the same. To the question: 'Where do you come from?' the patient will reply: 'From over there, where I was before.' He is clearly disorientated in space, and unable to name the place where he came from. Nonetheless, the internal representation of a change in place – place X before and place Y now – remains intact.

The following statements belong to the same category:

Q. 'Where are you?' A. 'Here where I was washing myself this morning' or 'Here where I have been for some time now.'

Q. 'What is this building?' A. 'It is the building where I have been put.'

Q. 'Who is this gentleman?' A. 'He is someone who is here.'

Q. 'What are you doing? A. 'At the moment I am staying here.'

If we put someone with general paralysis in front of a mirror and ask 'Whom can you see in there?' he will reply: 'Me.' But if we continue: 'But who is me?' he will not give his name or his job. This sort of reply is much less common in schizophrenics, even in states of deterioration, They will reply: 'Me' and then 'My activity, my personality', or 'It is energy', or, abandoning their delusions, simply state 'Me, the son of Claude Farrere'. One of our patients replied: 'I know who it is' but then admitted that she no longer experienced it in the same way: 'I know who it is, but this is merely an observation, there is nothing inside; it's a queer face; it has a fixed look, oblique and cold.'

The patient with general paralysis, even in the final stages of mental deterioration, retains some sense of awareness of self. The schizophrenic, on the other hand, does not, and is always affected by a sense of depersonalisation.

A sort of commonsense and a knowledge of where to find things is also retained in general paralysis. One such patient, when asked the date, picked up a newspaper. Another very demented patient on being asked 'What day is it?' replied: 'I have no means of knowing.' Another asked to give his date of birth, replied: 'I can't say; I haven't got a wedding ring.' On his wedding ring he would not find his date of birth but the date of his marriage[1] but that is not the point; he knew that there are ways of compensating for a failing memory and instinctively used them.

The behaviour of a schizophrenic is quite different. He usually knows the date, but the knowledge has no precise meaning for him; he cannot use it in a fashion appropriate to his circumstances. The *pragmatic* use of things is affected early in this condition.

A patient with general paralysis, in a state of profound dementia was asked: 'What are you doing?' He replied: 'I am waiting for something to happen and making plans.' Another patient, although so deteriorated that he could no longer speak, still noticed that I had left my hat in his room one day and laughed about it. For the schizophrenic such events or manoeuvres would pass him by.

These various comparisons establish what is a fundamental difference between the intellectual impairment in general paralysis and schizophrenic deterioration. We must not confuse them. In the former case the deficit is in static mental functions; in the latter dynamic factors bear the brunt of the morbid process.

This formula is obviously too schematic. The word 'dynamism' for instance is ambiguous. It can be given a physical interpretation. But here, as in the study of movement, as Bergson pointed out, time is already conceived as a straight line and assimilated within a spatial context.

True dynamism, as it relates to our actual experience of time, is entirely different. We can only glimpse its real nature in an imperfect and provisional way. A solid base for our ideas about it does not exist. To make some advance in knowledge we can only describe and group the phenomena in our life which have a bearing on real time and then see how they fit together in both normal and morbid states of mind. In this way we can begin to construct a psychology and a psychopathology of time as we experience it. This is undoubtedly a difficult task, but one which is indispensable for anyone who wants to understand the normal and pathological functioning of the human mind.

While awaiting further studies on these matters, I believe that my own formula provides a reasonable summary of current knowledge ... Let us examine general paralysis in more detail. In early cases the characteristics which I have just outlined are attenuated but can still be discerned. The appreciation of the passing of years, months or weeks, i.e. the notion of measurable duration linked to spatial events, is often lost, but this does not mean that such patients lose all sense of time. They may be able to give a correct account in chronological order of what they did during the war, but are no longer able to say when the war started or finished. Their memory for a succession of discrete events is preserved but their ability to relate this to a fixed point in time seems to be lost.

Spatial images to do with the passage of time also disappear. In their place, certain elements of the notion

---

[1] A French tradition. [**Translator's note**]

of time, now freed from the constraints of these spatial images, become more prominent and pervade the entire psychological apparatus. All the crazy ideas and plans of such patients have the quality of immediacy and have to be carried out quickly. Expressions such as 'soon', 'immediately', 'not long ago' and 'shortly' appear with surprising frequency in the things they say. One patient was always talking about how her husband, according to her, had to come and find her. She believed that he was already there, climbing the stairs or actually in her room. Or patients may talk about cars speeding at 500 miles an hour, or journeys they have made to Argentina which lasted only five minutes.

This dynamism invades the entire being of the patients, overwhelms them and appears to open up the entire universe to their stream of thought. These, then, are the symptoms of the delirious phase of general paralysis. The patient makes plans for the immediate future, grandiose schemes with no limits. He aims to go straight away to the racecourse and then make a world trip. He will blow up all the islands in the world and then collect the moon to put in a glass. He is all-powerful, feeling that he can do whatever he likes: undertake organ transplants, engage in cross-breeding animals, bring the dead back to life. He extends his extraordinary powers to all living things. He distributes his millions, wants everyone to be happy and invites all the doctors and nurses on his fantastic voyages. He is going to go to Rome to demand that all priests and nuns should be allowed to marry; he wants to set free all the fish in the world.

Everything has to do with movement here. There is nothing but vast rapid movement. No obstacle is considered, no distance is too great and no time limits are set. The patient interprets this state of affairs in everyday language, with the help of ideas which everyone knows are absurdly grandiose.

Let us now compare this picture with the way a schizophrenic, after several years of illness, depicts his state of mind:

> Everything seems immobile around me. Things present themselves in isolation, on their own, without evoking any response in me. Some things which ought to bring back a memory, or conjure up a thought or give rise to a picture, remain isolated. They seem to be understood rather than experienced. It is as if a pantomime were going on around me, one which I cannot take part in. There is nothing wrong with my judgement but I seem to lack any instinctive feel for life. I don't seem to be able to act with any vigour. I can't change from one emotion to another and how can you live like that. I've lost contact with all sorts of things. The value and complexity of things no longer exists. There no link between them and me. I can't immerse and forget myself in tasks anymore. . . . I've even less flexibility when I think about the future than I have about the present and the past. There's a kind of routine affecting me which does not allow me to contemplate the future. The creative ability in me has gone. I see the future only as a repetition of the past.

This account is taken from a patient who spent all her days in bed in a state of complete inertia and who, when she got up, behaved like an automaton. She had auditory hallucinations and delusions of bodily change, and on one occasion had set fire to her clothes in order, as she explained, to experience real sensations which were totally lacking under normal circumstances.

Do not such statements give a clue to the disorder underlying schizophrenia? They are so common in the histories of schizophrenics that we cannot avoid giving some weight to them. Time and again we hear them say: 'My ideas are immobile like a statue' or 'I feel static and lack a sense of reality.' These and other similar expressions reflect the fact that they are gradually being taken over by a sense of immobility, which, if they are aware of it, they find very unpleasant. Their posture and behaviour bear the stamp of this morbid immobility. It shows itself in their stereotyped movements, which are a kind of perpetual repetition of one movement.

It is hard to imagine a more extreme contrast between this clinical picture and that of general paralysis described earlier.

This contrast is also stressed by other writers on the matter. Kraepelin, for example, gave the specific nature of the terminal state an important role in his notion of dementia praecox. He talked in this case of 'Verblödung'. Nayrac, discussing the meaning of this term, wrote:

> Most writers have translated this word as dementia, but this has led to much confusion. In my view the word *Verblödung* means something different. I do not say this because of a desire to be pedantic. I genuinely think another word is needed. *Verblödung* denotes making someone feel shy and ashamed to such a degree that they look intellectually backward. For want of an equivalent expression in French, we have translated *Verblödung* as 'paradementia'.

Bleuler talked about *affective dementia* in schizophrenia, emphasising yet again the fundamental difference between the deterioration in schizophrenia and the intellectual decline in dementia. I myself am more concerned with factors underlying the disintegration of the personality, and I prefer to talk about *pragmatic dementia*. The juxtaposition of these two terms (pragmatic and dementia) is not altogether fortunate. I think that it would be better to omit the word dementia altogether, if this expression denotes a progressive decline in intellectual functions, and to talk instead of a *pragmatic deficit*. Whatever one thinks of this proposed term, it seems to hit on some grain of truth about schizophrenia. Claude and his pupils came to a similar conclusion in their study of schizomania, suggesting that in these cases there was an incongruity between intellectual and pragmatic activity.

Finally, I should like to draw attention to the definition of dementia praecox put forward by Dide and Guiraud:

> The condition is characterised by the sudden weakening, at an early age, of the instinctual drives of mental life, stemming directly from organic brain damage. Purely intellectual operations are only affected secondarily; they do not disappear, but are obstructed and made to work in a contradictory manner. The decline in vital spirit and strength of emotions is the necessary and sufficient element by which we can characterise the illness.

Dide and Guiraud suggested the term 'juvenile athymhormia' as a replacement for dementia praecox.

Putting on one side the organic interpretation of Dide and Guiraud, I agree with their ideas on the psychological nature of schizophrenia. They also confirm what Kraepelin and Bleuler have taught for some time, namely that dementia praecox is not a true dementia because spontaneous cures, impossible to predict, may occur years after the onset of the illness, in subjects who have had all the external signs of a complete and permanent deterioration.

Spatial Thought in Schizophrenia (morbid rationalisation and morbid preoccupation with geometry)

This is not the place to review all the psychopathological consequences of 'the primary disorder discussed earlier. I shall restrict myself to one or two examples, and indicate the direction in which I think psychological research should go. We shall see that schizophrenics, deprived of the ability to assimilate those aspects of reality which have to do with movement or time, tend to rely on the logical and mathematical side of experience. Life itself cannot be reduced to these latter factors, and any attempt to do so can only lead to a distorted view of it.

Consider the following case history which I have published under the title 'morbid rationalisation'.

The patient was a teacher, aged 32, who was referred to us at the Clinic for the Prevention of Mental Disorders. He complained at first of a 'physiological decomposition' which was causing him discomfort, and an 'emptiness in the head' which he attributed to excessive salivation. His voice, he maintained, was influencing him in a suggestive way; it seemed 'dead' and seemed to be a 'ghost voice'. His whole being had undergone 'a regression', and he felt as if he were again 15 years old, when he was a young student.

The patient had neither hallucinations nor delusions. There was no sign of intellectual decline, but from the first interview we were struck by his behaviour. This impression grew stronger in the course of subsequent interviews. His profoundly morbid attitude led to a diagnosis of schizophrenia, of a severe and well advanced form.

It is this attitude that I shall now try to describe as well as possible. The following incident was very characteristic. The patient told us that for several years now he had been interested in philosophical problems. He had been in the habit of writing down his thoughts and had amassed a considerable stack of notes. We asked him if he had read many philosophical works. He replied: 'No, on the contrary, I purposely avoided them so as not to spoil my own thoughts.' He shunned the company of other people, 'so as not to be disturbed in my reflections'. His morbid attitude is here shown in its clearest form. He was isolating himself from the world in order to keep within himself the source of his philosophical thoughts. We were not at all surprised to find that one of his theories concerned 'the way acid acting on nerve terminals gives rise to human behaviour'.

This strange attitude cannot be regarded as a disorder of judgement because then it would be necessary to ask why it takes this form rather than any other. In my view it has more to do with the morbid attitude which I have been discussing in this paper.

All of us need from time to time to withdraw from our surroundings and to commune with ourselves. In this way we draw strength to continue our mental activity and work. But we do not then totally reject all outside influence on our personality. On the contrary we allow our environment to interact with ourselves and recast our inner life according to the elements of this environment which affect us deeply. At the same time we do not allow our surroundings to dictate our entire life because we would then be enslaved by it. There must be some mechanism in normal people whereby the influence of one's environment and one's originality are kept in balance. It seems to me that this is an essential part of the human condition, and one which is difficult to describe in logical terms. We might designate it as a *feeling of harmony with life*.

It is essentially irrational, in the sense that our intellect cannot comprehend it completely, but this feeling enters into all the important situations which we encounter and is the source of most of our conflicts. Moreover, it is the basis for most of our decisions about the way we live because it gives *limits and strength* to these decisions which our intellect alone cannot provide.

Every major decision is determined by this feeling of *harmony with life* but, because the latter is not open to our scrutiny, its precise influence can never be quantified, and the decisions themselves may, therefore, appear irrational. As Pascal said: 'The heart has its reasons which pure reasoning can never uncover.' I am tempted to alter this to: 'Life has its reasons which pure reasoning cannot formulate.'

Returning to our patient's strange attitude, we can describe his psychological state in the following way. His mental energy, instead of being directed towards an integration with reality, entirely ignores the real world around him, and without any natural anchor for it to function the patient loses himself in the clouds. Not being a philosopher, even a second-rate one, our teacher ties himself up in knots with his own philosophical speculations. At the same time he rationalises his feeling of isolation by developing the notion that he does not want to be disturbed in his thoughts, and by doing so he cuts himself off from human contact.

The richness and variety of life disappears in the course of this process. However powerful an intellect may be, it cannot be entirely self-sufficient. Thinking and acting without taking into account the ideas of others or external circumstances is bound to lead to errors and absurdities.

We have analysed in some detail a single statement of this patient – i.e. 'I do not want to be disturbed in my thoughts' – because it seems to contain a distillation of his whole way of being and his relationship with the outside world.

Any act that we carry out can be regarded as an antithesis between yes and no, between good and bad, between what is allowed and what is forbidden, or between what is useful and what is harmful. We can talk in this sense of an antithetical attitude. It is the result of a lack of the irrational feeling of harmony with oneself and life, which we mentioned earlier, and indicates a total loss of ideas about the limits and strength of our intellectual activity. A person who follows this course will only behave in accordance with his own ideas and will become as a result doctrinaire and pedantic. It may be an advantage when it comes to solving mathematical problems, but it is morbid and dangerous when we are faced with practical issues and need guidance in our actions and our decisions. An example should make this clear. Our patient said that he 'always examined actions with a fine tooth comb' to see if they were in accord with his principles. His desire to be spiritually perfect led him to 'banish from existence all material work'. Before his illness he would devote all his leisure time to bee-keeping, but then, because he regarded it as material work, he completely neglected it. Whenever his parents, with whom he lived, brought up the question of money, he would see this as an attack on his ideals and avoid the conversation. He regarded his visit to the clinic as 'moral suicide', because he believed that 'man should be self-sufficient and should be under no other authority'. This is in itself logical, but is here taken to extreme lengths. His comment shows that principles can have absurd consequences by reason of inappropriate generalisation. Life is not made up of rigid and universal principles; there is always a built-in measure of irrationality which determines the limits of reason.

The patient's moral regeneration, he stated, began in 1918 while he was in a prisoner-of-war camp in Germany. He tried at that time to detach himself from material things and be directed in his behaviour by impersonal principles. He thought it right to achieve wisdom as the only true form of happiness, but for this purpose he had to be alone, removed from any disturbing elements. Under the influence of these ideas his personality was transformed. He devised a set of rules by which to live. These included temperance, silence, and the application of a new principle every week. He virtually ceased talking and would only answer questions when these were in conformity with his principles. His actions were regulated minute by minute. He believed that his problems only began when he allowed himself, against his principles, to talk impulsively. After the war he returned to his job as a teacher. At first he tried to apply to his teaching the principle of absolute indulgence, because he believed that his pupils were irresponsible. They laughed at him and had no idea what he was getting at. Next, at the suggestion of his headmaster, he applied a strict military regime. Then there followed a period of 'liberalism and gentleness'. He wrote in his diaries at this time:

> I put into practice, until last June, an impersonal discipline, firm and confident in my mind that I was encouraging a dignity in behaviour and thoughts. Inspired by logic, I had to stifle my idealist tendencies for a whole year in order to maintain military discipline. I carried out one or two manual tasks to please my parents, but this subordination of my actions to the wishes of two old people made me even more vulnerable to their sentimental assaults, which hitherto I had been able to withstand by my powerful humanitarian feelings. I soon found myself an obedient child. Any attempt at initiative seemed futile and I felt suffocated.

This, in brief, was the patient's attitude. In keeping with his antithetical outlook, he saw any outside force as an attack on his personality; if he succumbed to it he would be dragged down and engulfed. He could only register outside influences as having a hold on him or as a trap. How different he is in this respect from normal people! The bonds which attach us to our environment are infinitely more rich and complex. We may try to impose our will on others and dominate our immediate social circle; at the same time we know how to do our duty, to respond to love or pity, to recognise the authority of others and to follow their advice, without feeling any constraint on our freedom. Our teacher recognised only two categories: independence, which through his egocentricity he only achieved at opposite poles of his intellectual antithesis; and domination, which he continually suffered. He would only admit to being ill for two months, although in our view it had been much longer. He attributed the onset of his illness to his succumbing to suggestions from his parents which had affected his voice and made him emit ideas which went against his principles. He felt that he had lost control over himself and that he was behaving as if he were carrying out orders from another person.

Whereas before he had felt master of the way he looked or talked, now, when teaching in class, he felt in the sway of the sound of his own voice, and his gaze would fix, against his wishes, on the pupils. He had lost his desire to teach because he felt that his work and principles were being directly controlled by the headmaster.

It is unlikely that the way in which the teacher behaved was really a result of a conscious effort on his part, as he would have had us believe. It is more probable, as discussed earlier, that a regulatory factor in his life was missing and that the remaining elements regrouped to form some unifying whole. The patient then interpreted this intellectually as a coherent system, but it was in fact distorting his whole action and turning him into a 'stranger', we might almost say an 'alien', in his relationship with his environment and ourselves.

I should also like to comment on the way in which the world around him affected the patient's altered mental state. In this respect, his lack of vital contact with his environment and the disharmony of his mind are the main factors.

The patient's state of consciousness may be compared to that of a stage on which abstract principles enter and compete for attention. It was altogether a very impersonal stage, and he must have treated these principles accordingly. We saw that his pupils took no notice of his doctrines, probably because there was no warmth, no intimacy and no personal touch in the way he applied them. He had lost, one might say, the sensitivity which allows us to communicate with others, to feel with them and to enter into their concerns. The ability to make personal rapport was shattered and he no longer knew even how to look at people in a natural way. His sphere of interest might seem much wider than is usual, indeed almost boundless, but this is an artefact of the despair of a spirit deprived of affinity with normal concerns. He would tell us that he had become 'detached from material things and was only governed by impersonal principles', and that he was no longer under the influence of a *restraining milieu* but of the *entire* world. He lived for ideas and saw people as impersonal objects. He was kept going by thoughts, not people. He could appreciate a sense of humanity but always sought to achieve the absolute in this regard. His filial love was drowned by a much grander love. It is not surprising therefore, for someone who saw things in this way, that minor arguments between him and his parents became in his mind a veritable battle of giants. His parents, concerned at his bizarre attitude, tried to intervene. His father pointed out that if you cannot carry a load of 100 kilos on your back, you should try 50 kilos. In response to this and other such statements involving material topics, our patient only became more convinced that his ideals were under attack. His belief that his parents were trying to undermine his personality became stronger, and if he tried to make the slightest concession he immediately felt he was renouncing his ideals on a massive scale.

When recounting the story of his life he would merely give a list of the ideas and principles which he had adopted, as in the account of his teaching career – the periods of indulgence, of military discipline, and of liberalism. His whole life seemed to have evolved in fits and starts. It was not a continuous line, supple and elastic, but one that was broken in several places. The ideas which he had entertained seemed also to have appeared in isolation, with no links between them. This had also been the case with the rules governing his life, which were self-contradictory or incompatible with each other. Emotional factors and, even more striking, the sense of time seemed to have entirely disappeared from our teacher's existence. He was also continually in 'conflict with life'.

Let us compare this man with another patient who said that he could not be sure of the importance of money, because money did not take up much space. This patient had also said that he did not find change very interesting because everywhere he went he was always finding 'too much change, too much mobility'. Instead, his attention was completely absorbed in a project to enlarge the Gare de l'Est in Paris, which was in all the newspapers at the time. He invested it with enormous importance, exceeding all other events in his life.

In this case there seemed to be an abnormal generalisation concerning ideas about spatial order which had a morbid hold on his thinking and behaviour. This involved the application of mathematical criteria to determine the value of objects and events solely in terms of their dimensions or geometrical characteristics.

Do we not see here the first signs of what might be called a *morbid preoccupation with geometry*?

The same patient revealed that from the age of 16 he had been 'obsessed', as he put it, by the subject of construction. He would doubt the solidity of things and wondered if the walls of his school were straight.

'I was tormented,' he wrote in his autobiography, 'by the vaults in churches. I could not accept that all that weight could be supported by ribs, pillars and a keystone. I could not understand why it did not fall down. I could not see why the cement in the free stones did not crumble because it must be a particularly vulnerable pressure point. I concluded that houses stayed up only through some terrestrial attraction. I came to doubt my own senses.'

A 'mania for symmetry' then took hold of him, and also an 'obsession with pockets'. He wanted to know what difference there was between putting one's hands straight into a normal jacket pocket and putting them into the sloping pockets of an overcoat. He solved this problem by concluding that 'in the first instance you establish a feeling of parallelism between extreme things, arms and legs'.

He also had the habit of standing in front of a mirror, legs together, trying to place his body symmetrically, to achieve, as he said, 'an absolutely perfect position'. To this end, he would hold his breath as long as he could.

During his military service he had once been given an injection. The idea had then grown on him that a piece of cottonwool had entered his body along with the injected fluid. He then constructed a vast series of ramifications from this single idea, all following a geometrical and rational pattern:

The obsession grew and grew. It was no longer just cottonwool that had been inserted, it was the metal from the needle as well, the glass from the syringe; each organ in my body was systematically affected, until my brain was involved. I thought the substance which they had injected was poisonous, and so were all the injections I had had afterwards. And I also drew things which had happened before that into my obsession. Any treatment was useless. I had to uncover the cause of it all right down to its roots, right down to the foundations, and then build myself up again. It did not matter that an unpleasant treatment might have good results, because good results which stemmed from a bad event would be cancelled out by this event. I could not accept the illogical idea of a good thing emanating from a bad, for instance a cornerstone resting safely on rubble despite the evident fact that this could happen.

It is hardly necessary to point out the richness of architectural, spatial and geometrical images in this reasoning.

The patient wanted to put a bolt on his door. In case it would not fit the bolt-hole he replaced the latter with a bigger one. But he then noticed it was now higher than before, although of the same diameter. 'I said to myself', he reported, 'that logically, because it is higher, it ought to be wider and so I enlarged the hole.' There were more difficulties and more mathematical considerations, and eventually he ended up with a massive hole in the door and in the wall.

> 'Planning is everything for me in life', he went on, 'I wouldn't upset my plan for anything. I would rather upset my life. It is a taste for symmetry, for regularity that attracts me in planning. Life has no regularity or symmetry, and for that reason I manufacture my own reality. I attribute all my energies to my brain.
>
> What I am going to say may seem fantastic, but there it is. My state of mind consists of having no faith in anything except theory. I don't believe in the existence of anything until I have demonstrated it. For example, a woman's body has an effect on a man. Why? This is something that I doubt because I cannot prove it. I don't see myself giving way to such things, being carried away and relying only on my impressions. I would feel as if I were in the air, and that would be illogical.'

In the street, however, he was sometimes struck with the appearance of a woman. He would then return to his house, sit down on a chair, cross his arms and take up a position as symmetrical as possible to reflect on the event. He would try to solve the problem of why a woman's body made a particular impression on a man. He hoped that it could all be explained 'by mathematics, medicine and sexual impressions'. It was in this manner that he sought an answer. He wondered whether the human body cannot be reduced to geometry and therefore whether the highest form of beauty did not consist in having a spherical body, this being the perfect form.

He wrote:

> I want to examine my sexual impressions, even though this is a formidable problem, because the more I try to analyse these in terms of similar impressions, sub-impressions for instance, I only end up by deriving more impressions. And so it goes on.

He thought about what it would be like if he left hospital. He would become perplexed; his spatial thought, uniquely adapted to things which were durable and immobile, was totally incapable of taking in the slightest change. Here is his train of thought: 'I imagine myself leaving here. It is essential that I still keep some impression of being here and for that to happen I have to have something which represents my stay here.' And so when he left the hospital he took away with him all the bottles and all the empty boxes of pills used during his stay, and arranged them carefully in his house in order to have proof that he had been in the hospital and to have the impression that he was still there.

> 'I am always looking for immobility', he announced to us. 'I tend towards rest and immobilisation. I also have within me a tendency to prefer immobility in the things around me in my life. I like immovable objects, boxes and bolts, things that are always there, which never change. Stone is motionless, whereas the ground can move and inspires no confidence in me. I attach importance only to solidity. A train goes past on the embankment; the train doesn't exist for me: I want only to build the embankment.
>
> The past is a precipice. The future is a mountain. It occurred to me that it would be a good idea to have a buffer-day between the past and the future. On this day I would do nothing at all. In this way I once went 24 hours without urinating.
>
> I would like to recall my impressions of 15 years ago, to do away with time, to die with the same impressions that I was born with, to make circular movements, to stay in the same place, and not to be uprooted. All these things I would like.'

It would be hard to find a better example of the processes involved in purely spatial thought, which when liberated from the influence of the intuition which is indispensable to life tries to govern its own activity. We have seen the objectives which it sets out to achieve and the monstrous constructions at which it arrives. Can one imagine a better confirmation of those ideas of Bergson which were the point of departure of our analysis?

It should be added that when invited to write an account of all this our patient did so over numerous pages. Characteristically, he only mentioned objects, walls, boxes, bolts and bolt-holes; not one living person entered his description. One would say that his whole life was made up of solid and immovable objects.

It was equally clear that he never sought to combat his abnormal attitude. Not only did he accept it, but he continually tried to demonstrate its solid foundation with supra-logical and supra-rational arguments. He consulted us, not to be rid of his 'obsessions', but solely to 'rest', as he put it, in order to return to his bolts and other objects which were the mainstay of his life.

Madame Minkowska who examined this patient at length summarised her findings in the following way:

Life in his case is opposed to planning;
instinct to the brain;
feeling to thought;
the *faculty of penetration which synthesises* is opposed to analysis of infinite details;
whereas we rely on *impressions*, he demands proof;
movement is set against immobility;
events and people are opposed to objects;
realisation counters representation;
time is in opposition to space;
succession is contrasted with extension;
and the *end* is set against the means.

In this scheme the first element in each contrasted pair (in italics) is deficient, the second element hypertrophied.

I subscribe to this analysis. One can interpret them as an atrophy of those factors which have to do with instinct, 'modelled on life', and a compensatory hypertrophy of everything which concerns intelligence, or as Bergson put it 'has as its principal object things which are inorganic solids, dead, or not renewed at any moment in time and which are characterised by a lack of natural understanding of life'.

Here is an account by another schizophrenic:

Apart from my reason, which is intact, everything else is in complete disarray. I have suppressed my emotions as I have all aspects of reality. My body has an existence but there is no internal sensation in my life. I don't feel things any more. I don't have normal sensations. I make up for this lack of sensations with reason. Since my illness began I have suppressed the impression of time. Time doesn't matter any more. I can set aside an infinite amount of time to accomplish the most trivial act in my current life. I feel that I can reason quite well, but only in the absolute, because I have lost contact with life.

Another schizophrenic, in an advanced stage of her illness, passed the time making hats for herself. She had made 16 of them. One day, she lost two of them. As a form of retaliation against this she decided to break two of her mother's 16 cups.

Another patient, on being asked, after a visit to her mother, if she had been pleased to see her, replied: 'There was a lot of movement. I don't like that.' One schizophrenic that I saw showed none of these obsessional phenomena, but needed to give some durable

form to events in her life. She had collected newspapers and various scraps of paper relating to herself: 'This happened at this time and on this day (whereupon she indicated the exact hour and date) and I wrote this with a glass beside me which was exactly two centimetres from the paper I am writing on.' As she had done with the glass, on another occasion she took as her support, her witness as it were, any inanimate and immobile object which she found in front of her, e.g. a lamp.

*****

All these observations have also been made by other writers on the subject. But I hope that I have been able to view them from a new angle, to group them in a more adequate way and therefore to promote a better understanding of them . . .

We cannot imitate the states of mind described by our patients, and so, when we try to deepen our theoretical and practical understanding of the human personality, we need not be afraid of applying our own instincts and our own intuition to the task.

Binswanger, L. (1956), 'Extravagance, perverseness, manneristic behaviour and schizophrenia'

From (1987) *The Clinical Roots of the Schizophrenia Concept*. Edited by John Cutting and Michael Shepherd, translated by J. Cutting. Cambridge: Cambridge University Press. Originally published as (1956) *Drei Formen Missglückten Daseins: Verstiegenheit, Verschrobenheit, Manieriertheit*. Tübingen: Niemeyer: 188–97.

Editors' commentary

Binswanger wrote extensive case analysis of schizophrenia during his lifetime which take cross-sectional, longitudinal, clinical and existential perspectives. Some of them (e.g. the case of Ellen West) run to well over 100 pages. Throughout, there is a preoccupation with the notion of 'autism' or the inaccessible, ununderstandable qualities of schizophrenia that have been much written about. Binswanger's aim is to use existential analysis to extend understanding of schizophrenia beyond the limits that psychiatry has traditionally set. In this brief extract we can get a sense of Binswanger's approach in practice. For Binswanger autism appears in schizophrenia in three forms which he called in German 'Verstiegenheit', 'Verschroben-heit' and 'Manieriertheit'. This text has a stab at translating these terms. For Binswanger they are projections of an existential change, or form of life, which has become 'inauthentic' in Heidegger's sense.[2] *In Ver-stiegenheit (extravagance) inauthenticity manifests as a kind of artificial going over the top or flight of fancy. In Verschrobenheit (perverseness), it manifests as a tendency to reduce any situation to an idea, to a concept, or to a definition, which then becomes binding, rigid and solid. In Manieriertheit (manneristic behaviour), inauthenticity manifests as an artificial version of what is intended, or as a set role play reflecting the intellectual side of human nature rather than the 'free play' of individual life forces. For Binswanger taking description of schizophrenic autism toward phenomenological–existential analysis makes it more understandable. Although this understanding operates at an existential or metaphysical level – i.e. at a level which clinicians may not regard as part of their remit – Binswanger thinks it has practical consequences for how clinicians make endeavours on behalf of people with schizophrenia. How far Binswanger goes beyond a mere redescription of schizophrenia in new terms (and terms which to a modern ear may sound derogatory) and quite how existential understanding of schizophrenia, if it can be gained, aids clinical practice we think remain important debating points.*

Extravagance, perverseness and manneristic behaviour are forms of *existential failure* in the sense that an individual's sense of the flow of life has come to a stop or been frozen. At such a point, it is no longer possible for him to continue within the framework of love and friendship. This, as I intend to show in this article, is more typical of the schizophrenic's world than of a normal person's experience. These three aspects of their existential state – extravagance, perverseness and manneristic behaviour – correspond respectively in the areas of psychopathology to *rigidity, stupor* and *splitting*. For this reason the studies I have made on existential aspects of schizophrenia should help us to understand in greater depth the phenomena of splitting and stupor. I have shown in

a number of detailed case histories that, whenever the flow of a person's life is threatened or arrested, that person can no longer realise himself, no longer mature, and will lose the capacity to make rapport and emotional contact with others. This arrest of the flow of existence does not mean that an individual can no longer make sense of his present world, but it does mean that his concept of a future for himself is severely impaired. One might say that the 'way to the future' is barred.

This state of affairs is illustrated in several of the cases that I have described. Ellen West was torn between an urge for gluttony and the ideal of being slim. In her own words, she saw 'all exits from the stage as barred'. In her ensuing despair she went to pieces at this stage, and the only 'exit' remaining open to her, the only way forward that she could see, lay in a decision to take her own life. In the case of Jürg Zünd, the arrest of true self-realisation took the form of seeking anonymity in the crowd. For Lola Voss the 'arrest' occurred when she abandoned herself to superstition and amateur soothsaying, prior to the development of frank delusions of persecution. In Suzanne Urban's case it was a surrender to a feeling of terror and fear.

Of the three characteristics of the existential state of a psychotic individual, extravagance appears at an early stage. It can be regarded as representing an extravagant or exaggerated concept of an ideal existence. *Perverseness*, on the other hand, is a manifestation of the contrariness of the world as it is seen, and is a preliminary stage of the schizophrenic 'arrest' of self-realisation. A normal person views the world as consisting of stable, symmetrical and natural relationships; it is a world where everything is straight, not crooked or awry. Not so the schizophrenic. For him it is contrary, distorted and disconnected: a sense of the future no longer appears natural, but is somehow unattainable and removed from the self. The connection between *manneristic behaviour* and schizophrenia is a particularly close one. It can be regarded as a 'loss of sparkle', a freezing and repetition of present existence, and a reflection of the intellectual side of man's nature rather than the 'free play' of individual life forces. It is as if there is an 'iron net' round the free expression of gestures, an invisible and incomprehensible force which is stifling the natural flow of life.

It should be pointed out that, when we talk about a 'preliminary stage' of schizophrenia, this does not mean that the characteristic triad will necessarily

---

[2] See Arthur Tatossian's 'Phenomenology of psychoses' (1979) for an historical account of Binswanger's approach. Available in English translation at http://maudsleyphilosophygroup.org/resources.html. **[Editors' note]**

evolve into a florid schizophrenic illness. The existential and clinical points of view should always be kept separate. The clinical approach deals with hard *clinical facts* and the *course of an illness*. The existential analysis is concerned with unravelling what it is like to *be schizophrenic* and what it is like to change from one *mode of being to another*. For this purpose we are justified in using the language of metaphor, and to talk about the power of the 'iron net', the meaning of 'ceremony' and the role of the 'mask' and the 'grimace' in the experience of an individual. How else can we understand what it must be like to be gripped by despair and cut off from human love and trust. It was these experiences which led Ellen West to commit suicide, Jürg Zünd to seek permanent institutional care, and Lola Voss and Suzanne Urban to develop delusions of persecution.

Although I have emphasised that clinical and existential analyses should be kept separate, the existential approach can sometimes shed light on the clinical. For example, one might regard schizophrenic autism, as it is understood clinically, as a state of extreme self-sufficiency, where an individual is impervious to social influences. In fact, existential analysis has shown this to be false. It is in fact an exaggerated dependence on some aspect of the rules of society. An individual will either accept some set of rules with avid obedience, or fight against them. Either way, the nature of autism is best viewed, not as a rejection of the world of others, but either as exaggerated conformity or exaggerated opposition to it. This is clearly illustrated in the case of Jürg Zünd, who changed from being an angry fighter for society to being an extreme imitator of current social fashions.

There is one exception to the rule that schizophrenia merely causes an exaggeration of the prevailing social norms. This concerns cases of schizophrenia with a stormy onset, particularly those that begin with the 'end of the world experience'. In such states, the 'world', as an individual knows it, disappears, and with it all the social institutions that one may live for. Even in these cases, however, the individual must rebuild his world, when the acute state is past, and he then chooses models or images which are part of his culture. This shows that schizophrenics can never 'break away' permanently from what is regarded as a 'normal' life, or achieve extraordinary artistic skills. The most that they can achieve is an extravagant, perverse and manneristic distortion of all that is typical of human existence, all that is mundane.

Bleuler mentioned that one of his schizophrenic patients 'expressed trivialities in the most lofty, affected phrases, as if he were dealing with the highest interests of mankind'. Minkowski's patient, a school-teacher who rigidly applied certain pedagogic principles without regard to whether they were appropriate, is another example of how schizophrenia desiccates and denatures existence, leaving only a shell or a mask of what life is really about.

One might say that schizophrenic existence is not only a mask of all that is real and vibrant in life, but that a schizophrenic lives behind this mask. In doing so he surrenders himself to anxiety and despair, and the world is then emptied of meaning. At an intermediate stage, when there is neither complete immersion in the normal flow of life nor complete arrest of this process, an individual may achieve, temporarily, a precarious existence. There is no sense of happiness in just being alive, however, and no capacity for love. Instead, the individual experiences a pervasive anxiety and emptiness, and looks, to an observer, as if he is numb or distracted. Later, he can no longer 'hold out' against the power of the anxiety and dread, and sinks into the abyss of a new world, warped and denuded of all the usual landmarks. The most characteristic feature of this new world which the patient has entered is its abnormal *temporal* quality. Time virtually comes to a standstill: there is no notion of a future, and the present becomes detached from its past.

Psychopathological and existential, accounts of schizophrenia differ in particular on the question of what is known as *splitting*. Bleuler used the term 'split mind' to mean a loss of associative connections. His theoretical model was that of association psychology. The term is also used in psychodynamic formulations. From an existential point of view, 'splitting' means that an individual's existence is losing its personal quality and uniqueness and becoming a mere copy of some general way of life. A person loses his individuality and becomes typical of a certain class of people. The terms 'emptiness' and 'arrest' express a similar concept, the former emphasising the loss of potentiality for participation in life that ensues, and the latter the standstill in time which occurs.

To illustrate these concepts I shall now describe the case of a 39-year-old married woman, Ilse.

> Her illness and her existential change began when she put her right hand into a burning stove in order to show her father, whom she loved passionately, 'What love can

do', and in order to move him by this proof of love to alter his tyrannical behaviour towards her mother. This act was indeed *extravagant*: she climbed too high. We might say that 'she went over the top'. [Binswanger's term *Verstiegenheit*, translated here as extravagance, literally means 'climbing too high', Tr.] she lacked the necessary psychological experience to see that she could achieve nothing lasting by this heroic deed in the face of one as tyrannical as her father. To pursue our metaphor, an experienced 'climbing guide', someone who knew his fellow men, would have dissuaded her from such rash mental 'scaling of the heights' and would have assured her confidently that with her lack of experience in this unfamiliar and extremely difficult field, such heroic measures would get her nowhere. He would have told her that she was 'climbing much too high'.

The action may also be described as *perverse*, in that the daughter wants to make a loving approach to her father, but estranges him immediately by her choice of method. The tortured logic of her theme, namely that she will move her father and make him change his attitude and behaviour, is apparent when we consider that the action, instead of being a pure proof of love, becomes something tyrannical or violent, exercising pressure or compulsion on the father. She wants to force her father to treat her mother better. 'If I take such pain upon myself', she wants to say to him clearly 'then you must treat mother better.' The rationale that equated proof of love with change of attitude on the part of her father is thus perverted into its exact opposite – into an alarming shock.

The clinical development of the case consisted in a sudden transformation of her love for her father and her sacrifice for him into acute delusions of love, reference and influence. Recovery saw a restoration of her love. The ordeal by fire, the sacrifice, was in fact the preliminary stage of a schizophrenic psychosis that lasted a year. By this I do not mean that the perverseness went on to become, in the clinical sense, a schizophrenic psychosis. I am trying to show, in existential terms, how a change took place from a world that was distorted or upside down to an actual delusional world, how an existence which was threatened by alien powers became one in which existence was overwhelmed by these powers.

Turning to the ordeal by fire viewed as *manneristic behaviour*, I should first point out that an individual who follows the traditions of his culture is not necessarily being manneristic. An artist may emulate a certain style in painting because he admires it and wants to make others acquainted with it. Ilse's behaviour, however, cannot be seen as a personal statement freely communicating her beliefs or values in this way. It was merely an act calculated to produce an effect, to appeal

and even to alarm. Nor was it a freely made decision, but to a large extent carried out under the compulsion that she had to play the role of a martyr. Yet she explained to her husband, who knew of her intention, that she had to free herself of an overwhelming compulsion to carry out the ordeal by fire. What we have here is therefore a desperate attempt to play a role of her own within the confines of an existential threat caused by her fear of madness. It is this role-playing which is the essence of manneristic behaviour.

The content of her subsequent delusions support this analysis. She mentioned at this later stage that doctors were using the 'tools of martyrdom' in her treatment, that she was being exposed to the scorn and mockery of others, and that her arms were becoming cold like clay. This shows that the development of delusions can be seen as the martyr's role having, so to speak, 'got out of hand'. Whereas in the preliminary stage of the psychosis she surrenders to the mask or role while continuing to exist behind the mask, in the delusional stage it is only as a mask or a role that she does exist.

I hope that by this example I have succeeded in demonstrating the psychiatric meaning and purpose of our three concepts. I hope that I have been able to show how an existential analysis can elucidate the clinical concept of autism in terms of the flow of events that is human existence. And I hope that I have been able to explain the mechanisms whereby disturbances in this flow lead to the clinical condition known as schizophrenia. A thorough knowledge of what is happening to an individual who is overtaken by these events should help us in our practical and theoretical endeavours on their behalf.

Blankenburg, W. (1968), 'First steps toward a psychopathology of "common sense"'

From (2001) *Philosophy, Psychiatry and Psychology* 8(4): 303–15. Translated by A. L. Mishara. Originally published in 1968 as Ansätze zu einer Psychopathologie des 'common sense.' *Confinia Psychiatrica* 12: 144–63.

Editors' commentary

Mental illness is often grasped by the layperson as a departure from 'common sense'. The concept of 'common sense' has attracted considerable philosophical attention but is little discussed in psychology. In this text, Blankenburg reviews the philosophical literature on common sense and argues that rather than it being lost in all forms of psychopathology, only specific forms (e.g. OCD, schizophrenia) highlight its loss. He selects a case of simple schizophrenia as an example of a mental state that shows us what it is like to lose common sense.

The phrase in our title, "Psychopathology of Common Sense," may seem strange to some readers. How can the disturbance of what is obviously a banal ability have significance? However, we find here something that is frequently true: The deepest human problems lurk behind the obvious.

One dictionary defines common sense as "practical understanding; capacity to see and take things in their right light; sound judgement. Ordinary mental capacity" (Funk and Wagnall 1964). In this definition, an understanding governed by practice and the ability to see things in their "right light" is considered most essential. Healthy judgement is simply equated with normalcy.

In general, our current understanding of the term, "common sense"[3] predominantly derives from Anglo-American usage. The conceptual history of "common sense," however, extends back to ancient times. Our present term is a translation of the Latin *sensus communis*. The Aristotelian definition of common sense ... from which the Latin *sensus communis* is derived is the organ that orders and sums up sensations.[4] However, we will not concern ourselves with the Aristotelian definition. In Anglo-American usage, the definition of common sense, such as the one above, more closely resembles that proposed by the stoics. Although it will not be our emphasis, it is still possible to trace relationships between the two definitions.

Many modern thinkers have addressed the problem of common sense. Descartes (1953), Vico (1966), Shaftesbury (1711), Thomas Reid (1846) and the Scottish school, and Kant are some. We need not enter here into a debate with the philosophical tradition. Gadamer (1965) has already done this with masterful subtlety. From these modern thinkers there spans a sweeping arch which extends to the more recent philosophy of life, Bergson's views, Husserl's approach to the life-world[5] and Heidegger's (1927) analysis of the everydayness of Dasein. It also extends to Marxist conceptions of practice, pragmatism, Moore's (1969) approach, and various sociological and anthropological trends of recent times.

The problems connected with the concept of common sense become particularly salient for us under the following conditions:

1. When the scope of an exclusively cognitive approach to the relationship between subject and world is critically examined; this is when one questions the human subject as merely being a subject of cognition and, with this, questions the rift between theory and praxis; this manner of questioning leads to a concept of praxis in a wider sense, which is no longer seen as the opposite of cognition but is rather included as a part of it. Praxis is now seen as a form of coping with world and, with this, its function of opening up and interpreting world only properly comes to light.

2. When the relationship between mediacy and immediacy, as it pertains to our ability to make judgments, becomes questionable.

3. When our attention shifts away from major human problems to the basic, apparently banal assumptions of everyday life; these are seemingly obvious, taken-for-granted assumptions, which do not lose any of their fundamental importance even as we strive to go beyond them.

4. When we raise the question about the social underpinnings of our cognition and knowledge. This touches, perhaps, the most important condition. It is the question of a relationship between cognition and the social world.[6] If we speak about common sense, then we are speaking about a "sense" that is common to each of us. That means that either it has its origin in this commonality or it aligns itself to such a commonality, which then becomes binding for it. This problem becomes particularly critical in Husserl's examination of the intersubjective constitution of the life-world.

---

[3] English in the original. [**Translator's note**]

[4] Aristotle, *De Anima* III a. More precisely stated: as the actual perception enables the relation of sensations to self and world. [**Original note**]

[5] In doing so, one is able take into account the entirety of Husserl's late work, especially *The Crisis of the European Sciences and Transcendental Phenomenology*. [**Original note**]

[6] As each of the above four points are closely connected with one another, 3 and 4 may be considered in tandem. [**Original note**]

In conclusion, we come across the following themes in our investigation of the phenomenon of common sense: 1. the relationship between cognition and action or practice, 2. the relationship between mediacy and immediacy, 3. the questionableness of the obviousness of what seems obvious, and 4. the intersubjective constitution of the world.

We see that the topic of common sense is a legitimate philosophical problem. For the philosophical sociological thinker, Natanson (1963, 909), common sense is "potentially the most productive topic for our philosophical investigations." We now must ask: What can we know about it empirically, and what kind of empirical studies have been undertaken?

The concept is barely mentioned in psychological handbooks. It does not seem to play much of a role in contemporary psychology. This is not to say that it is not pertinent. It is rather to acknowledge that the appropriate methods, which could tackle these problems systematically, have not yet been explored. With the current trend for psychology to be ever more concerned with sociological questions, however, this lack will presumably change.

Admittedly, this concept, which has been so variously accentuated in its history, requires sharper analysis. There is no consensus, for example, of whether common sense involves a unitary "function." For the time being, we must leave open the question whether, indeed, it may be that heterogeneous factors preserve its intactness.

In a first step, we should not allow ourselves to interpret the concept's evanescent quality and lack of contours merely negatively. We may be tempted to do so for the sake of greater conceptual clarity. While such clarity is often a desirable goal, it will in the present case make our concept dissolve into nothing. The very "sponginess" of the concept, rather, is connected with its richness and vitality. We should not presume that its vagueness signifies a lack of clarity on our part. It says at the same time something about the peculiarity of the matter itself. It withdraws from our efforts to conceptualize it unambiguously as an object. However, we must not simply yield to this withdrawal. In our very striving to overcome this resistance, we should take heed of it. We should take this withdrawal as an indication of the mode of Being of common sense itself.

For the empirical research of this function, it is best to start with examining when it fails. In doing so, we enter the realm of psychopathology. Descartes had expressed the view that nothing in the world is so well apportioned as common sense (cf. the first sentence in his *Discours de la méthode* [1637] (Descartes, 1953). We cannot agree. Even among the mentally healthy, there is great variability. This range of fine variability for the most part recedes from efforts to objectify and measure it. Any quantitative variations can be attributed to random chance or accident.

The situation changes when we come to neurotic and psychopathological developments. The loss of certainty with regard to common sense in the various disorders can no longer be overlooked. Von Gebsattel (1954) and Goeppert (1960) have demonstrated that patients with obsessive–compulsive disorder do not place into question, doubt, enumerate, continuously monitor, and repeat those things that are usually taken as problematic by others. They concern themselves rather with "small, everyday things." These are things, which are normally taken as matter of course or "understood in themselves." They are things that a healthy common sense usually considers taken care of and does not bother with.[7] In 1938, Straus described "an insistent need to powerlessly question" in such patients, which emerges in the place of the spontaneous "being able to live one's day" (Straus 1960, 208). These patients require certainty in areas of life in which "mere opinion (doxa)" should prevail. Still, even in this example, our attempt to discover what is specific to the function of common sense remains incomplete. Therefore, we should turn in our analysis to even greater symptoms of loss of this function.

How does the function of common sense appear in the endogenous psychoses? Notably, we do not find a disturbance to common sense in cyclothymic patients. They experience, rather, an enveloping loss of affective relationships to their world, which is something different. On the contrary, we could ask whether patients with major depression are not, in their pre-morbid personality structure, too strictly attached to their common sense. Older psychoanalytic investigations, such as the one by Cohen, Baker, Cohen et al. (1954), support such a view. In any case, the preserving of this ability in cyclothymic patients is an important criterion for differential diagnosis with

---

[7] Blankenburg uses the German expression for common sense, *gesunder Menschenverstand*, for the first time in the essay. The German expression contains the word for "healthy" (*gesund*) and implies mental health in its ordinary usage. [**Translators' note**]

schizophrenic patients. In manic patients, the common sense of their wit enables an astonishing accuracy in their ability to provoke, even hurt those around them. Their manner of "coming too near" others and ability to "be on target" would not be possible without access to common sense and differentiates them from manic-form hebephrenic patients.

We will now turn to the other group of patients with endogenous psychoses: those with schizophrenia. In turning to schizophrenia, we enter the proper domain for the psychopathology of common sense. For example, Strindberg writes, "It is not the logic of the merely given that prevails here" (Inferno, 423). Or in another place, "This is not a matter of the proper things. It is not natural, not a logic of events" (Entzweit, Einsam, 85). It becomes clear that there is an abdication of common sense. (For a discussion of these matters and Strindberg's psychosis, see Binswanger 1963, 1965; Hofer 1968a, b.)

We are able to study the loss of this ability not only in paranoid psychoses. This loss is even more pronounced in the slow and insidious course of hebephrenic schizophrenia or schizophrenia simplex. This frequently begins with a barely noticeable decline in the ability "to take things in their right light." This subtle loss or atrophy precedes the emergence of other symptoms. What becomes striking for those around the patient is that there is a withering away of a sense of tact, a feeling for the proper thing to do in situations, a loss of awareness of the current fashions or what is "in," and a general indifference toward what might be disturbing to others.

We also find a loss of tact and shame in manic patients. This indicates, however, that when we use the same terms, we are actually meaning quite different things. Manic patients and, in a clearly different way, sociopathic as well as healthy individuals can all be tactless and shameless. Each of these groups may disregard the basic considerateness that others expect from them. Nevertheless, they are still in possession of what they disregard. This ignoring or disregarding is fundamentally different from the "clueless groping" of the hebephrenic patients.

It is not only the loss of the feeling for what is suitable, but also for what others may think, or what the situation demands. That is, there is a loss of the sense for what is nearest and what is less so. They lose a sense for what can be understood as a matter of course as determined "by the matter itself." This is all a matter of common sense. What first emerges for many patients is a being unable to play along with the rules of the game of interpersonal behavior. Conrad had described this as "trema" to indicate a prodromal stage of schizophrenia. The judgments, emotions, reactions, and actions, which thereby result, no longer have relationship to social reality.

This process can sometimes have effects in the sphere of sensory processing. For example, a young craftsman reports that "it" (referring to his illness) began in the following manner: He lost his sense of proportion at the same time that a nearby young girl lost her "taste" for a meal. Drawing upon Tellenbach's (1968) investigations of sense-psychology, we could make reference to Aristotle's definition of common sense by taking into account the ambiguity of the word "taste."

As far as judgement is concerned, it is less a matter of differentiating true from false than of distinguishing the probable from the improbable. Vico had emphasized that just as science is concerned with the truth, so common sense is concerned with the probable (verisimile). It is precisely those errors and derailments at the beginning of the hebephrenic psychoses that make evident for us the fact that the significance of the probable is in no way a deficient mode of cognition of what is true. Rather, the probable is encompassing and provides the basis for what is true, which is here meant in the sense of what is correct and demonstrable. Vico (1963, 27) described an "infima vera," the scope of which is not to be underestimated. The proper thing to do in life is to be judged according to the weight of the circumstances and things at hand and thus, it becomes a matter for common sense. This faculty should be developed in young people as early as possible so that they do not fall prey in later life to all kinds of deviancies and folly. Common sense is here viewed as the ability to put things in their proper place. Without this, all manner of correctness simply hangs in the air.

This brings us to the ancient distinction between logic and topos. This distinction becomes relevant when we examine the school essays of our hebephrenic patients before they fell ill. There is a frequent being off key when it comes to the topic (the topoi). This is the case although the logic remains intact, even if overemployed. In Husserl's sense, we are able to state: The formal logic is embedded in a "world-logic." The question about the manner of this embedding has the greatest interest for psychopathology.

The logic that we are talking about is a logic of the "life-world," to which common sense belongs.[8] To put it more precisely; the life-world is to a large extent nothing other than the intentional correlate of common sense.

It is not uncommon for the relatives of the patient to report that the illness began with the patient raising questions about "the most ordinary things." These are things, which, to the common sense of the healthy person, are the most obvious, naturally understood things in life. In contrast, the patients still manage to solve difficult, intellectually more demanding tasks without considerable effort. These are tasks, however, that do not require much interpretive skills. In this early stage, some patients retreat to the study of mathematics or physics. They try to replace the "natural successiveness or consistency" of experience that rests on common sense with what are sometimes more – and sometimes less – ingenious logical constructions.[9] These efforts are only temporarily successful. There follows a rigidity and consistency that is maintained with painstaking efforts. Binswanger (1956) has shown that such efforts result in a becoming "extravagant" (Verstiegenheit) and exhibiting highly mannered eccentricities.

One might think that all this might be easily established by psychological tests. But that is far from the case. The Wechsler Intelligence Test has little to say about the functioning of common sense. We have seen schizophrenic patients in our clinic who have a massive disturbance to common sense functioning and yet whose IQs exceed 130. The profile of subtests sometimes gives indications but not always. The Rorschach test is more informative but still lacks specificity. Recent efforts in clinical psychology to propose a hypothesis of "overinclusive thinking" still have not been particularly applicable in the practical domain but have considerable theoretical interest. (For reviews, see Payne [1966] and Fish [1966].) "Overinclusion" indicates a loss of contours in thinking, or to put it more precisely, a lack of the ability to distinguish between the relevant and the irrelevant. It would seem that the concept of relevance is a particularly tangible term, and for that reason, it is rarely reflected upon. What actually allows us to recognize something as relevant or irrelevant? Whatever this may be, it is, without question, not formal logic. It is also not some empirical criterion. On the other hand, however, it is also not something that is simply irrational, or purely dictated by feeling. We refer, rather, to what the older tradition describes as the "faculty of judgement," which in turn provides a basis for common sense.

So far, relatively simple methods of clinical investigation have proven to be most effective in investigating this problem. The patient, for example, is requested to retell fables, explain proverbs and sayings, interpret picture stories, etc. What is being examined in such procedures? I think that it is basically – although not exclusively – common sense. These procedures are usually conceptualized in terms of the search for the presence of a latent formal thought disorder. Every psychiatrist knows from experience that thought disorder only becomes a concern with the more severely disturbed patients. In such cases, Beringer (1924, 1926) described an abridgement of the patient's "scope of intentional arc." By way of contrast, in a still significant analysis of the father-and-son-image test with patients with schizophrenia, Kühn (1943) found an "impairment of the patient's cognitive sympathy function."

---

[8] For Husserl, the "life-world ... is the world that is concealed in the horizon of our shared humanity" and thus serves as "the continuous basis for our experience of validity, an always ready source for self-evident, taken for granted assumptions." (1954, 124). [Original note]

[9] Binswanger's concept of "natural consistency," which he developed in close relationship with the phenomenological philosopher, Szilasi, needs to be further developed both with regard to what he means by "natural" and by "consistency." What common sense actually preserves is the balance of what has been called by Binswanger the "anthropological proportions." This balance is maintained by dampening the tendency to ascend vertically in one's perspective. It also means not merging or melting into the horizontal dimension of existence. (We are now more readily able to understand the ambivalence of Goethe or Hegel towards common sense.) [Original note] This difficult but critical footnote for understanding Blankenburg's definition of common sense requires some clarification. It may help to cite a similar passage by the same author (Blankenburg 1971). In describing Descartes's methodological doubt and the inherent danger of losing common sense, Blankenburg writes that there is a "possible endangering of what Binswanger has called the 'anthropological proportions.' This is determined by the relationship between height and breadth. In relation to Descartes, this means: in order to accomplish the pure cogito he must ascend into isolating heights. This radically precludes the healthy habituality of natural experience" (1971, 66, my translation). [Translator's note]

In spite of his reference to the philosopher Max Scheler, who is known for his phenomenological studies of emotions and sympathy, however, the decisive question of how sympathy could have a "cognitive" component remains unresolved. Indeed, when dealing with a so-called disturbance of "empathy" (Einfuehlung) function in the actual patient, it is often impossible to decide whether the disorder is primarily one of thought or affect.

The very alternative of disturbance to cognition or affect is itself questionable. We find ourselves rather thrown up against what turns out to be a circular structure. One is able to say that in the ability to judge, feeling has become the organ of cognition. But even this formulation is not sufficient. Affectivity and the ability to judge, as we find it in common sense, refer back to an original unity of thinking, feeling, and willing in human existence, which is primarily related to an intersubjective world (mitweltbezogen).

In view of the above difficulties to put such structural abnormalities into objective form, the phenomenological analysis of the introspective descriptions of those patients who are able to give them remains the method of choice. Patients of the subtype, reflective schizophrenia simplex, are particularly suited to this purpose. Wyrsch (1940) was the first to describe and point out the theoretical importance of this disorder. Clinically, it is rare. From the 455 patients examined for this disorder in our clinic, only twenty-seven were in a prolonged condition of pronounced reflectiveness. Of this group, only five could be classified as having schizophrenia simplex.

The following are extracts taken from statements made by a twenty-year-old female patient. Following a serious suicide attempt, she was admitted to the Freiburg University Psychiatric Clinic:

"What is it that I am missing? It is something so small, but strange, it is something so important. It is impossible to live without it. I find that I no longer have footing in the world. I have lost a hold in regard to the simplest, everyday things. It seems that I lack a natural understanding for what is matter of course and obvious to others."

She then explains what she means:

"Every person knows how to behave, to take a direction, or to think something specific. The person's taking action, humanity, ability to socialize ... all these involve rules that the person follows. I am not able to recognize what these rules are. I am missing the basics ... It just does not work for me ... Each thing builds on the next ... I don't know what to call this ... It is not knowledge ... Every child knows these things! It is the kind of thing you just get naturally.

See, for instance, how difficult it has been for me. I was admitted to the clinic and everyday – how all this took place in this space – I tried to absorb how others, as people, behaved in front of me. I had to disappear like a child ... this just isn't normal. My soul is sick ... what else could it be?"

In order to take what is expressed in the patient's stammerings on its own terms, psychiatrists are required – according to Kisker (1960, 10) – to become more philosophical. This does not mean, however, that we need to interpret these statements metaphysically or engage in metaphysical speculation. Statements by patients such as the ones made above reveal, in a kind of immediacy, the conditions of possibility of our existence that otherwise remain concealed. The patient states that what she lacks is "something so small ... something so important. It is impossible to live without it." She herself considers it "strange" that something so small, something so unapparent, should prove to be so important and necessary for life. This amazement – born from a desperate perplexity – is our starting point. We must allow ourselves to be drawn into this amazement to fully comprehend the implications of such statements. The patient's stammering and struggle for words need not merely be seen as the expression of a thought disorder. It could be caused by the incapacity of our colloquial language to provide ways of expressing what, as it were, lies beneath such a disorder, that is, a pre-predicative, nameless understanding and communicating. This small and important thing, which the patient thinks that she lacks, is not only the knowledge of the naturally understood and matter-of-course things of everyday life, it is also the manner in which she understands things to be this way or that. The "what" and the "how" of this knowing are inextricably interrelated.

A twenty-four-year-old, male patient with schizophrenia clearly had something similar in mind when he wrote in a letter addressed "to a stranger":

"I do not know whether you are happy. Let us just put it this way so you will understand. Whom do you thank for this being – let us just call it – unburdened? Your childhood, your youth, your family? Perhaps. Your experience of protection and security, your being unburdened or your happiness are all indebted to something in relation to which you are barely conscious. It is this something which enables the being unburdened as well as these other things. It is what forms the first foundation."

What we find expressed more awkwardly and, therefore, seeming at first to be more genuine in the first patient, we find in more reflective and self-conscious form in the second. In terms of the matter described, the two descriptions really involve the same thing. With the consciously patronizing expression, "... well, let us just put it this way so you will understand ...", the second patient is indicating that he has something very specific in mind. Indeed, he continues, "This mysterious 'something' appears to obstinately oppose conscious awareness. It furnishes the greatest resistance – and this has its reasons." In his reflection about what he is missing, the patient is able to obtain essential (anthropological) insights into the human condition.

Our first patient spoke about "something so small." She lives in the belief that what she is missing is something entirely unapparent and worthy of disdain. She finds it hard to grasp that it should have such great importance. She says, "It is so small. One comes upon it, as it were, in passing. There is really not much in it. It is just naturally there as self-evident for everyone. Other things have much more importance." Then she says rather derogatorily, "It is just a matter of mere feeling, sensing what is appropriate. One has this from nature." That is, one should have it "from nature" as a tacit possession, as the necessary prerequisite to accomplishing one's daily tasks.

In the face of their experienced deficits, our patients assume a mask of seeming banality and disdain. Behind this mask they conceal how what is naturally obvious and self-evident for healthy persons has withdrawn from them and been denied them. Healthy common sense is based on this seeming natural obviousness. Kant (1799) writes, "Common human understanding, which, as mere healthy (not yet cultivated) understanding, which, as the least to be expected from anyone claiming to be human, has therefore the doubtful honor of being given the name of 'common sense' (sensus communis); and in such a way that by the name 'common' (not merely in our language, where the word actually has a double signification, but in many others), we understand 'vulgar,' that which is everywhere met with, the possession of which indicates absolutely no merit or superiority." (156–67). But this is precisely what our patients are

missing. They state over and over again that they are missing the most banal and mundane of things.

Our female patient states, "It is such a strange feeling, when one does not even know the simplest of things." Indeed, these are, seen objectively, the simplest of things which seem to slip away from her: how to behave in certain situations, how to dress, how to grapple with everyday problems, how to speak with the people one meets, or what one is supposed to think about them, and so on. It was possible, however, to discuss with her abstract, theoretical questions about her experience in an unimpeded and rather differentiated manner.

Let us take a concrete example. The patient asks herself which dress she should wear for a particular occasion. This becomes a tortured asking herself which material the dress should have. She tries to make clear to herself up to the smallest detail why it should be precisely this color and this material for this occasion. It is quite easy to see how this becomes an endless undertaking. After all, the particular qualities that one finds pleasing in the material of a dress are, in part, complexly determined by processes of social judgment. We should not suppose that it is possible to completely analyze – i.e., without remainder – these processes into their component parts. We may attempt to enumerate them by listing the bourgeois conventions, prevailing fashions, striking aesthetic qualities, possible relevant personal memories, one's will to have a personal style, personal preferences, and so on. These are precisely the kind of experiences that becomes problematic for her. They are also the kind of experiences that resist being subsumed under unambiguous, rational definition. They are based on assumptions, which are rooted in the interpersonal, intersubjective realm. They are a matter of a certain delicacy and subtlety of feeling.

In this regard, it is interesting to read in Kant (1799): "Taste can be called sensus communis with more justice than sound (healthy) understanding can ... aesthetic rather than intellectual judgment may bear this name of a sense common to all" (160). Vico, Shaftesbury, and others had already made suggestive statements in this direction. At the beginning of the twentieth century, Simmel (1909, 26) employed the term "imitation" to indicate "the transition from the group into the individual's life." He developed this concept especially for its application to fashion. He wanted to grant to practical life the same kind of feelings of satisfaction that one experiences in theoretical thinking. The experience of transition to individual life by means of imitation in fashion might be likened to the feeling of satisfaction one experiences when subsuming the individual appearance under the general concept. Our patients, however, are unable to take any solace in such feelings of satisfaction. The ability to dwell healthily in a habitual and customary world is based on the ability to be consoled in this way (Wyrsch 1949). The healthiness of common sense rests on habituality. The natural self-evidence of everyday existence draws its nourishment from just such a habituality.

We are now confronted in our analysis by the problem of the relationship between the logical and the social significance of what is universal or presumably common to each individual. We must ask how can that which has been found to be generally valid for those who belong to a particular ethnic and cultural group be built, as it were, into the particular person's spontaneous understanding of things and integrated into the personality? This same commonality is to be found again on the outside of the person with a certain independence as taken for granted and naturally self-evident in the person's social environment. We may ask how the person from this basis in common sense (which spontaneously emerges as naturally self-evident within the person) comes to be an individual, i.e., taking an independent position in the world. The unity between common sense and being an individual is a natural developmental process in the healthy person. For many of our patients as we have seen, however, this whole process becomes problematic. As a result, they constantly alternate between a stereotyped assuming of maxims taken from their environment and an autistic retreat into themselves.

It would certainly be an error to assume that this could be explained in these patients as a morbid relationship to self, what Conrad identifies as a "cramp" in the ability to reflect. On the contrary, things would improve for such patients if only they could reflect less. When this was suggested to our female patient, she responded vehemently:

"One always measures oneself in terms of other people ... Everybody does that. This goes on unnoticed in others" [i.e., in healthy people]. "What I am talking about everyone does or has done at one time. It is what one calls a developed sensitivity or feeling for situations. Everybody needs it."

Our patient refers to a basic need to compare. The healthy person has it as part of an available repertoire,

what Heidegger (1927) calls an "a priori perfect" (in the Latin sense of what is already accomplished). The patient makes this very clear by constantly stating how strange it is that she is missing this ability to compare:

"This is what is so strange for me. What is missing for me is even more fundamental than what is missing for others. Many people do not know how to dress well. Even if they know that they do not have any taste, they are not particularly bothered by it. But I am missing something even more fundamental. These people do not even sense the necessity of common sense because they do not lack it. They simply have common sense. Then they are able to put two and two together. It is no longer so critical for them. They are able to create a connection with others and enter a realm in which everything functions from itself. Then, one is able to find a way. Then, it is natural and obvious. One is unable to live without it." In despair, she continues: "Without it, one cannot manage at all!"

Kant (1799) writes, "But under the sensus communis we must include the idea of a sense common to all, i.e., of a faculty of judgment which, in its reflection, takes account (a priori) of the mode of presentation of all other persons in thought, in order, as it were, to compare its judgment with the collective reason of humanity" (157; translation by Bernard 1951, 136, slightly modified).

In contrast to this, our patient complains, "I have no inner standard of comparison by which I could see whether I am able to sympathize with others." This is in marked contrast to that which bears an a priori character in the healthy person. As an inner, or respectively, internalized standard, it serves as an indispensable basis for being able to place oneself in the other person's position. It also serves as the presupposition for judgments shared with others, which have a universal character. For our patients, however, this is accomplished each day anew only with the greatest effort.

Blankenburg, W. (1965), 'On the differential phenomenology of delusional perception: a study of an abnormal significant experience'

From (1965) Zur Differentialphänomenologie der Wahnwahrnehmung. *Nervenarzt* 36: 285–98. Translated by M. Symmons (2009).

Editors' commentary

Blankenburg states that he will address 'The most exciting issue', namely, 'how to differentiate between "healthy" and "sick"'. He laments that these two terms are often taken uncritically from 'pre-scientific experience' and used further without being given the necessary scrutiny in psychiatric research and practice. Blankenburg's bold aim is to use 'phenomenological explanation' to distinguish between normal and pathological. He describes in rich detail the commonalities between a patient's experience of delusional perception and a poet's transforming experience – the latter he sees conveyed in a poem by Rilke. However, do Blankenburg's attempts to distinguish between the two experiences escape preconceived notions of what is poetic experience and what is psychiatric symptomatology?

Müller-Suur begins his work on "Schizophrenia as Event"[10] with the sentence: "Every psychiatrist is familiar from the descriptions of schizophrenic patients with those events that in a flash can fundamentally change the meaning of a person's life. Their fleeting nature means that their meaning largely escapes one's grasp, but nonetheless, grounded in these events, as madness, as 'in-sanity', is the new meaning of a life changed in its very essence."

The following is a discussion of the nature of such eventful experiences and the manner in which they descend on a person. In psychopathological terms, they can take quite different forms. They do not by any means have to bear the mark of delusional perception; yet it is in this form that they stand out particularly strikingly. For that reason it makes sense to use the example of a delusional perception to investigate what it is that in accordance with its nature strives to escape "its meaning being grasped". The subject matter almost inevitably calls for a phenomenological approach. Of course, the phenomenological methodology can be defined as just that practice of aiming to describe in visible terms and thereby making accessible to research those things that escape definition in the scientific cognitive process of unreflective objectivisation. The nature of this form of "escape" is itself an urphenomenon,[11] something that phenomenology is concerned with. The methodological foundations of phenomenology must be presumed here.

However, another question also arises in relation to this task: are there not also healthy people who experience "events that in a flash can fundamentally change the meaning of a person's life"? There is, for example, much scope for consideration in the field of the psycho (patho) logy of conversion.[12] It is true that it is generally not difficult for psychiatric experts, for the so-called clinical gaze – if necessary with the help of the observation of process – to make the necessary distinctions by way of the individual symptoms and the overall impression, in other words, to commit to conclusive diagnoses. But do we really fully understand the criteria that we generally accept uncritically as given?

Time and again the question arises as to whether or to what extent the phenomenological approach could gain in importance in daily clinical routine, and in particular for differential diagnostic questions. Of those who have expressed positive views on this matter, mention must be made above all of J. Wyrsch. He was already attempting over 15 years ago to demonstrate how phenomenological existential analytical experiences and insights could be used productively in the clinic. It is certainly possible to have theoretical misgivings about this practice, and whilst these might not actually rule out the diagnostic relevance of phenomenological experiences, they do allow us to question its premises. It is by no means clear if what the phenomenologist extrapolates as the unique Eidos and what he tries then to make discernable as the Logos of the appearance was without further ado equal to the clinical pathological entities, which direct our diagnoses – or even with pathogenic and aetiological wider boundaries, which in terms of causal research may turn out to be necessary. The cleft that opens up here originates in the different points of departure. The existential analytical phenomenological approach on the one hand and the conditional analytical approach on the other presuppose methodologically opposing developmental directions; yet sooner or later their paths must cross. Where, at which points, and how has not as yet been established.

The most exciting issue is how to differentiate between "healthy" and "sick". These terms are taken uncritically from pre-scientific experience and although diversely articulated and at some

---

[10] "Psychopathology Today", Commemorative Publication for K. Schneider, Stuttgart 1962, p. 81ff. [**Original note**]

[11] Literally a 'primary phenomenon'. [**Editors' note**]

[12] Cf. among others Weitbrecht 1948, Heimann 1956 and 1961. [**Original note**]

points even fundamentally questioned in the process of objectively directed research, this is not done in any sort of scientifically transparent or even scientifically based way.[13] All findings that relate to the morbidity of an event – whether or not this involves specific theories about disorders or defects in certain mechanisms – necessarily remain dependent on the pre-scientific experience of the human being as a whole. It is important to stress the importance of this fact, since it is so self-evident it is easy to overlook, and in fact it indicates the place at which phenomenological investigations must begin.

In the field of psychopathology the claims made in the pre-scientific [pre-operational] understanding of the subject – particularly in questions relating to the clinical diagnostics of schizophrenia – were allowed to stand for longer than in other areas. To some extent they still do. A well-known example of this is the "praecox feeling" or "praecox experience" (Rümke). If one looks at the publications relating to this from recent years, one does become aware of a tendency to restrict this concept to within scientific perimeters. Nevertheless, as a survey carried out by Irle has revealed, the concept does still play a considerable role in day-to-day clinical psychiatry, along with other terms such as "glass wall", "schizophrenic cold", "curtain", and similar roundabout descriptions that come from the nuanced impressionability of pre-scientific consciousness. The expert knows how to handle these ideas, and the canny diagnostician can give himself a significant qualitative advantage by mastering them. But the more one tries to elevate what is meant in these descriptions to the level of an actual symptom, the more it eludes diagnostic application. In the end all that is left as a formal indication is what Müller-Suur calls "definitive unintelligibility", the abstract acuteness of which is sacrificed to the fullness of its content. It is the task of the phenomenologists to give a more clear definition of what is meant by "definitive" in relation to this "unintelligibility"; in other words, it is important to find a corresponding intentional correlative even for the negative forms of "intelligibility", and where possible to illustrate/demonstrate them. … It is a question of using these subtleties that are to a great extent still part of the clinical diagnostician's repertoire of instinctive feeling, and developing them in such a way that they can be made to bear fruit as the source of phenomenological understanding of character. For that, what is needed is an articulation of terms that do not only formally define and register characteristics – that would be the task if it were a case of furthering classical psychopathology [descriptions of signs and symptoms] – but that are also able to turn these nuanced, but vague, impressions into an equally differentiated concept. … The ability to be competent with both experience and with terminology, to be familiar with both facts and character, these things are in a relationship of mutual concealment but also of dependency. Instead of playing them off against one another, what is needed is to bring them into a mutual relationship whereby each is furthered and intensified by the other. But it is difficult to further both these sides at the same time. The principle aim of the following discussion is the clarification of an eidetic concept [i.e. this is an investigation of a clinical phenomenological kind rather than a clinical psychopathological kind].

It is in this sense that an attempt is made at a "differential phenomenology". This stands in a similar relationship to differential diagnosis as the whole phenomenological existential analytical research does to clinical psychopathology. Any transposition in one direction or another brings with it certain problems that cannot be debated here.[14]

Out of the host of psychopathological occurrences, delusional perception is here selected as an example – in fact as an extreme pathological example – of an eventful irruption into the natural self-world-relationship of "healthy normality" (Wyrsch). Delusional perception has always been viewed as particularly characteristic of

---

[13] This paradox, that the scientifically orientated field of medicine always presupposes, but never actually pins down, its most inherent theme (the difference between healthy and sick), is principally to be found in the nature of it as an unreflexively objectivising single science. Heidegger (1954) established this paradox as the "non-appearing content" which pervades and defines the character of all modern science. – This has always been sensed and expressed by individual researchers, for example when the pathologist G. Ricker demanded in a methodologically systematic manner that the concept of disease should actually be eliminated from pathology. [Original note]

[14] Wherever the terms healthy, sick, abnormal, schizophrenic etc. appear in the following discussion, they should actually be placed in inverted commas to make it clear that they are not to be understood as naively employed predicates of clinical empiricism but simply as the main threads of a phenomenological investigation of an eidetic nature. [Original note]

schizophrenia. K. Schneider described it as a "primary symptom" [or first rank symptom]. Despite many objections, it is generally still seen as such in normal clinical situations.

It is not possible to spend time here setting out an historical account of the term, but we can remember the foundational descriptions which Jaspers applied to the abnormal consciousness of meaning; Gruhle's rightly controversial general definition of delusion ("delusion of reference with no cause"); K. Schneider's emphasis on the two-part nature of delusional perception; and further, the gestalt-psychological and gestalt-analytical approaches of Matussek and Conrad as well as Kulenkampff's work on the anthropological meaning of delusional perception as an expression of a disturbance related to the order of the world around or a "loss of position" ... Without entering into any debate with these numerous approaches and theories, the following discussion will nevertheless take them into account. Its aim is to contrast the particular delusional perception of a schizophrenic patient and a liminal experience in a healthy mind, and thereby to discuss some issues relating to the phenomenological constitution of inner life in a healthy and a sick form.

In order to undertake an analysis of the modes of being, the first approach will be to give preference to examples that most clearly illuminate the diversity within what is to be distinguished. However, should the phenomenological approach prove successful not only in working out general structures but also in making further differentiations, then it is better to choose examples where the differences are less obvious or even prove to be problematic. Therefore, the first description will be of the delusional perception of a sick person, emphasising those moments that could still be partly understood from the perspective of the limit experiences of the healthy person. Then, as a comparison, an example from the borderline of normal inner life will be set alongside this, one that appears to share significant characteristics with the psychotic syndrome. By accentuating what is close to psychotic in the healthy mind and what can be sensed as normal in the psychological makeup of the psychotic, we do not need to obliterate the borders between the two. Rather, this method can act as a device to win phenomenological ground, from where the modes of being can perhaps be worked out in a more precise, differentiated and phenomenologically based manner.

The central psychotic experience in the clinical history of the 21-year-old plumber Albrecht M. will serve as a good example of a delusional perception:

It is known from the family history that the father was killed in the war in 1944, when the patient was 6 years old. – During the menopause, the mother temporarily suffered from a psychosis, which according to the clinical history from the Psychiatric State Hospital of Emmendingen was "characterised by thought blocking, alien thoughts, acoustic hallucinations, persecution complexes with sporadic attacks of extreme anxiety".... After pressure from relatives, she was allowed to return home with a "tolerable improvement noted". In her opinion she was only completely cured some weeks later "by hormone injections given by the family doctor". The patient was at that time 17 years old. The mother had felt well since then and had had no further attacks ... In the rest of the family, there was no history of any nervous or dispositional condition.

The patient grew up as the only child of this woman, who had been widowed at a young age. Something of a "stay-at-home" and "mummy's boy", as he himself admitted during the exploration, he had nevertheless not been a loner, but by virtue of his warm-hearted, good-natured temperament had always had many friends. He was described by his mother as a happy, lively, occasionally even boisterous child. – The birth was a difficult one. When the patient came into the world he was "blue" and "appeared dead". Apart from the usual childhood illnesses, swollen glands, tonsillitis, there is no record of any more serious illnesses. – The emotional development seemed to have proceeded in a harmonious and unremarkable manner. It was only the lack of a father and the adverse post-war conditions that were cause for any suffering. In school he was extremely assiduous and always one of the best. This obviously stemmed not so much from over-ambition as from a genuine interest in various subjects, above all in the natural sciences. From a young age he had a tendency to brood over difficult fundamental issues and was by then obviously already recognised as a thinker by his school friends.

After leaving school he completed an apprenticeship with Daimler-Benz, where he had a good relationship with his colleagues and superiors. Whilst it is true that he was more critical to those above him than his peers were, in general he was, as he said himself, still "a bit of a ruffian" at that time. He passed his final apprentice examination with very good grades, and managed to qualify additionally as a welder.

*****

At the time of the admission for treatment the patient was 21 years old. He had been complaining for 3 or 4 years of occasional stomach pains, which had been assumed to be "welder gastritis", related to his job . . . These gastric complaints later carried imperceptibly over into the preliminary hypochondriac stage of the incipient psychosis. More obvious symptoms only appeared in the last half a year before admission. These consisted predominantly of hallucinations of an acoustic and physical nature: of a monotonous humming in the ears, changing between different frequencies, for which the patient – without exactly stipulating this – sought physical explanations; in addition they consisted of "waves" that he experienced passing through his body. At the same time a striking change, described in very differentiated terms by the patient, had occurred in his spatial and "optical" experience, which cannot be gone into in any more detail here.

Among the psychotic experiences that appeared subsequently, one was absolutely central. Whilst it must not be described as the initial experience – too much had already happened before it – in the following period it achieved such a central position that one can say that in the patient's understanding this one experience tore his whole biography into two parts, a before and an after. Everything in his life subsequent to it was lived, viewed and valued in the light of this one single experience. His experience serves as a particularly clear example of what Müller-Suur calls "schizophrenia as event". As it also portrays a delusional perception, it seems particularly suitable for the purposes of our task.

As the psychosis intensified, the patient was referred by his family doctor to a neurologist in Baden-Baden. There, as he entered the building, he caught sight of a picture in the back courtyard that captivated and compelled him from the first moment he set eyes on it, and from then on did not loose its hold over him. For a while he could scarcely talk of anything else. Again and again he would become caught up in what could be called eulogistic descriptions of this picture and of what he had experienced in relation to it. He could never have enough of it.

According to the description that he gave in various versions, partly in written form, this picture hung "perfectly discreetly" between other pictures in the back courtyard. There were frames all over the place, just as if it was a perfectly normal workshop where pictures were framed per order. However, he had known immediately that it was a picture of a sick soul hung up to convince a sick person that he was also sick. It was the "prognosis of a soul", to his mind, "conceived by Dr. X. or internationally". The picture had simultaneously influenced and disturbed him. Previously, he said, he had never "thought about the soul or anything like that". But now suddenly it had become clear to him that he was mentally ill. – He elaborated at great length what he understood by the term "prognosis of the soul", namely something along the lines of a specifically projective test; a test that did not only make manifest the fact that there was a mental illness, but that also had an effect in reality. For he felt from then on that he was "bound" to the picture – or more accurately, to its colours, above all to the blue with its strangely shimmering effect; this seemed to be so "endless". He could not rave about it enough. – His relationship to the picture was strangely ambivalent; on the one hand he felt absolutely drawn to it, fascinated by it, but on the other hand, at the same time – indeed essentially as a result of feeling so bound to it – uncomfortably influenced by it. He felt as if he were being dazzled by the hues of the picture in both a positive and a negative sense.

When he stepped into Dr. X.'s waiting room after seeing the picture in the yard, he felt as if he were being stared at by the other patients in a very strange manner. The thought came to him that perhaps "they were also bound to the picture". A panic attack with heavy sweating drove him outside. He hurried home and took to his bed for 3 days. – After that he had become "more scientific". At home he had even looked up "sensuality" ["Sinnlichkeit"] and "psychiatry" and seen from the content of what he had read that he must be mentally ill. In fact, though, the realisation of this change in him had already hit him as he stood in front of the picture during his visit to Dr. X.

What was the nature of the patient's own experience of being changed? He talked of being bound to the picture or to the colours of the picture. Because he was compelled to think constantly about these colours, the rest of the world felt insipid and empty to him – insofar as it did not remind him of the glimmering luminosity of those colours. The expression "bound" had become a solid terminus for him, a way, so he believed, of describing his condition in the most succinct manner. He understood it to mean not a coincidental nor temporary connection, but one which would of necessity demonstrate how fundamentally senseless it was to try to escape or free himself from the picture. To him, this connection represented a complete deprivation of power of the self; he suffered terribly from it and considered it to be abnormal. Nevertheless, it also possessed the character of finality for him. He often referred to how he was bound to the picture with the word "suggestion" and compared this notion to the influence an Indian fakir might wield – he himself had once been present at such an event – over a crowd of people as he suggested whole scenes to them. When asked if he felt in any way spiritually connected to the picture, his reply was serious and emphatic: "No, not spiritually, but organically!" With these words he gave expression to the incredible facticity that the connection held for him. These words expressed something we describe as being endogenous or processual – almost in a form of self-interpretation – with a conciseness and succinctness we have rarely heard otherwise from a patient. Any other attitude other than this absolute fatalism in response to such a feeling of being "bound" was unthinkable to M. He described arrestingly how the rest of the world lost its radiance when compared with the intensity of this experience: "Earlier I felt as if everything was more alive, but now it feels like I am being displaced, as if something were brushing past." Prior to that, he had been interested by everything that occurred, but now all that was just a "brief moment, nothing but a passing incident", and so forth. Only the picture continued to hold anything of interest for him; in his eyes nothing else could coexist with it.

Before he was discharged, when all the other psychotic symptoms were for the most part already fading into the background, he still spoke about his altered "attitude" to the world and still expressed a preference for his "illusions" (those engendered by the picture); these were just too beautiful for words, he said, and he could not cope with them. For a brief period only, he succeeded in undertaking a type of double bookkeeping, in silent resignation. After his discharge from the clinic he returned home and carried on working at his old workplace, as before. As the mother later reported, however, he soon started complaining again that he was having difficulties concentrating; he increasingly shut himself off

from the world around him, and in an unguarded moment committed suicide.

Let us concentrate entirely on that one psychotic experience described above. It is a typical case of delusional perception. We hear about a picture hanging quite discreetly, indeed "perfectly discreetly", in a framing workshop. The patient saw it – and this is surely no coincidence – on the way to an appointment with the neurologist. As is so often the case, here the way that something not conspicuous becomes conspicuous is a first important signal of the world "losing its innocence", and represents the first approach towards the schizophrenic metamorphosis of the world. Things appear to be unmoored from their everyday referential connections, emptied of meaning or overloaded with strange new meanings that the sick person feels at the mercy of. This experience has often been described and does not need to be discussed again here.

When the patient was asked what had been so remarkable about the picture, the answer would be something like this: it had been the shimmering of the blue,[15] there was something "so endless" about it, "as endless as the universe!". There was something so quiet and serene within it that had spoken to him, something "so eternal"; it was "greater than everything" that he had seen or experienced up to that point. From then on he was unable to escape this picture, it was like "paradise". His discussion of it always circled around a few particular expressions, and with these he attempted to encapsulate everything that made him harried, and that made him feel like he had been struck by a spell and overwhelmed. Often he would summon a form of lyrical pathos to his aid, which did not seem to be put on in any way. A number of phrases meant to bring out what was unnatural or supernatural about the picture were used almost identically over and over again. He constantly stressed the fact that the real impression had come not

---

15 It is perhaps not entirely coincidental that it was the colour blue that had this effect. Goethe writes about the sensory-moral effect of blue: "This colour has a remarkable and almost inexpressible effect on the eyes. As a colour it is an energy; but it is a negative energy and in its absolute purity it is simultaneously an alluring nothingness. The sight of it engenders a conflicting sense of allure and quiet . . . " (Theory of Colours 779). "Thus we enjoy looking at blue, not because it presses itself upon us, but because it pulls us after it" (781). [Original note]

so much from what had been painted but far more from how it had been painted. The luminescence of the colours, the shimmering blue, had taken him captive.

It was therefore far more difficult to find out from the patient anything about what was represented on the picture than about its painterly qualities. All the details of the picture had to be virtually dragged out of him. According to his description, it depicted a brown girl with flowers, floating on a blue background: around this girl – as "the chosen one" were grouped some other girls and dark-skinned servants. It was not possible to ascertain the composition of the picture with any clarity.[16] The girl looked, in his words, like a "Hawaii girl". He had already heard some things about the South Pacific; the girls there were "morally corrupt". An element of expectancy, something like "temptation", resided in the picture. It may well have excited him, he said, but in a way that was quite different from, say, his response to pictures of girls in magazines. In that case it is "worldly", but here "unnatural", since the girl is floating on a blue background. The blue suggests something gaseous, and that is not natural; whereby he began talking about the qualities of the colours again. It was clear that for him the whole impression had merged into something representing the promise of fullness itself.

At the same time, he said that because he was "naturally" bound to the picture, he could not find his way to the girl, he could not reach her. That is why he was here. The patient's statements appeared to contradict one another. At one moment he seemed to be describing the effect of the picture as sensual and sexual, at the next supersensory, disconnected from the earth, and supernatural. What was fascinating for him was clearly the coincidence of the two. His descriptions vaguely recalled the representation of the song of the sirens in the Odyssey or the sensual over-sensuousness of some mystics . . . .

When he could not find an answer to the question of what exactly was so special about the painting, he would say that it was the art that had had such a singular, irresistible and overwhelming effect on him. It was clear that the word "art" had thereby taken on a quite specific, numinous meaning for the patient. He was obviously attempting to use the word to capture what was emanating from the picture as picture. He spoke of art as if it were an independent, substantial being, which in the face of the picture had overwhelmed him, taken him captive and monopolised him forever. It had struck him as "strange", although he had already seen a lot of art, read books about the subject and even bought a painting from a Nuremberg artist (in a young man of his background such an interest would surely have been quite unusual). Nevertheless, when he talked so seriously and emphatically about the "art" overwhelming him, one did not get the impression that what he understood by it was really qualitatively different to what a healthy person would understand by the same thing: namely, in broad terms, that it gives illusory form to real elements, reveals the illusory as true essence and so allows the deeper unity of the two to be illuminated in the work of art.

Asked in more detail what he meant by "art", the patient said that painting represented a "glorification", although he was hardly able to say what it was that was being glorified. He would simply return over and over again to the shimmering blue, in which he felt its "supernatural" quality to be concentrated. The picture signified a "glorification" in itself; no explanation was deemed necessary. It made no sense to him to be asked any further question.

*****

This . . . character of revelation to be found both in human nature and in the nature of all appearances has been seen elsewhere, too. Of the poets, after Hölderlin it was above all Rilke who was affected by it. When we therefore place alongside our sick person's experience of "art" one that is similar from the normal psychological range, it is no coincidence that it is a poem by Rilke on which we draw.

. . . It was a question of selecting a particular type of poetic statement, one which manages to embody the phenomenal aspect of being overwhelmed by the essence of art and go some way to unravelling what is compressed into the phenomenological analysis. This task is particularly suited to a poet like Rilke, whose concern is to "say things", in other words, to find a way of expressing things that appear in language in an essentially transparent manner.

The poem reads as follows:

Archaic Torso of Apollo
We did not know his legendary head
With eyes ripening like fruit. But
His torso glows still like a candelabrum
In which his gaze, though dimmer now,

---

[16] It is possible that the picture in question is a Gauguin reproduction. [**Original note**]

Is held steady and shines. Otherwise the curve
Of the breast could not blind you, and in the soft turn
Of the loins a smile could not cross
To that point deep within, where new life springs.

Otherwise this stone would stand defaced, hacked short
Under the shoulders, transparent as they drop,
And would not glimmer like the skin of a wild beast;

And would not break out of all its boundaries
Like a star; for there is no place
Which does not see you. You must change your life.

Each declaration in the poem is strongly orientated towards the end. The sentence "for there is no place which does not see you" concisely summarises the elements that have previously been described in detail, one after another, giving each individual phrase its relative importance in the whole poem. In this sentence it becomes clear why the eyes are significant right at the beginning ("We did not know his legendary head, with eyes ripening like fruit"). Only because he failed each time he tried to treat the torso like any other thing, only because the observer becomes the one observed from the very start, can he ask where the gaze comes from that overwhelms and penetrates his being with such force. Since he does not find the head with the eyes ripening like fruit, the poet than scans the stone, looking to see where this immense power of the gaze is coming from. With the exception of the final sentence, the whole poem depicts nothing other than the arduous attempt to trace the point where the gaze could have been "dimmed". The poet goes into detail about the "glow" and "shine" of the torso as a whole: he is blinded by the curve of the breast, a smile dazzles him in the turn of the loins, there is a glimmering on the surface of the stone, an explosion like flashing stars from the limits of his own self, until finally he sums it all up with: "for there is no place which does not see you". The gaze strikes him from all angles. The torso is not simply the remains of an artificially cut stone, which one could observe with a connoisseur's expression, but rather from out of the being embodied within it there streams forth a power encapsulating human existence in its overwhelming entirety; the power of "beautiful semblance", as one would have called it in the classical period.

*****

The appearance of essence becomes a glance and this essential glance meeting the observer is experienced . . .

as one that does not just look . . . but looks through us and exposes us. Firstly there is an overwhelming surge, a physiognomic impression of power in the form of a "penetrating gaze" and then, the consequence leading directly from it: "You must change your life".

Each of the five words in this sentence can be made the focus of emphasis, lending it a different meaning each time: this ambiguity is what gives it its peculiarly shifting character . . . Only by hearing the combination of all the different possible emphases does the full meaning of this command emerge, with the pressing force of a categorical imperative: "You must change your life". (It could also have read "man, become your essence!" or in the words of the Delphic Apollo, which Rilke must surely have had in mind: "Know thyself".)

Let us for a moment envisage the situation described from the narrower perspective of a psychiatrist in the process of exploration. Then, it seems, the situation presents itself in the following way: someone is walking around amongst the antique sculptures in the Louvre, looking at the variously dated pieces of art that have been excavated. Suddenly he stops in front of an early archaic torso and – there – he is suddenly somehow "different". He feels unexpectedly as if he is being looked at by this headless torso, looked at through and through, yes, looked through. He believes that he has been "blinded", thinks that he can detect a smile in the area of the missing genitalia, sees the boundaries "breaking", is overwhelmed by a glimmering sensation. And not only that! This glance emanating from the torso flashes through him with the sudden certainty: you must change your life. The historical continuity of life seems to have been abruptly broken apart. An event has occurred which has introduced something new into the life of the observer. – Seen thus, the psychiatrist can say: what is that if not a delusional perception? According to Kurt Schneider, two things happen: someone sees a normal Greek torso – apparently no differently from any other visitors – and all at once he feels as if it is looking at him and he is pervaded with the certainty that he must change his life. Is that not a "delusion of reference with no cause" (Gruhle), the "ultimately rationally and emotionally incomprehensible path" of a delusional perception (K. Schneider)? . . . Are there really any significant differences from the experience of the sick person who felt art revealing its essence in the shimmering blue of the picture? And if so, what do they consist of?

By rendering the poem profane in the prose language of the psychopathologist, the content is clearly subject to considerable distortion. The description has deliberately been somewhat exaggerated as a way of provoking and demonstrating how difficult it is to make essential differences sufficiently comprehensible within the conceptual range of psychopathology, even when these differences appear to be perfectly obvious to experts in the field of psychiatry and to the clinical gaze.

*****

If one looks first of all at what the two examples have in common, the following points of comparison can be identified: both times it is the intrinsic appearance of a work of art, of art itself which descends upon existence with an overwhelming impression of power, threatening to displace and capture it. What is imposing itself in each case is a piece of world that in the process of appearing has managed to acquire substance and autonomy through the power of the gaze.

*****

What this is about in essence is a transformation of the whole relationship between self and world. That is why both of these people, the sick person and the poet alike, experience alongside the change in the external world a simultaneous transformation of their own self – of their inner-worldly state. In response, both are not only capable of reflecting on this, but they also see in this event nothing less than the culmination of the whole event. The transformation of the constitution of the world in the consciousness therefore indicates – in both these cases for the person experiencing the event as well – a change in the constitution of the self. It is not only the over-powerful physiognomy pressing in – the supernatural shimmering of the blue or the god Apollo – which informs the experience, but rather it is the fact that the manner of the physiognomisation sinks deep into the mind, and leads the attention back to the one experiencing it himself. In other words, it is not the external experience but the experience of the self formed in this experience which is crucial both for the poet and for the patient. The interlocking of the transformation of the constitution of the world and the constitution of the self is what defines the character of the event taking place here.

And so for the patient the picture does not have the meaning that the world is about to end, that a great happiness is about to befall him, or that he should do this thing or that thing, but rather that he is mentally ill. The fact that the picture gives the patient the immediate certainty that he is mentally ill is what sets our example apart from other common delusional perceptions. What is particular about this case is that the subject matter of the patient's delusional perception is ultimately his own altered state. Its content, the significance of which weighs heavily on the patient, is not, say, the imminent end of the world or some other numinous event, whether it be of a terrible or uplifting nature. The picture leads him rather above all to the understanding that he is mentally ill. This is the certainty that it dictates to him. Formulated in more exaggerated terms, the dialectic consists in the fact that the abnormal meaning of this awareness of meaning purports to its own abnormality. The manner in which the picture signifies this to the patient is invested with such intensity and revelatory character that he feels exposed to the whole world. It is not just he who is aware of being changed, but the whole world. The picture is in his eyes thus a "prognosis of a soul"; one, however, that does not simply make manifest once and for all that he is mentally ill, but which at the same time also exerts a corresponding effect on him. For in his eyes the illness consists precisely of the fact that he feels himself "bound" to this picture. – The impression of being overpowered, laid bare, exposed, the experience of the abnormality of being affected in this way, feeling at the mercy of something else, disempowered, and therefore bound: all these sensations are intimately linked to one another. In his perception of the picture the patient believes that he has been imprinted with the mark of mental illness, not only in an ideal sense, but also in a real one. One can view the individual moments in this interrelationship as elements of an interlocking, self-sufficient Gestalt-circle (V. Weizsäcker). Therein is founded the strangely shifting, uncontoured condition, rupturing all discursiveness, which the patient was able to understand well enough to articulate clearly in his own descriptions. The interplay and interaction of the individual moments of the Gestalt-circle are in themselves enough to reveal the relative stability of the whole experiential complex. The manner in which all discursiveness is ruptured, allowing a new relationship between self and world to be established, can be used to define and clarify more precisely the specific nature of the "definitive unintelligibility" (Müller-Suur) of this psychological event.

We do not often come across cases of schizophrenics where a perception of illness or – if one would prefer to call it that – even an insight into an illness appears to be integrally part of the delusional experience in this way, although this does occur more often than one may think if one does not specifically look out for it. The benchmark of the healthy person, according to which the morbidity of the transformation can be measured, is here unusually integrated into the psychosis. In M.'s case, the capacity to transcend his condition went so far that despite all his psychotic enthusiasm for the picture he could still with tears in his eyes innocently lament how "childish" – in other words "mentally ill" – he had become. Even that was something that he reflected upon still further: the patient, in amazed incomprehension, said that he could not grasp how his "brain was able to understand anything about psychology" (that is, understand what was going on with him) "and still be mentally ill". This aspect of the case is something that raises a problem for the patient and for psychopathological research alike.

Is it possible to come by way of this special case to the bold conclusion that a certain perception of one's own transformation is a constitutive moment of each delusional perception, even in those cases where it seems far less tangible than in our example? Is this something that is simply more concealed and less clearly expressed in other patients? Does the delusional perception necessarily involve a consciousness deep within of one's own transformation, in such a manner that it also in some way becomes constitutive of the eventfulness of this happening? If these questions could be answered in the affirmative, then the constitution of the delusional perception would also include the more or less latent self-experience of the patient of his own transformation.

*****

As with the sick person, for the poet the eventful experience does not result in the certainty about some objective fact, for example about the origin of the torso or about Greek art, but it is the order "you must change your life", which is communicated to him through the work of art. What strikes the observer with such visual intensity is actually not so much and not only the essence of the god or youth represented, but more the purity and immediacy with which it is made to appear. This appearance has been condensed into a very particular reality. It is this that speaks from within the work of art and that compels the observer in the form of an inner demand. ... Out of an impression of "essential characteristics" (Metzger, Conrad, Matussek), as particularly marks out the artistic experience, comes the demand: "You must change your life". A factual encounter invites a factual response, but essential encounters, by contrast, invite the essentiality of the human in a response that as yet remains unexplained.

What is demanded of existence here is not a normal psychologically interpretable effort, but a transcendental achievement. It has to do with a transformation of the constitution of the self and the world. Life as a whole, as a condition of the possibility of all individual acts carried out – that is, the whole basic plan of this existence – must change. However, one must also consider the manner in which such a change is necessitated, for the poet on the one hand, and the sick person on the other.

What we have described up to this point is what is comparable on the part of the sick person and the poet, as something belonging in quite general terms to the nature of a heightened significant experience. This is also reflected in its formal structure. Even in 1948 Matussek had already convincingly argued with reference to K. Schneider that in purely formal terms unusual significant experiences do not have to show up defining differences between healthy people and schizophrenics. Here, as there, a certain two-part quality becomes apparent.

As an example of an "abnormal consciousness of something significant" from the sphere of the healthy mind, Matussek mentions a student who at the sight of a gate suddenly experienced the instruction to refrain from making a certain visit. If viewed in act-phenomenological terms with respect to intention and fulfilment of what is significant, an individual symbolic experience such as this one did not seem to indicate any real differences when compared to the classic model of delusional perception. An analogous situation is present in the case of our observer of the torso. The demand "you must change your life" corresponds to the second element of a delusional perception or an abnormal consciousness of something significant.

It is true that K. Schneider (1949) objected to Matussek (1948), saying that by a "second element" he only understood the "final part of the process, which can be understood in neither rational nor emotional terms", and which leads from perception to delusional significance, to madness (non-sense) in response to what has been perceived. In a non-schizophrenic symbolic experience one cannot talk about a "second element" like this, because in the final analysis it is always understandable. The delusions of reference, he said, always presuppose secret anxieties on the part of the one experiencing them or something similar – in our case, for example, the readiness to experience art as an order directed at humanity. Thereby, however, the supposedly formal two-part criterion is reduced to the question of how understandable or deducible the second element is, a question that according to Matussek is unanswerable in psychological terms.

The only criterion that then remains is "being personally affected by a 'higher reality'", as K. Schneider, in reference to Zucker, formulates it; albeit doubting whether the quality of being affected is conceptually comprehensible and reliable in a differential diagnostic respect. – "The extraordinary sensation of the self being overwhelmed, the 'transverse' to all that has come before it so far, the colour of revelation" are also characteristic of the delusional intuition, according to K. Schneider.

*****

Up until now we have predominantly emphasised the common elements in the experience of the poet and the sick man. These elements have to be fully considered, because only by making the most substantial comparisons possible are we then in a position to ascertain what is not comparable, and it is this that we intend to turn to now.

"The 'basis', the affliction, may well be the same for the poet as for the 'metaphysically broken' schizophrenic, for genius as for madness", says Binswanger,[17] but only for the poet, for the artist, for the mentally creative person generally, is this "a basis" on which the "flower 'of the spirit'" will blossom. What can be meant by this now requires a phenomenological explanation.

*****

For the patient the impression that the picture makes on him leads him to the unshakeable certainty that he is mentally ill. The change is something that he senses is irrevocable, a fact that cannot be reversed – one that

is beyond his control or even influence – and an event with the character of finality about it, untouched by temporary clinically-induced improvements. For the poet, on the other hand, an inner transformation is only really touched upon. The impression, like every other normal impression of our daily life, issues him with the command to find his place within the rest of the connections in the world. This classification seems not to be possible, however, without a fundamental alteration of his whole "being-in-the-world" ("you must change your life"). An assimilation of the experience is not only possible, but becomes an immediate undertaking. In the case of the sick man, by contrast, this possibility is excluded. For him the experience bears from the very start the sign of something unprocessable and becomes therefore a happening that ruptures the continuity of meaning ... "Whilst the sick man reconciles himself to the transformation that has happened to him, and proceeds to lose himself in an autistic world without adapting to the world around, the artist does not fix" what has been experienced "into a failed structure, but actively exposes himself to the experience and reorganises it" (Spoerri). If this ability exists, or rather, if a certain room for manoeuvre remains to exercise it despite the overwhelming nature of what is pressing upon it, then the eventful experience signifies an impact upon day-to-day existence that, however, does not interfere with the life line, but – taken up and integrated within it – perhaps simply suggests a new direction for it to take. In contrast to the sick man, the poet is not at the mercy of the event ... In the case of Rilke the changed state is not fixed in this way, even though he does speak of a change .... In the case of our patient, by contrast, it means something fundamentally different when he says that he is bound to the picture, that it represents a "prognosis of a soul": "I know that I will be focused on the picture for the rest of my life." It is not in his power to turn his focus to the picture, rather he is focused on it, in the sense of once and for all.

*****

Whilst we can talk – in metaphorical terms – of an "irruption" in the transcendental organisation in the case of the sick person, when it comes to the poet we are dealing with an "expansion" of the same thing. The stabilising impregnation of a "prognosis of the soul" in the first case, which signifies a summons from the world, contrasts with a summons in the second case to a new experience of the world, to a

---

[17] *Selected Papers*, vol. II, p. 251. Bern 1955. [**Original note**]

heightened openness to it. Here what we have is rigidity, in which the impressions that have been received stabilise, leading to a permanent restructuring of the categorical organisation to the point where it is, as it were, "cataleptically numbed". There, we have access to a freer mobility and new elasticity.

*****

1. Finally, though, one more essential difference between poet and patient is to be emphasised, and it is one that should not be passed over. This difference lies in the communicability of what is experienced: to what extent does the possibility exist – the need and the ability – to make what has been experienced into something communicable? In the case of the poet we see this possibility developed to a high degree. Even by simply being able to begin the poem "We did not know ..." he shifts the personal affectedness into the realm of the intersubjective, universal experience of man.

Each essential experience is an isolating one. It singles the person out from their assumed commonality with others and throws him back on himself. One can even exaggerate and say that the essential experience leads through a form of autism – one that is dissolved in a healthy person in *statu nascendi*[18] just as every real perception of the other – if one takes seriously the Sartrean analyses of gaze – crosses an ego disorder that is similarly dissolved in statu nascendi. These are theses that cannot be substantiated further here. In any case, it appears that the definitive moment of "dissolution in statu nascendi" is more or less absent in the sick person.

It is true that many schizophrenics also struggle – particularly in the initial stages of their illness – to find ways of helping themselves and others understand their incomprehensible experience, in order to bring the experience safely back into the realm of intersubjectivity. However, the question arises as to whether we are not only dealing with what are (for the moment) still healthy elements of the personality. Ultimately, what is critical is how far that does or does not succeed in the long term. Over the course of time we are almost always able to observe – as something essentially part of this type of illness – that so called "contraction of the relation to the self" (Kisker), which simultaneously signifies a contraction

of the possibilities of coexistence and of relating to the world altogether .... After it seemed, at the outset, that there was a threat of obliterating the boundaries between a psychotic and a non-psychotic significant experience, in the course of our phenomenological investigation these became more and more distinguished in terms of their essential polarity. What is important is that the differences, indeed, oppositions, which crystallise along the path of a study of what is fundamentally comparable, are not of a static but a dynamic–dialectical nature. At the basis of a dynamic–dialectical process of differentiation such as this, which becomes more and more clearly demarcated the more intensively comparable elements are elaborated, is a phenomenological concept of achievement ... of a transcendentally "achieving life". To demonstrate and substantiate this more fully is no longer within the scope of this inquiry.

Conrad, K. (1958), 'Beginning schizophrenia: attempt for a Gestalt-analysis of delusion'

Selected excerpts taken from (1958) *Die beginnende Schizophrenie.* Stuttgart: Thieme Verlag. Translated by A. Mishara (2011).[19]

---

[18] Literally 'in the state of being born' in the sense of more or less immediate. [**Editors' note**]

[19] Any attempt to translate selected passages from Conrad's remarkably rich monograph runs the danger of distorting the original unity of the work. This translation is meant to give more the flavor of his approach rather than a comprehensive rendering. Conrad develops a stage model of beginning schizophrenia in which among other symptoms, delusions are formed and maintained: 1) Delusional mood: Conrad calls this initial expectational phase "Trema" as the patient has the feeling that something very important is about to happen. Conrad describes different kinds of delusional mood but they all suggest an underlying pernicious neurobiological process; 2) Apophany (Greek apo [from] phaenein to show/revelation): in which the delusional meaning is experienced as revelation (Aha-Erlebnis); 3) Anastrophe (Greek, ana- (back) + strephein (to turn)/ turning back) whereby the patient feels the self to be a passive middle point (subject-directed complement to world-directed apophany); 4) apocalyptic-catatonic; 5) consolidation (or partial remission), and 6) residual defect state. See Mishara, A. L. (2010). Klaus Conrad (1905–1961): Delusional mood, psychosis and beginning schizophrenia. Clinical Concept Translation-Feature. *Schizophrenia Bulletin* 36: 9–13. [**Translator's note**]

Editors' commentary

Conrad combines phenomenological description with Gestalt psychology to interpret a wide range of schizophrenic symptoms and signs. The excerpts range from the prodrome of schizophrenia to the 'end state' and give insights into the structure of classic symptoms such as delusional perception and delusional misidentification. Conrad is probably most famous for his account of the prodrome of schizophrenia for which he coined terms with unclear etymological roots, 'trema' and 'aphophany'. However, Conrad's clinical descriptions give a particularly lucid account of aspects of the schizophrenic prodrome.

A. The Gestalt-Analysis of Schizophrenic Delusions

When perusing the innumerable psychiatric textbooks out there, one sees that beginning schizophrenic illness is represented so variously that it is no wonder that many psychiatrists view only the "defective" end-state as what is specific to schizophrenia and what alone justifies classifying the disorder in its diverse forms under the same name. The doubt that psychosis indicates anything unitary is so widespread that few today dare to express the view that schizophrenia comprises a single illness. One speaks rather of the "group of schizophrenias." Gruhle remarks aptly that this amounts to little more than an excuse with little utility because the "task then becomes to indicate what is common to this group." Very different modes of behavior are then gathered together as harbingers of illness during the prodrome period. For example, clinicians will report inexplicable and sudden journeys, alienating preoccupation with mystic or anthroposophic writings, detachment, eccentricity, tactlessness, and bouts of crime as indicators of illness. Still, such reports take into account the patient's external behavior as peculiar and little or no effort is made to take into account the patient's subjective experience or what is going on in the patient during such reported behaviors.

I. The Trema

Mistrust as a Form of Trema

Mistrust has its own effects on consciousness as a subjectively structured experiential field. These become evident when we consider the related example of anxiously trying to walk alone through a dark forest at night. In such circumstances, nothing is "taken for granted" anymore. Nothing is experienced as "natural." In the darkness, precisely where one cannot see, there lurks something, behind the trees – one does not ask what it is that lurks. It remains undefined. It is the lurking itself. In that area between what is visible and what is "behind" the visible (e.g., the particular tree), what we call the background, where what we cannot grasp becomes uncanny. The background, from which the things we do grasp stand out, loses its neutrality. It is not the tree or bush which one sees, nor is it is the sound of the wind shaking the tree tops, the owl's shriek, which one hears, that makes us tremble. Rather it is the background, the entire surrounding space, which remains even after disentangling from the individual tree or bush, the sound of the wind, or caw. It is precisely the darkness as background which makes us tremble.

It is the same with mistrust. It is not what people say or do that disturbs us. It is what they do not say, what they do secretly behind our backs. It is what they intend to do, the destruction they plan, and what they say to one another when we are not present to monitor them. Once distrust enters, the experiential background acquires entirely new characteristics it did not have before. Prior to the mistrust, we did not pay any particular heed to the background. The very nature of background is to be overlooked. Normally, we pay attention to what is distinct or salient with regard to the background, the figure. *Now the neutrality of this background is lost.*

When the background of the subjective experiential field changes so fundamentally, we may start to encounter spatial "barriers" which as now comprising this field. For example, when walking in darkness, one's lamp or flashlight casts a weak flicker around one. Beyond the shifting flicker, darkness forms an impenetrable wall – full of threat and animosity – but pushed off with each step. It is similar with the mistrust for all that falls just outside one's current scope of attention. Everything which lies in the periphery, what is behind, not part of one's current thematic focus, becomes a barrier. It is not simply openness to world as neutral possibility, something to which one could orient in the next moment. Rather, an aggressive character has taken over. It is directed against the subject, shields itself against him or lurks about, seeming to follow him everywhere. From this initial trema (taking the form of mistrust or other emotional forms), result numerous sequelae which we examine in the next sections.

In cases where the delusion grows out of a mistrust-stage, it is difficult to demarcate precisely where the mistrust ends and the delusion begins. In our view, the boundary lies in the subjectively experienced phenomenal-field and cannot be determined "objectively." It lies precisely at the point where the individual loses the capacity to transcend the experience (*nicht mehr des Überstiegs maechtig ist*).[20] As long as the patient is still able to achieve an exchange of reference frames or perspectives, to consider the situation – even if only temporarily – with the eyes of the other(s), and therefore, find himself in a world shared with others, that is, as long as he is still in the realm of mistrust, he is not yet ill. Although we are able to define this boundary theoretically, we are unable to pinpoint it in our clinical practice. No individual (including the psychiatrist) has the capacity to look inside the mind of another and the patient himself is unable to report this to us. He is not conscious of this loss of the ability to transcend. It is only in the most inexact manner that we are able to infer this sudden shift into delusion from the patient's behavior. The proposed criteria for delusion in the older (classical) view, i.e., its incorrigibility or our inability to persuade the patient otherwise through argument, are indeed very closely connected with this loss of ability to transcend. In this context, corrigibility means the ability to exchange frame of reference or perspective (see below).

Delusional Mood

We have already made reference to the delusional mood. This is classical psychiatry's most important concept for determining the boundary between "normal" and delusional experience. It is a fine or subtle "transformation which nevertheless penetrates everything" (Jaspers). "There is something in the air," says our patient Rainer N. (case 54, not included in this translation), who uses precisely this same descriptive phrasing as Jaspers.

II. The Apophanic Phase

For those kinds of experience which classical psychiatry labeled the "delusional perception" or "delusional idea," we introduce the term apophany. These experiences have been variously characterized as an "abnormal consciousness of significance" (Jaspers) or the "positing of a relationship without cause" (Gruhle). At any rate, I attempt with the term "apophany" to make available a useful and clearly defined concept for a form of experience which – in agreement with Jaspers, Gruhle, K. Schneider, Mayer-Gross – is central to the process. I have coined this term on the basis of Jaspers' observation that "the immediate, obtrusive knowing of significant meanings" occurs as a revelation. The "revelation" as the manifestation of the delusional meaning is the essential feature which characterizes primary delusion.

1. Apophany as a Being Stricken (external-space)

This concept is illustrated by the following example. From my home, I hear someone call out for me from the street. Upon looking out the window, however, I see that I was not the person intended but someone else. This requires that I, for the moment, step "outside myself" and place someone else precisely at the "place" I just occupied. Here, I must "step beyond" my own world to enter this world of others, to have the experience that "the calling out does not concern me." We perform this exchange of reference-frames without the slightest effort thousands of times each day – as when I experience the calling out on the street as a shifting to a different contextual meaning and, as a result, the original experience becomes perceptually transformed. We are constantly shifting from the one attitude to the other. This resembles what happens when we view an experimental Gestalt-figure (see Figure 1). Although to a certain extent we are able to shift at will, we also shift involuntarily as indicated by the fact that we are unable to stick with one view of the shifting figure for very long.

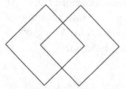

Figure 1. If I interpret the two above proximal figures as two squares intersecting one another, then the small rectangle formed in the middle "signifies" a common region for both. However, if I interpret them as one overlaying the other, then the small square becomes part of the background of the underlying figure. Although nothing has changed 'objectively', the same figural component slips, by means of a shifting attitude, into a different contextual meaning with a completely different perceptual appearance.

---

[20] As his contemporary Binswanger, Conrad (1958) applies the concept of a loss of ability to transcend one's current perspective (*sich übersteigen*, literally a stepping over) as a characterization of acute psychosis. [**Translator's note**]

The delusional patient is unable to become conscious of his inability (often very sudden or abrupt) to "naturally" change reference frame in a manner that he has done up till now. This however should not be surprising as generally, we are not aware of our shifting reference-frame but only the changes in the perceptual Gestalt.

Another example helps illustrate this point. Let us consider a passenger riding on a train who for the moment convinces himself that he (and the train) are at rest and the landscape is moving rapidly past him. However, let us further imagine that due to some sudden change in his brain-organization, he is no longer able to shift back from this experimental consideration to his previous frame of reference in contrast to the healthy individual who realizes that he only momentarily suffered this common illusion while riding the train. In fact, strictly according to the principle of relativity, each view-point is "correct." What one experiences as "rest" and "movement" depends on one's current frame of reference.

Nevertheless, we consider the "normal" view to be that the earth is taken at rest and serves as relative reference-point for movements which take place on its surface. If someone adopts the counter-position by taking his own point of view as the only standard of rest, we would certainly consider him abnormal, if not insane. The patient resembles Ptolemy[21] sealed off in his own microcosm.[22]

Admittedly, this imaginary form of insanity (*Verrücktheit*) could not exist, as the individual is never able to experience him-/herself in movement. Rather, the relative displacement between oneself and the objects – let us say in the ongoing changing of one's own location – would still have to be registered, for example, in terms of the movement of one's own eyes. If there were such an illness, however, we would have a very fruitful analogy to delusion. To pursue the analogy further, there would be a fixing of the reference-system such that each experienced movement in external space would only appear to move with reference to the experiencing subject. If this person moved, for example, from one room to another, it would seem to him that he is at rest while the apartment wanders past him, as if it so to speak "revolved" about him. If he wandered onto the street, then the houses in their rows and lined up trees would just appear to roll past him. If the patient knew nothing about his disorder, he would not be able to grasp why such movement occurs at all. In short, the patient remains a captive of the Ptolemaic world-view.

Up to this point, we have been considering the movement of things in space as standing in relationship to subjectivity at rest. Taking our analogy a further step, let us now consider that the very meaning of things, in their being in the here and now, stand in exclusive relationship to the subject. In terms of the Ptolemaic fixing of the reference frame, each component of the current experiential field, i.e., wherever one's regard happens to turn, is found to have relationship to the self. In fact, nothing is exempt from this relationship. Everything has somehow changed. Things are "no longer the same" as before. They appear the same externally, but have somehow transformed in their meaning. Now appearing in a different contexture of referential meaning (*Bedeutungszusammenhang*), they are altered in character. Deprived of neutrality, they now jut forward from their place in the background. Each and every detail or aspect now means something, although admittedly, it is at first unclear what this meaning is. Now we are getting very close to what in the apophanic experiencing is *specific* to schizophrenia and we may return to our analysis of individual cases . . .

In the next case, a full-blown apophany is exhibited with particular clarity. This case is of particular interest because: 1) The patient experiences the changes in his environment with uncharacteristic

---

21 Conrad's point is that the modern Copernican view that the earth revolves about the sun requires *relinquishing* the older Ptolemaic view that the earth (or self) is motionless (passive) center of the universe. [**Translator's note**]

22 Both Conrad and Binswanger were indebted to their contemporary V. von Weizsäcker, a sense-physiologist and founder of German psychosomatic medicine. By experimentally inducing vertigo, von Weizsäcker discovered the Gestalt-circle, the forming of the Gestalt (as preserved coherence) in a hidden unity between perception and movement. Experimental vertigo models the delusional "Ptolemaic" position because the patient experiences the self to be at rest but everything else (in his perceptual field) as revolving about him as its center-point. See Mishara, A. L. (2012). The "unconscious" in paranoid delusional psychosis: phenomenology, neuroscience, psychoanalysis. In *Founding Psychoanalysis Phenomenologically*, eds D. Lohmar and J. Brudzińska. New York: Springer: 169–98. [**Translator's note**]

affective neutrality; 2) The apophanic change nevertheless spreads completely to all aspects of his environment; 3) For the time being at least, the patient's entire inner-space (including mental images, thinking, memories, etc.) remains preserved from apophanic distortion.

Case history 10. 32-year-old first class private, Karl B., reports a long developing Trema phase with attendant delusions developing insidiously. By questioning further during interview, we obtain the following account: "Things begin," as Karl B. puts it, one morning as his unit breaks to leave camp. When the sergeant asks him for the key to his quarters, it is immediately clear to him that this is a ploy to "test" him. While traveling in the bus, he notices that his comrades are behaving strangely. They obviously know something he is not supposed to know. One of his comrades asks conspicuously if he has some bread. At mid-day, they arrive in town A to relieve units positioned there. A few in his company are charged with finding quarters for the rest of them. This is only a ruse, however, for the few to receive instructions in how to deal with him, while he waits with the others in the motor coach. One after another, groups of men leave the coach only for the others to return. Upon meeting the soldier who is leaving the small quarters now assigned to him, he sees immediately that the soldier also has been instructed in how to deal with him. The patient is unable to explain how he sees these things. He simply "sees them." He straightens the quarters and then goes below to buy cigarettes. Proceeding through a garden, he observes some non-commissioned officers, the staff sergeant and a woman sitting there. Showing surprise to suddenly see him there, they are clearly planning that the woman fabricate something with him that evening. Upon seeing him, one of the officers gets up and drives off to inform the superiors about this recent turn of events. In the pub that evening, the music, the young woman selling cigarettes, the conversations have been prearranged to "test" whether he notices. Everyone is instructed and knows exactly what to do. As he sits there drinking beer with his comrades, each person has the task to insure that everything seem as inconspicuous as possible. In this way, everyone has been very precisely instructed how to behave. Even as the soldier-colleagues speak with one another, the conversation always has some special relationship to him.

He senses that something very special is going on, but is not entirely sure what this is. He has no anxiety as he is free to act as he likes. He is free to state at any moment he chooses, I am not going to participate in this. Actually, he is quite flattered and proud that he is entrusted with this special task. Something magnificent and unique is happening to him ...

Due to Karl B.'s failure to follow orders, which is merely another "test," the staff sergeant transports him by car back to V. Everything along the road – for example, the haystack which had no business being there, piles of stone for a construction site when in fact the road was in good condition, sheep barely noticeable on the side of the road, men passing on bicycles – all this is arranged to test whether he notices. There was so much going on, he could not report everything. Every 100 meters or so there is something new. In fact, literally everything which he encounters on the road stands out. Everything has been arranged for his benefit. While looking out the window, he is also able to see from the manner in which the staff sergeant is observing him that the latter was checking whether he correctly notes all of this ...

On the next day, he is supposed to report at a specific place. As he is waiting, he notes that each person becomes anxious as they pass by him. He notices this from their contorted, tense, and artificial facial expressions. Their bodily movements are not natural. Even the dogs turn around quickly with their tails between their legs. "They were all quite glad when they could get away as quickly as possible." He thinks, "There must be some kind of peculiar effect emanating from me. Other people are under my influence as if under a spell."

... For many of our patients, the entire scenario in the apophanic process becomes transformed into a kind of film-studio or theatrical-stage. Similarly, the above patient, K. B., his entire experiential field transforms into one meant to test him. For others, it becomes an "ambush" or "trap."

2. Delusional Perception

Jaspers and his followers (e.g., K. Schneider) place the delusional perception in the middle-point of their treatment of delusion. Animated debates followed. It was disputed whether the delusional perception is understandable or not understandable, primary or secondary, one or two-tiered, and to what extent the perceptual object is itself changed in meaning. Despite a rather long history, this discussion has not lead to any satisfactory clarification. What had once been a boom of interest has in most recent times become an object of derision as an example of how classical psychopathology has taken a false path.

Nevertheless, Matussek recently made an important contribution on delusional perception. I emphasize two points from his work: 1) In delusion, there is a loosening or respectively, complete dissolution of the natural perceptual context; 2) There is in delusion an increased and expanded prevalence (beyond the norm) of the perceptual object's "essential properties" (*Wesenseigenschaften*). These two observations clarify (at least partially) much of what classical psychopathology held to be "non-understandable" in the delusional patient.

In my opinion, the classical approach has been unable to progress on the delusional perception problem because it merely focused on individual examples forcibly removed from their context in the patient's perceptual experience. For example, Gruhle, who is perhaps the most vocal representative of the view that the perceptual object in the delusional perception remains unchanged, does precisely this ... In contrast to these so-called "intuitions" of the classical school (e.g., as articulated by Gruhle), the patient experiences the objects as fundamentally changed in a highly specific manner. It is not the classical problem here of "understandability" but rather the objects are perceived from within the apophany. If a patient – to borrow from one of Matussek's examples – experientially lives the meaning of "purity" and "innocence" simply seeing this in the white bark of the birch tree, then we have grasped something very typical of the schizophrenia's experience of the perceptual field. By referring to the Gestalt psychologist, Metzger's (1940) concept of "expressive-essential properties," Matussek performed a great service.[23] Still, we should not stop

with this insight in stating what is specific to the transformation of the experienced Gestalt in delusional perception. As we are about to demonstrate through the following case examples, the actual "essential qualities" – as Gestalt psychology refers to them – do emerge and prevail in the delusional perception. However, these are not the only qualities to emerge. As in the case reported above,[24] the patient, upon seeing the doctor's white coat speckled with blood spots, all of a sudden "knows" that he is to be slaughtered. Still, the atmosphere of the slaughterhouse may not be said to belong to the doctor's white coat. Additional properties attach to the object's meaning. The lab coat somehow emits or "releases" the delusional certainty as an apophany for the patient. It is as if the object, "white lab coat," mysteriously contains essential-expressive meanings related to barbering, i.e., handling sharp instruments, but now also the "slaughtering house atmosphere," with blood being sprayed. With the work of cutting open by the surgeon, there is now a world of slaughter and being slaughtered.

Our everyday language is too poor to grasp this qualitative fullness. Moreover, there is no scientific expression for this "halo of qualities," which surrounds our everyday experience of things. Still, we need to find our way. I persist in using the term "essential-expressive qualities" – but with certain caveats – as the concept we use here contains considerably more than Metzger's original definition. The word "essence" is appropriate because it actually concerns the "essential." That is, the slaughter-house atmosphere "exists"[25] in the very perception of the white coat, just as enumerable other things, and under circumstances, the precise opposite, e.g., the hygienic-germ-free, the friendly-wanting-to-help, etc. Therefore, I describe a "cloud of essential properties," which is captured in each thing but, as I elaborate below, is "released" in the delusion. At no point in our

---

23 The Gestalt-psychologist, Metzger (Matussek's and Conrad's source) classifies the *Ganzeigenschaften*: 1) "Structural properties" contribute to the Gestalt's overall organization or goodness (*Prägnanz*) (e.g., round, jagged, color, course of movement, or melody for tones); 2) "Textural-material properties" (e.g., transparency, rough, smooth, soft, hard, and shrill); 3) "Expressive-essential properties" (sometimes referred to as "tertiary qualities") whereby both animate and inanimate beings are experienced as having physiognomic character (e.g., friendly, sinister, stunning), and are evocative of feelings. W. Metzger, *Psychologie*. Dresden, 1975. The physiognomic-expressive properties are not the result of attribution, predication or judgment imposed on the

perception but are (following Scheler and Klages) part of the perception itself. As von Ehrenfels' Gestalt-qualities, the global-properties remain "invariant in transposition," e.g., a change of key of a melody. See Mishara 2010, 2012. [**Translator's note**]

24 This case is not included in the present translation. [**Translator's note**]

25 Conrad employs the verb "*wesen*" to play on his reference to the object's essential properties (*Wesenseigenschaften*) in the previous sentence. [**Translator's note**]

treatment is it so obvious as here that what we are looking for here evades academic psychology so far as it continues searching for "elements." It is precisely because classical psychopathology relied on the "elemental psychology" that it became stuck in its analysis of delusion. When psychology proceeds from the human mental totality, it opens entirely new horizons. What we have been calling "perceptual delusions" as individual or isolated events now becomes clearer in terms of their total-context within delusional themes.

In many of our case histories we have seen that a specific meaningful interconnection exists between the object and the content of the delusional perception. This had been overlooked in the classical approach, which saw only a complete "non-understandability." After all, the fact that the perception is "abnormally interpreted," i.e., precisely as apophany, and therefore not "understood" by the clinician is prosaic . . .

If I describe here a certain quality, intonation or metaphoric meaning in the holistic-properties (Ganzeigenschaften) of the object, then I mean that a "qualitative cloud" of meaning is already contained in each given perception, which may include particular intonations or expressive movements of the person misidentified in the delusional perception (see below).

From our phenomenological analyses, we distinguish three stages of delusional perception:

1. The perceived object indicates to the patient that it concerns him, but the patient is unable to state in what sense it does so (pure apophany).

2. The perceived object indicates to the patient that it concerns him and the patient 'knows' immediately in what sense. In Karl B.'s case, everything is arranged simply to test whether he notices. Alternatively, everything is "arranged" to fit into entirely new contexts, as if a film or stage production is being made (what K. Schneider describes as passivity experiences of things "being made or done" to the patient).

3. The perceived object signifies something entirely specific (now the perception is completely dominated by its expressive-essential properties)

For the moment, let us assume that these three forms represent the fundamental degrees or gradations, if you will, of the apophanic transformation of the Gestalt-meaning. In the first stage, the apophany is weakly developed. The abnormal consciousness is abated. The loosening of the perceptual context and obtrusiveness of the "essential-expressive properties" are still not particularly evident. One finds this apophanic form only at the beginning of the delusional process, but slowly becomes more developed as it progresses from the delusional mood to its other forms.

The second apophanic stage already exhibits some of its more pronounced features. This is particularly well documented in Karl B.'s case in which the apophanic experience never extends beyond this phase. During his transport, he examines the various events along the road as having been staged only for his benefit. However, these events never take on a "metaphoric" meaning as in the more advanced form. In this stage, the loosening of the perceptual context and the obtrusiveness of "essential-expressive qualities" is more noticeable.

With regard to our analyses so far, the third stage is the most pronounced expression of the apophany. Here also, the delusional perception is most evident. The obtrusiveness of the expressive-essential properties serves as a sign that there has been a change of the entire perceptual-structure. In the next section, we will discuss that with greater increases of apophany, catatonic experiences (reactions) may result which I call "apocalyptic." In this stage, the entire perceptual field dissolves into a purely qualitative nebulousness and thereby resembles dreaming . . . Only through our taking note of the "setting free of the essential-expressive properties" in the delusion are we able to actually "interpret" the subjective experience of the patients.[26]

In a tortured need to find clarity in the apophanic field, the patient is formally compelled to look about for solutions . . . With the loosening of the perceptual context, there is a "release" of the qualities, i.e., that "cloud of qualities" which lies concealed in each perceived thing. In a further step, the sense-continuity of the field itself tears (Sinnkontinuität). Whereas up to this point, there are still "objects," albeit derealized, which appear in relation to a meaningfully interconnected "background," and a situational matrix has

---

[26] We refer to H. Ey's important concept (in reliance on H. Jackson) of the 'liberation' ("release") of deeper meaning-levels. [**Original note**]. For Conrad's relationship to H. Jackson and H. Ey, see Mishara 2012. [**Translator's note**]

been properly grasped, now all components of the field have become dissolved into their expressive-essential properties. At this point, the apocalyptic stage of catatonic "world-design" is achieved (see below) ...

3. Experiences of Delusional Familiarity and Absence of Familiarity

In my view, delusional person misidentification belongs to the discussion of delusional perception. Providing one has obtained enough material from the patient, delusional misidentification is nearly always present during the apophanic phase. Jaspers treats this phenomenon all too briefly, calling it a "disturbance of achievement" (Leistungsstörung) in the various respective cognitive domains. This paltry interest indicates how little classical psychopathology is able to consider anything that cannot be immediately viewed in terms of its atomistic approach.

I also find it remarkable that none of my predecessors have pursued the role of physiognomic similarity (universally present in the above cases previously presented in this monograph) as decisive for the delusional misidentification. The person with whom a stranger is mistaken is not accidental (nor "un-understandable"). There is always a certain similarity present and it is precisely that which contributes to the misidentification. The decisive point, however, is that the "similarities" emerge in the most forceful manner, and impose themselves all at once. It is possible that such similarities are registered in everyday cognition, but they are usually unconscious. Such similarities only achieve their delusional obtrusiveness, however, when, precisely as physiognomic (expressive-essential) qualities, *they dominate over the originally present structure-qualities*. In previous studies, I found this to be a cardinal symptom of the organic syndromes. We need not call the feature which the patient finds in person A (a stranger) to be a similar in person B (already known to the patient) an essential-expressive property in the narrow sense. The problem is rather the following. For the patient with schizophrenia, there is within the physiognomy of stranger A a certain feature – in fact, it may merely be a detail, a jagged scar or arrangement of the teeth – that protrudes to such a degree that the physiognomy of the person known to him, person B, now appears in the stranger's face. This negates the epicritic function and as a result,

the physiognomic-expressive takes precedence over the structural.[27]

If we now base our analysis of delusional misidentification on this moment of physiognomic similarity, then we are are closer to our solution. Classical psychopathology's so-called "subtle" distinctions about which cases of delusional misidentification should be more regarded as a perceptual illusion vs. one of judgment, or more due to disrupted conceptual thinking vs. disrupted memory or even *déjà vu* seem – in my view – lead to a dead end. Rather, what is psychologically relevant is the insight that during acute delusions the patient reports perceiving in a manner similarly as to when healthy subjects are exposed to conditions that lead to a loosening of perceptual binding. These impoverished conditions include perceiving during darkness or low illumination, with reduced purview (either too close or too far away), when the stimulus is presented very briefly (as in tachistoscopic displays), or accessible only to peripheral vision. Moreover, there are physiologic states that lead to the same results, for example, extreme fatigue.

We thereby obtain a model for delusional misidentification. Moreover, we find analogies between the delusional experiences and what happens in certain organic disorders. It is not trivial that delusional misidentication, in which there is a so-called disruption of cognitive achievement (Leistungsstoerung), is found in both organic disorders and schizophrenia.

In connection with this discussion, the following patient's report indicates that merely how a person

---

[27] Conrad borrows the term "epicritic" from the British neurologist, Sir Henry Head who allows the surgical division and suturing of the radial nerve of his own forearm. For 5 years, he and his colleague, W. J. Rivers, carefully document the returning sensibility and discovered two underlying systems: 1) protopathic; 2) epicritic. The protopathic (Greek, proto-, 'first, primitive' + pathos, 'suffering, feeling') returns first and is more "primitive" phylogenetically. The epicritic innervation (Gk., *epikritikos* 'giving judgment over,' from *epi* 'upon or over' + *krinein* 'to judge') is more recent evolutionarily, producing localized, gradated, and proportionate (tempered), fine spatial descriminations. Inspired by their predecessor, Hughlings Jackson, Head and Rivers conclude that the more evolved, epicritic functions are more vulnerable to disorder (*dissolution*) and thus, the first lost in pathological conditions. See Mishara, in press. [**Translator's note**]

moves, the "physiognomy" of the movement can lead to the misidentification:

Case 50. The patient reports, "The housekeeper gave me a key with the same movement that my young girl would. Each person makes their own very specific movements. And that is exactly what the housekeeper did. I could catch the meaning right away that my daughter was intended."

We find in this case what our previous cases have also indicated but now with regard to movement. The physiognomy of the housekeeper's movement (as result in a general reduction in level of the patient's general ability to grasp perceptual figural stability of the structural goodness of Gestalt) is experienced suddenly and as surprisingly similar to the movements performed by the girl. The similarity emerges because the essential-expressive properties have obtruded over the other holistic perceptual properties.

In a final case of this sort, I indicate how the quality of familiarity can spread to real components of the surrounding perceptual field. These are in fact parts of the perceptual field in relation to which one would ordinarily not ascribe any physiognomic properties.

Case 12. Before transport to the military hospital, the patient (a carpenter) is confined to a small guard-house. There were simply no other facilities available to contain his confused and restless behavior. The patient reports that he notes right away that this small room was made exclusively for him. In fact, it is quite clear that everywhere in the room were things he had previously made as a carpenter. The doors appeared so familiar. Yes, they are the same ones he made when he was a carpenter. There were definite scratchings on it which he had made when he first constructed the doors. They had probably obtained these doors from his old workshop in Leipzig. The floor-boards were loose and under them there lay some burned matches. The window was also so familiar, made either by his acquaintances or by himself. He could tell from its abrasions in several places. Still other things appeared so familiar. The porthole was red from being so born through, it black rim was scratched precisely in the manner he had done previously with his own fingers. Even the windowsill had the same scratches he made on it as a child in his parents' home. They have taken the sill from his home. A new pane of glass was placed in it. One could see that right away. When he arrives at the hospital, he sees that there are three beds. Judging how familiar they are, they have also been taken from his home, partially belonging to his brothers and in part belonging to his friends. He has the feeling that everything revolves about him.

Generally, we do not recognize the degree to which even everyday objects can have "physiognomic" character. It is different with regard to human faces, where we are all experts and have evolved an ability to recognize and distinguish them with great detail. In Gestalt-psychology terms, we have at our disposal the richness of many levels of structural detail or goodness of fit. It is no accident that the former carpenter is able to "recognize" the wooden objects in his cell given his prior expertise. Now in an individual with such expertise, a sudden reduction of ability to determine the structural details coupled with a sudden obtrusiveness of the expressive-essential properties will lead to delusional misidentification. Just as a shepherd is able to recognize each of his sheep, who appear to us to be all more or less the same, so the carpenter has at his disposal so many levels of structural meaning in his material that, once compromised, they decompose to the above misidentifications.

Finally, the same phenomenon, person misidentification, is able to spread to the entire experiential field. The landscape itself takes on a physiognomic quality. Rather than saying that a person misidentification underlies the experience, it is more appropriate to say that it is a physiogonomic misidentification.

Case 10 reports that "everything looks so familiar." It seems as if he is in Kobenzl (a small village outside Vienna). The patient is reminded that he is in Marburg. "Yes, certainly we are in Marburg. But that complex of buildings is Kobenzl. That is, here in Marburg. It was perhaps earlier the region down there but now it is rechristened in Marburg."

The patient's formulations are similar to the confabulations one finds in Korsakoff's syndrome. These reports are highly significant because they suggest the involvement of the brain in the subjective experience of delusions, which I pursue below.

Now I present cases which appear to be precisely opposite to the delusional misidentification of familiarity. Here, the patients experience what had hitherto been familiar as now unfamiliar, strange or no longer recognizable. While this effect need not directly concern the recognition of faces, it does involve persons, objects or even landscapes.

Case 37 is taken back upon seeing his neighbor's wife who suddenly looked so different.

Case 43 sends the letters from his wife back because they have been counterfeited.

Case 56 reports that nature now appears completely different as if the landscape were in some different part of the world. Looking out the window he exclaims: "Everything seems so blown around, as if in a film with animals, birds, everything ... Even as I turn my eyes to some point and then return to it some 10 minutes later, it is as if everything has changed ... something is just not right."

In these reports, the apophanic transformation plays a critical role in that things now appear "fake" or "nongenuine." Many of these reports indicate a transformation of the perceptual Gestalt, which may be characterized as "quality of familiarity" or "unfamiliarity, alienation." In both cases, there is a domination in terms of the expressive-essential properties in the perceiving. It is important to be very clear that if the physiognomic properties become overly weighted over against the previously important objective (structural, material) properties, then the perceiving itself is deprived of any certainty. A precise and certain "recognizing" in the perceiving is just as much ruled out as its precise differentiation. I have addressed this issue in my prior analyses of aphasia. The essential-expressive properties are insufficient to either distinguish what is different in the apparently similar or conversely to recognize what is the same in encountering it again. That is, when the expressive-essential qualities become dominant, then the unfamiliar is taken to be familiar or similar, and the familiar taken as unfamiliar (in re-encountering it).

The obtrusiveness of the expressive-essential qualities can lead to either the delusional experience of similar physiognomies as the same or what is the same now taken as no longer alike. That is, our proposed obtrusiveness of expressive-essential properties accounts for how what is identical may be doubted and how truly different things can be thought to be identical.

4. The Subjective Experience of Omnipotence

As reported above, it sometimes happens that the patient experiences him-/herself in the middle of a world which has changed fundamentally in some peculiar manner. In this world, everything seems constructed as if it were scenery on a stage arranged especially for the patient in order to somehow test or deceive him. Here, what has been familiar is now reversed into the strange and what had been strange is now familiar or known. Nevertheless, the patient him-/herself is condemned to a complete passivity in the face of all this. A nearly omnipotent impresario, manager, or godlike director are received by the patient without the slightest doubt and who is then given the responsibility for the theatrical play, or game the patient finds themselves in ...

It is only in very specific cases where the direction of agency or effectiveness is experienced as emanating from the patient onto the world whereby the "I" is not damaged or reduced but experienced with full "weightiness." This tendency is already evident in such cases at the beginning of psychosis. While such experiential-forms may also be seen later in the course in so-called end-states, we must be very careful in making any inferences given the reduced reliability of the reports from such patients.

5. Anastrophé

In examining the apophanic moment of the delusional experience, I cited patients who express the feeling "as if everything revolves about me." Even when the patients do not express this explicitly, it does not require much exploratory effort on the part of the clinician to elicit an inclination to completely give oneself over to such experiences. Notably, classical psychiatry has not attempted to name or find the appropriate terminology for such an important feature in the patient's subjective field of experience. This should not be too surprising as psychiatry for the longest time has been merely the description of behaviors. However, it is not possible to decipher what I am describing here merely from observing the patient's behavior. To describe it as "delusions of grandeur" is to miss the point entirely.

It is only by means of further exploration that Case 56 reports, "the entire world is quite crazy. It seems that everything is a film, everything is so positioned and made that way ..." Upon further questioning he becomes silent and then, suddenly, "I will tell you quite precisely. It is a means for a purpose, more than that I will not say. The entire matter revolves about me ... after all, am I not useful to you? The whole thing with the war revolves about me ... more than that I will not say ... "

Case 28 is convinced that everything in the military hospital revolves about him. The other patients are only actors who are here because of him. However, he is not concerned with the question of why this takes place in a hospital.

Case 30 does not understand why everyone wants to make him the middle-point. Everything in the room revolves about him. He is not an ape nor is he Christ. He really comes from a very modest background. This is not a reason for everyone to constantly ape after him and imitate him.

The patient registers all this passively. He is the passive middle-point of the world. It is important to consider how the apophanic transformation plays a role in this. The patient sees how everything around him looks at him. This does not refer only to the immediate people around him, but also strangers on the street. Wherever the patient turns, things have already been arranged for him. They are somehow meant for him and it does not really matter whether he hears this on the radio, or reads it in the newspaper. The conviction results that everything, the entire world, takes up specific relationship to him.

At any rate, we require a term for this turning back on oneself, a being captured in one's own I, that is, the experience that everything revolves about the self. I have chosen the term, anastrophé, which means in the ancient Greek, a turning-back.

Anastrophé and apophany and belong together as subject and object, i.e., the I and what it stands over against, the object. While apophany concerns the transformation of the world and its objects in their relation to the subject, anastrophé is the mode in which the I appears to itself, namely as standing in the middle of the world. The mutual dependency of the two concepts may be stated as follows: wherever the patient apophanically experiences a world, there is, at the same time, anastrophic transformation of the I. Conversely, wherever the anastrophic transformation has prevailed (even if only in rudimentary or scarcely noticeable form), the objects have also been transformed apophantically. This reciprocal relationship also applies to the degree of disruption: whenever one is strongly pronounced, it follows that the other is also so. The two concepts are only two sides of the same state of affairs, namely what is specific to schizophrenia, the structural change of the patient's subjective experience.

6. Temporal Structure and Attunement of Mood

Notably, the patients in my sample did not provide detailed reports of abnormal experiences of time. However, this may be due to the nature of the material provided by my patients at their time of illness. My impression is that such deeply penetrating transformations only occur after several acute episodes, or after longer enduring chronic processes come into play.

Despite Fischer's (1929, 1930) observations, I have rarely been able to obtain accounts of specific structural changes to the experience of the course of time either during the patient's first break or for that matter, later in the clinic. It is probably not accidental that it is only in those patients who very rapidly decline to a so-called severe end-state, who report change of the experience of time, and then this experience is very peculiar. The pre-history of the following case had already been briefly reported in the previous chapter.

Case 76. The patient states that he is already acquainted with everyone present in the room (including the interviewer). Upon being asked who is in the room, he answers: "Everyone here is already dead. I have already come upon everyone's corpse. I recognize everyone here as those who have been shot ... " Are we dead? "No, now everyone is alive again." How is this possible? The patient becomes agitated: "Now everything is different." Do the dead come back to life? "Indeed ... everything is going backwards in time, everything happens in reverse ... You can do with me what you want (now crying) ... you may martyr me as you have already done. Let me see my wife. She knows that everything goes backwards ... I remain so old as I now am. I have eternal life, but the others become always younger, not older ... Yesterday, I received a bullet wound in my chest (shows his chest) and I died. The entire world seeks me. I am Christ. Therefore you may do with me what you want."

Case 30. The patient has the impression that time stands still. Through hypnosis, he is able to experience in 5 minutes what others experience as occurring in 4 months ...

In my view, the temporal structure of experience is only then first compromised – and then in a short-lived manner – following a pervasive destruction of the Gestalt-meaning of the entire field. This apocalyptic mode of experiencing (described below) has for the patient in retrospect the suggestion that the patient had perished at that time. Since the patient is now living again, there emerge ideas that one is reborn, or the sensation that time is going backwards, or at least standing still. Once again, these experiences depend on an impaired ability to shift reference-frame, which in the anastrophic reorganization is characterized by the I as ultimate reference point. As precisely our analyses of the experience of schizophrenia indicate, there is a relativity principle in temporal experience (relative to the self in total field). However, as already indicated, it is only by taking into account reports from patients with chronic or longer enduring illness that we are able to make headway on this problem.

This is a good point to revisit themes only broached upon in our previous discussion of the prodromal Trema phase. Namely, to what extent does the delusional mood continue or develop in the apophanic phase which follows it? Generally, we can track a further development of the delusional mood initiated during Trema well into the subsequent psychosis. The patient who experienced "neutral" anticipation during Trema becomes a neutral observer in the psychosis. The depressive–anxious prodromal patient, who anticipates being condemned to execution, continues to be so but with severe exacerbations, and being trapped in their own anxiety, often attempts suicide. The hypomanically agitated patient, who, mecurial and hyperkinetic, exhibits flight of ideas, often transitions to a catatonic-scattered clinical picture.

Our numerous cases [not presented in these excerpts, A. M.] indicate a great diversity in initial mood. There is always an initial fundamental mood which is preserved during psychosis. If there are fluctuations, these are usually cyclothymic in character. However, just as small, accumulating waves may eventually lead to a tidal wave, the patient's extreme susceptibility to environmental influences builds on the initial fundamental mood. This suggestibility is at any rate much stronger than what we sometimes see in healthy individuals.

Even for healthy individuals, the landscape may take on a friendly or oppressive atmosphere. Its space is experienced as inviting or repulsing. That is, we are dealing here once again with the essential-expressive qualities, which can dominate massively. Such qualities are feeling-toned in the sense of Felix Krueger's "complex-qualities." While passing under a train-viaduct, one patient exclaims with remarkably deep insight, "I always had the belief that I was striving for light but it was really a fear of the dark." Who could bring a healthy person, while passing under such a bridge, to have similar metaphoric insights into themselves? There is no other disorder in which the environment, the situational field, including its illumination, current lay out, even slight gestures, voice-tone or other aspects of the persons who happen to be around, has so much significance as in delusional schizophrenia. The healthy person is incomparably more insensate, more resilient against environmental disturbance. The patient is disproportionately sensitive to registering the essential-expressive qualities, as locked into his situational field, and reacts by lashing out with the slightest changes in this field. The deeper the original mood, the deeper is this susceptibility to the outside. Here psychotherapeutic intervention is possible. Treating the patient in a kindly respectful manner is therapeutic. Since this has been known to phenomenologically-oriented psychiatrists for decades, I am surprised that current researchers regard such observations as new, promoting them as their own discovery.

7. Apophany of Making Imaginatively Present (inner space)

As already reported, we are able to observe numerous cases in which the apophanic abnormal transformation of conscious meaning is restricted to aspects of the patients experience of external space and the patient's "inner space" remains intact. However, apophany can also impact components of inner space, of what Metzger called our ability to make imaginatively present to ourselves. There is clearly a natural difference between the first being stricken by something in fresh impression and our reproducing it imaginatively which the illness process to a certain extent also respects. On the other hand, we also see cases in which both realms are overpowered from the start.

There are indeed cases in which only the inner space or inner mental processes are impacted. Sometimes, this may be limited to that aspect of inner space we call having an idea or thought. Some patients may have this as well in their dreaming.

Case 102 reports that someone sends him his dreams. He knows very well that his dreams are not his own for such things he never dreamed before: "One simply knows this. One senses that it is completely different here. There is some foreign being who wants to penetrate me with strange feelings into my body, which are meant to weaken my nerves, precisely because it is a foreign being. When sleeping, it is possible to experience his penetrating into my body, so leaden, so heavy, it is just like I am supposed to be steered off my course."

Here we see how penetrating apophanic dream-experience must be. However, we should also be clear that it is only in the subsequent reflecting on it that the apophanic meaning enters when remembering of the dream. Even healthy individuals only experience their dreams by subsequently reflecting on them in their memories. More frequent than disrupted dreaming is when the apophanic transformation otherwise takes hold of inner space, where everything appears as already imbued with the radiance of the abnormal consciousness of significance as in delusions of thought control, hearing one's thought (thought sonorization) or thought broadcasting. [Conrad then provides case reports and phenomenological analyses for each of these impairments of "inner space".]

8. Thought-Structure

Disturbances of thought in schizophrenia play a definitive role in classical psychopathology and comprise one of its greatest problems. However, I believe that the Gestalt-analysis can also be helpful here. I begin with a brief examination concerning the role of experiencing "insinuations" which generally refer to a processing of the delusional perception.

Case 54 states emphatically that the others are making insinuations and hints that he has two illegitimate children who are both five months old. But that is nonsense and is untrue! No one said this to him directly but it was intimated in various indirect ways.

It was only by very persistent questioning that we are able to recount the particulars that lead to his experience of the intimations. During rounds the previous day, the patient had been standing on line. When one of the patients before him on line had been questioned how many children he had, the patient answered, "One five month old child." The next patient, who had epilepsy, was asked how much is 2x5? In apophanic transformation, the delusional patient (Case 54) had related the question about the children of the first patient back to himself. It was if he were being asked in a circuitous fashion how many children he himself had. The question reverberated still further when the epileptic patient was asked the multiplication problem. The second question appeared to be related to the delusional patient, and at the same time to the first question. The 2x5 question interfered with the previous question, which was experienced as the insinuation that the delusional patient had "two children who are five months old." The illegitimacy of the children was indicated by the way that the questions were so indirectly posed to him through questioning the other patients. In the apophany, the references to the patient emerge insistently and are processed for a while, filed away, ad acta, as it

were, and make room for similar questions which are experienced as the same type. This example demonstrates a certain "agglutination" of the delusional meaning. That is, things in the field having nothing to do with one another, apart from the fact that they follow one another successively, reciprocally interfere with their respective meanings, become fused and are experienced as forming one totality. In my view, this process underlies the peculiar "agglutination" thought form, which we find in severe thought disorder.

9. Bodily Sensations

Classical psychopathology leaves unanswered the question of where do delusional bodily sensations come from. Where do the feelings of electricity, or the effects of poisoning, as lived-bodily experiences come from? Do the patients suffer from the same sort of parathesias, which we find in neurologic patients? One hears the story that an old psychiatrist had placed the bed of a patient under electric current. The patient laughs at the psychiatrist's incorrect assumption that this should have anything to with the actual electric current he feels all the time.

The various remarks of the above cases presented [omitted in this translation, A. M.] suggest that parathesias in the neurological sense are not experienced. For example, the mere pressing of clothes on the skin can press to the foreground in the erupting apophany.

Case 32 reports that the electric tensions change continuously as if one could change a loudspeaker from soft to loud.

Case 91 feels a magnetic pulling on his entire body. When the apparatus is actually turned on, he also feels the humming inside his skull.

The above examples do not provide any clear indication how these sensations are first phenomenally interpreted. Once again, the clinician feels the inclination to ascribe some kind of underlying neurologic sensation. But this is incorrect. I present a case that clearly indicates that the lived-bodily experience of standing under electric current is solely an apophanic transformation.

Case 10, Karl B., reports that for the last days, he had been suffering the effects of an apparatus. Just a while ago, he was in town. Along the entire path everything had been prepared. The people on the street stood in formation, emitting signs and directing him along the path. This is regulated by an apparatus from which the whole process proceeds. The apparatus produces electronic waves and can be adjusted as being "more strong" or "less strong." When set at higher strengths, the patient loses his will and he must do everything the apparatus inputs. Even his slightest movement is directly controlled, steered by the apparatus. When adjusted to weaker magnitudes, he for the time regains his free will. On the path in the town, he was steered the entire way and was therefore without will. It also happens that the two counter-influences mutually criss-cross, and lack attunement to one another. Usually, however, the whole process runs like clock-work, down to the smallest detail. He writes a birthday letter to his wife, but the act of writing just as much as the content were steered from without. He notices immediately. It was not his manner of phrasing things and the calligraphy was not his own. "I know my own writing!" Each small movement in the writing was without remainder steered from a distance ...

These cases suggest that when patients describe bodily influence, such as by electric current, there is an underlying apophanic transformation of the lived-bodily experience. At the same time, the skin as sensory surface imparts a tactile sensory field in a highly differentiated and articulated manner with its own complex topology in each moment of waking consciousness. There is the pressure from supports, the clothes, feelings of temperature, tension, joint and muscle sensations, which are constantly changing ... all these components comprise the tactile sense-field. The fact that each of these components can alter in the apophany and may be experienced as controlled, non-genuine, artificial – requires its own study. Recently, G. Huber has described the clinical pictures when such sensations prevail, as coenesthetic variants of the schizophrenic process. These bodily sensations appear to play a particularly important role in the apocalyptic phase, to which we now turn.

III. The Apocalyptic Phase

Up to this point, we have considered patients with whom we were able to conduct interviews, who were able to report with astonishing detail the pre-history, beginning of illness and their various subjective experiences. That is, we have considered primarily cases generally called paranoid schizophrenia.

In describing the catatonic clinical picture, however, we enter a realm in which the phenomenological research method very quickly encounters its own limits. We have an excited or apathic individual before us who expresses incoherent, incomprehensible, or

often a complete absence of spontaneous statements, who does not respond to questions in any meaningful manner so that when we receive an answer we do not know it was intended as answer to our question, or happens to correspond coincidentally at the time of asking it ... If the patient recovers from this psychotic phase and again establishes contact with the outer world, we rarely hear anything about this previous time. It would be particularly valuable but probably rare to find out in retrospect, what the patient subjectively experienced during the catatonic phase. What we do learn are always fragments, just individual pieces. However, every response is valuable, not unlike shards for the archaeologist.

In the following, we must leave the path of empirical phenomenology in order to now bridge the missing areas with interpretations, deductions and hypotheses. We do not do this impulsively or ill-advisedly but because it is our only alternative.

Case 24. After undergoing an operation to his glands, the company leader reported that he did appear to be mentally fit. However, medical examination was negative. The patient neglected himself, did not follow commands. Due to washing himself only when instructed, his fellow soldiers complained, leading to the patient's punishment several times. Then suddenly, early one morning, he grabs a rifle from the stand and runs in night-gown down the stairs while carrying blank-cartridges in his other hand. Stopped by the military police, he is brought to the company commander, where three sergeants are being tried for treason. He comes upon one of the greatest espionage cases. He is brought to bed after which he throws his various gear out the window. He is placed on watch where he becomes mute. He greets the commander with a handshake, however, identifying himself as the new captain of the airforce on his way to Berlin. However, the three sergeants must be shot before he undertakes his journey. He was diagnosed with mania and sent to us in a state of great agitation, flight of ideas and mannered gestures. We were unable to interview him as he generated meaningless phrases, commenting on whatever happened to be in his visual field. He states, "I am one and two would I let things happen, three is you, four is nothing, five is my meal, six the soap, seven I leave ..." but all the time whispering so that one cannot really hear what he says. One had the impression that he experienced a whirl of thoughts or thoughts in his mind to which he could not give expression. There were many sterotypies, constantly in movement, grimacing, winking, arbitrary gesturing, playing. The agitation reduces over time leaving a severely transformed residual state with echolalia, echopraxia, and gestures of embarrassment. The patient gave the impression of "emptiness," euphoric state, scattered, and lacking motivational drive.

As in the other catatonia cases presented here, there is a long prodromal period. Although we learn nothing about his subjective experiences, we may assume their inner transformation. In an acutely arising apophanic phase, the espionage themes lead him to intervene by grabbing the weapon in hyper-active manner. Then his state intensifies abruptly into a manic-like agitation but with a complete disintegration of his experiential field into fragments of meaning.

In these cases, the uniformity of the psychosis, or rather what is typical in their uniformity clarifies the underlying matter: after a long trema phase, which may be distinguishable from our previous cases merely by the emergence of a greater sensitivity to transformed lived-bodily experiences, which may seem reminiscent to some as a kind of "hypochondria." We see, no matter how briefly or acutely, an apophanic phase run its course, with its abnormal consciousness of significance, thought broadcasting, delusional perceptions, etc., with the usual themes of hypnosis or espionage. If it happens that we interview one of these patients during this period, we consider the patient to be experiencing paranoid schizophrenia. However, this phase very quickly declines into a catatonic psychosis with severe agitation, mostly followed by a stuporous phase with catalepsy. So far as this phase remits, the patient may run through a paranoid, i.e., apophanic phase. This typical course which clinical experience has supported time and again brings us to view catatonic psychosis as a deeper level of that which we described in the previous chapter as apophany.

Although I do not regard this conclusion as particularly controversial, I am unable to find appropriate discussion of these topics in the textbooks. Although the two clinical pictures are placed next to one another, we never see this decisive point: the one form, paranoia, must run its course in lawful stages before the other (catatonia) may occur. This appears to be essential for the understanding of the patient's experience of catatonia.

We now make the attempt, purely contemplatively, to imagine what it would be like to take all that we have said about apophany in the previous chapter but now increase it to a deeper level of severity. In attempting to visualize or deduce the catatonic experience, any effort to reproduce it in the "light of rational consciousness" must be abandoned. In the previous chapter, we had seen that the perceptual and cognitive contexts are considerably loosened in the apophanic stage. That is, everything already becomes dreamlike. I am convinced that catatonic experiencing is even more similar to the experience of dreaming: each present phase glides into the next, something new always emerges, there is a relentless stream of images, which, however, unlike the dream have their source solely from the inner realm, but are related to the environment, which has dissolved into a world of discontinuous images. The patient feels himself to be at the mercy of this, marvels at what unfolds before him, agitated, anxious, in once again an exacerbation of the original delusional mood.

It should not come as a surprise then that the continuity of the I is temporarily lost. Here results subjective experiences that the "I is no longer I" or one's consciousness has died. Connected with the nearness to dreaming – for dreaming is a pure experiencing of the Gestalt-qualities – is the problem of reestablishing the continuity of meaning in memory. Only shreds, individual pieces or images can be recalled. No continuity of meaning has been established and therefore cannot be reported. Similarly to an amnesia, only the most flighty dreamlike images can be recalled.

If the catatonic patient retrospectively reports some self-enclosed continuity of meaning, I always have my doubts. Much poetry can fill in the gaps of our memory as is often the case in many dream-reports.

IV. Consolidation (Partial Remission)

When patients report in this phase or in recollecting it we often hear phrases such as the following:

Case 10. In the last days, the central power station has slowly stopped its operations. Still their observing continues . . .

Case 11. As his bride came for a visit, the patient suddenly "sees everything clearly." He is therefore comforted. "I used to have a delusion of persecution but it was a true one. That is, I really was persecuted and therefore developed the delusion."

Case 28 reports after his delusions have subsided: "Because I have the good Lord's protection, I believed that God protected me. Now I see that I am just as much self-important and snooty as the next person. I was previously in a dream-state. Now everything has returned to normal as it always has been. The illness consisted of false impressions and imaginings . . . everything seemed arranged like a film." Upon answering the question how does he explain all this, he remains with the conviction that indeed everything was so set up. "In films, it is also so that everything is set up or arranged." A few weeks later he states: "Everything is like it never was. I just can't remember what happened."

Case 56 states, after what appears externally to be very good remission, "I don't know. My body must have somehow changed. Try as hard as I might, I am unable to reproduce my thoughts of being persecuted."

These cases indicate that a complete re-structuring may occur either gradually or surprisingly quickly, whereby, from one day to the next, the Copernican turn is accomplished: It is not the patient who now stands in the middle of worldly occurrences but rather things proceed as they always did, and he is just a small unimportant part of this process. The ability to transcend current experience is re-established. The apophany can stop as quickly as a neurologic symptom, e.g., a parathesia during acute attack from multiple sclerosis, seeing double, or vertigo following vestibular stimulation.

V.   Residual State

The entire delusional process can become resolved as it were without remainder, even with complete correction and insight into the delusion(s). And yet, it is often possible to detect a residuum. This often is more salient to the patient than the surrounding world.

Therefore, we rely once again on the phenomenologic method.

Because of this abiding remainder, the second acute psychosis often impacts an already changed personality, which is not the same as the premorbid one. That is, the newly acutely disease state impacts an already transformed structure. Therefore, what is specific to these residual states is most apparent immediately following such acute episodes. Also, with later psychoses, we are able to obtain very good depictions to the extent that the patients are able to recount the difference with their premorbid personality structure.

In the history of our discipline, there were many attempts to grasp what is specific to the schizophrenic

defect. Berze described a hypotonia of consciousness, Beringer a relaxation of the intentional arc, Stranski of an intrapsychic ataxia. Actually, it is arbitrary which metaphoric image one selects to describe the defect. I prefer the provisional concept, "residuum," since it has less assumptions and is more apt than "defect," which is objectionable for additional reasons. In our sample, we have many very good depictions of patients, who themselves, must know better than anyone else, what is specific to what they now experience as opposed to earlier.

Case 108 reports that now he is now able to see things quite differently and is able to take "considerable distance" to the things that preoccupied him. He has shifted from one extreme to another. Now, he is anxious and questions whether he is doing things correctly in a manner that he has never done before. The ability to act naively is completely gone. He used to be described by his teachers as calm, naive and modest. Since from the very beginning he complains of indecisiveness, the interviewer requests that he give an example: "I wanted to get some matches since I had run out. I wanted so much to get them, for example, from the train-station (which is 8 minutes away by foot). But something held me back. Something prevented it from being realized. I could not do it. The desire remained in its initial rudiments, as a mere seed. Now, it is better. But even now, I want to go into the shop to buy cigarettes but start having misgivings that as a soldier I should not do it. Every time I pass the shop I want to go in but am unable. When I want to write a letter and finally have some peace and quiet to do so, I am so easily distractable. Previously, I could sit at the desk and despite the radio playing, I could concentrate. At times, this has been worse. I could hardly finish a sentence because everything around me would right away break my concentration."

This and the other protocols [not included in this translation] describe what Beringer called the "relaxation of the intentional arc." For example, many schizophrenics in the residual state like to go to the movies, because the suspense from outside carries the patient along. The patient needs this prod from outside because the patient is unable to provide it for himself. It is for this reason that residual patients are able to work relatively efficiently in business settings which place them under persistent but evenly applied external pressure.

In addition to the typical indecisiveness and attentional deficits, we also find in these protocols a consciously experienced reflectiveness. Along with the reductions in the ability to concentrate, it is this attending to only specific aspects of field, which appears to be relict of the apophanic phase. However, at this stage, no delusions may be discerned. What is most striking in these descriptions is that in every case there is a loss of tonicity or vigor. The patient's comportment may be described as loss of any vigor in one's self-presentation, bodily attitude, the ability to formulate and pursue goals. It is what Beringer described metaphorically as a reduction of the intentional arc.

It is striking that during psychosis such complaints were nowhere to be found. The agitated patient often demonstrated enormous ability to make decisions. We need only consider the suicide attempts, the intense pursuit, forceful deeds and resistance the patients are able to muster. It is only with the consolidation phase that we first hear complaints of feeling that one has irrevocably changed in a loss of energy. One has the clinical impression that this transformation has already insidiously taken place but unnoticed by the patients during the acute psychotic phases. Still one does find hints that this has taken place already during psychosis whereby one has the clinical picture of the reduction in energy potential in statu nascendi. Already in psychosis, the patient experiences this energy decline, but mobilizes all remaining volition to rebel but proceeds as one already transformed, depleted, to this battle. The reduction in energy is particularly apparent in the catatonic stupor.

Each person has at his or her disposal a relatively fixed energetic potential. To put it still more precisely: each individual is his/her energy potential. This is experienced as the measure of tonus in the force of one's own will, in the intensity of one's own wishes and desires, ability to be engaged, and in the ongoing dynamic of orienting to or disengaging and turning away from things. The reduction in energy potential may be slight or severe in the residual phase.

C. Summary and a View to the Future

Our analysis of the patient's subjective experience very quickly yielded two salient points. Both concerned the transformation of Gestalt-perception in the patient's experience and both were found to be related to one another: 1) the experience of emergent awareness of abnormal meaning – which we labeled apophany; 2) the experience of being in the middle-point as if all the world's happenings revolved about the patient – which we labeled anastrophé. Moreover, we found these two moments of subjective experience, interconnected with one another, to be at the core of the schizophrenic disturbance. That is, they are the result of a deeply reaching disruption of the ability to shift frame of reference.

By turning to the example of movement, we are able to illustrate what we mean with this last concept. We are only able to subjectively experience movement from the standpoint of rest, that is some situated reference-point which is itself at rest, as, for example, when we unwittingly presume the earth's surface to be at "rest." This requisite reference point of stability usually does not usually enter our awareness. Rather, it is taken for granted and becomes evident only when we consider various illusions of movement. While moving on the earth's surface, however, it is thoroughly indispensable that we always have something at rest as our presumed reference-point. Not infrequently, however, we do come into situations where we must deliberately reorient our reference point. For example, while walking from cabin to cabin in a train, we naturally take ourselves to be the reference point of the movement but then, upon looking out the window, we are once again taken up into the train's own movement (and forget about ourselves as movement source). Following Binswanger, we call this shift of reference-frames, which we perform unceasingly, even at times with a kind of skilled playfulness or elasticity, an ability to "transcend" (überstieg) the current situation. At any given moment, we are able to displace, as it were, the reference-point (as, e.g., with movement as in our train example) into ourselves or back out into the world. Practically speaking, we are able at any given time, to experience ourselves at rest or in movement.

What we are here able to illustrate with the movement example holds in the widest sense for experience per se. Although each individual is indeed middle-point of his own world, he is also able at each moment to transcend his perspective: to consider himself from outside, from above or some bird's eye perspective, as one being among others. He is able to voluntarily shift his frame of reference more or less at will.

The schizophrenia patient has lost this ability to transcend. He is no longer able to shift frame of reference. Apophany and anastrophé belong together as two sides of the same process. They are not separable from one another, even if they do not always find equal expression in the same patient. They are indications of a deeply lying transformation of the structure of subjective experience.

If one adheres in the concept of schizophrenia to rigorously demonstrated phenomenological criteria, e.g., the apophany, anastrophé, and the loss of energy potential, then in our view the diagnosis of schizophrenia could eventually become uniform practice. Certainly, there will be cases where we will not be sure but this will depend on not getting enough clinical material. As long as one bases the diagnosis on behavioral criteria rather than subjective experience, and includes all kinds of "crazy" behaviors, indifferent to whatever the underlying subjectively experienced phenomenology, then there will never be uniformity in the diagnosis.

The subjective experience of delusions exhibits all the features of transformation of the Gestalt-meaning, i.e., a loss of the epicritic function and resultant release of the protopathic forms of mental achievement. The resemblance between the apocalyptic and dreaming also supports this view. Nobody would resist the view that dreaming involves a transformation of brain function. Finally, the reduction of potential energy also bears the character of an organically based disturbance and is similar to cases of frontal lesions where there is also a reduction in motivation.

*****

Therefore, the problem of researching schizophrenia in terms of the underlying physiological pathology does not seem to be completely irremediable. The current investigation supports the view that physiological–pathological substrate of the illness may be eventually found.

Rümke, H. (1948), 'The nuclear symptom of schizophrenia and the praecox feeling'

From (1990) *History of Psychiatry* 1: 331–441. Translated by J. Neeleman. Originally published as (1948) Het Kernsymptoom der Schizophrenic en het Praecoxgevoel. In *Studies en Voordrachten over Psychiatrie*. Amsterdam: Scheltema & Holkema: 53–8.

Editors' commentary

In this article, the Dutch psychiatrist Rümke discusses the diagnostic value of the praecox feeling, which he describes as the specific feeling that a clinician

experiences when encountering a patient with schizophrenia. Rümke attributes this to a diminished 'rapprochement-instinct' in the patient. This notion is based on phenomenological work on empathy (e.g. by Karl Jaspers) and sympathy (e.g. Max Scheler). The idea of including the interpersonal relationship between doctors and patients for diagnostic purposes (for example by including it as a disorder criterion) is alien to current approaches in diagnostics and taxonomy. Indeed, even Rümke himself recognizes how using the interpersonal realm to inform diagnosis could be unreliable. However, even today's clinicians seem to rely on their intuition and on the feeling that there is a schizophrenic coloration to their patients' symptoms (though there is no supporting evidence base for the use of such feelings for diagnostic purposes in clinical practice). An intriguing possibility is that such feelings in clinicians are evoked by a systematically different social interaction pattern specific to patients with schizophrenia

How does the psychiatrist diagnose schizophrenia? This question remains of crucial importance, in spite of the fact that schizophrenia is one of the commonest mental disorders about which there is a wealth of literature, and which is diagnosed daily by most psychiatrists. No answer is available as yet, and in this essay a definite solution cannot be given either.

The difficulties surrounding the clinical diagnosis of schizophrenia crop up repeatedly during the clinical process, and disagreement between clinicians is not at all uncommon.

*****

It is remarkable that it is rare for a diagnostician to be able to indicate exactly how he arrives at a diagnosis of schizophrenia. He might point out widely accepted symptoms such as schizophrenic thought disorder, the loss of awareness of own activity, ideas of influence, 'intrapsychic ataxia', affective stiffness, the impossibility of empathy, the absence of a vital contact with the external world, autism, the schizophrenic smile or even the delusions of persecution or world destruction. His opponent, however, distinguishes such phenomena in various other illnesses as well, e.g. in confusional manias, schizoid psychopathies, atypical involutional states, degenerative psychoses and various uncertain cases which definitely do not warrant a label of schizophrenia. Alternatively, the opponent might claim that 'splitness' does not exist at all, he might find the smile quite appropriate, he might be able to empathize with this patient without difficulty, or he might think of autism as a ubiquitous phenomenon. The conclusion will often be that the proponent has sensed a specific schizophrenia or praecoxfeeling during the interview of this patient – he has noticed that this patient's mental state has a specific schizophrenic colour. It will become clear that this is decisive for him. The opponent would have diagnosed schizophrenia with all these symptoms and signs but he has not sensed the praecoxfeeling.

Here we have arrived at today's question: 'What is the praecoxfeeling?' I feel that this term is preferable to 'schizophrenic colouration', as it implies that a feeling, induced in the clinician, is the final and most important guideline.

As it plays such an important role in diagnosis, it deserves some further analysis and in this study I will try to work out on which basis I diagnose schizophrenia. I should first point out that the above-mentioned symptoms in themselves almost never justify a diagnosis of schizophrenia; they are useful to illustrate the diagnosis, but for me they lose all their pathognomonic value if what I consider as essential is lacking.

If one tries to put one's finger on what it is that gives the aforementioned symptoms a schizophrenic colouration, then the conclusion must be that it is something that cannot be classified in the usual way but that it is comprehended in all the categories of the conventional mental state examination.

The phenomenon is most clearly interwoven with the affective disturbances, the anomalies of thought and with the psychomotor symptoms. This undefinable attribute that surrounds all the observed symptoms induces the praecoxfeeling.

Can we define it more accurately? Even after a very brief mental state examination it becomes clear to the psychiatrist that his empathy is lacking. It is not only the patient's affect that cannot be empathized with; it is impossible to establish contact with his personality as a whole. One becomes acutely aware that this is caused by 'something' in the patient; the 'directedness' toward other people and the environment is disturbed. Somewhat pathetically one could say: 'the schizophrenic is outside the human community'. This lack of intercourse with people is not merely an affective disturbance; something is affected that determines the relationship between people, and this cannot be exhaustively described by the

conventional mental state examination, which after all deals with patients who are observed in isolation.

One of the most fundamental attributes of man as a social creature is his inclination to establish contact with others, and this is not an act of will but a purely instinctual drive. This urge remains below the level of awareness as long as it can be satisfied; it reaches consciousness if its goals cannot be met. (There is a human instinct to avoid contact as well, but I will not discuss it here; it exerts a polarizing influence which calls for separate investigation.) The weakening of this instinct which I will call the rapprochement-instinct, is probably the fundamental phenomenon in schizophrenia and I know of no other condition in which this instinct is so thoroughly affected.

As interpersonal relations are not one-sided, the investigator examining a sufferer from schizophrenia notices something out of the order within himself; he cannot find the patient. The one-sidedness of the attempts to establish a relation induces feelings of despair in the healthy investigator, who often starts to make manoeuvres that irritate the patient and may even cause additional active withdrawal. Only very delicate intuition can indicate successful avenues that might be left available.

The importance of two-sidedness in interpersonal relations not only shows itself in the case of schizophrenia; it is important for the understanding of other illnesses as well. The doctor's internal attitude induced by the patient is a very sensitive diagnostic tool, and it would be helpful if we were more skilled in recognizing changes in our own internal attitude; it would certainly make us more self-confident in making diagnoses. Patients suffering from schizophrenia, mania, hysteria, psychopathy or dementia are approached by us in radically different ways. For instance, one of the strongest arguments in favour of a diagnosis of incipient dementia in a gentleman of high cultural standing, was for me a slight touch of over-joviality which I noticed within myself, a slight verbal sloppiness; my own disinhibitions indicated to me my patient's dementia. The patient's illness strikes, almost unnoticeably, equivalent chords in the doctor. How many of us are a bit manic when confronted with a manic patient, somewhat psychopathic with a psychopath or neurotic if our patient is neurotic. If we do not control this, then, taking the last example, a shared neurosis will establish itself which can cause a great deal of confusion. It is hoped that this digression has highlighted the importance of the doctor–patient relationship, and it may be clear that the praecoxfeeling is a special example of the doctor's reaction to his patients.

Of crucial importance is the way in which the doctor's urge to establish rapport is affected by the schizophrenic's decrease in rapprochement-instinct. This central factor is linked up with various phenomena which can be shown to be related to the diminution in rapprochement-drive in the schizophrenic. I consider the latter as the fundamental phenomenon in schizophrenia.

Often the praecoxfeeling is felt even before one has spoken to the patient; the condition is recognized by mere observation of body-posture, facial expression, motor behaviour – the whole of the patient's expressivity. It is intuitively felt that all these are disturbed, i.e. changed with respect to the norm. Motor behaviour is stiff, bizarre, ceremonious; there are tic-like movements and the queerness of the smile is beyond description – the famous empty smile. I do not believe that this smile is empty, as it does express something; irony, inappropriate shyness stemming from an inner world which is unfamiliar to us.

This smile is a specific example of the above-mentioned disorders of expression. I am convinced that many of these are intricately related to the diminution of the rapprochement-instinct; many typically schizophrenic motor disorders are really examples of motor behaviour of thoroughly isolated persons. Remember, for example, the weird grimaces and movements, the stereotypies, tics or even catatonic postures of a man who, in his isolation, knows that he is not being spied upon, e.g. in the toilet or the bathroom. I feel that the schizophrenic motor and movement syndrome is caused by the disappearance of movements which are geared towards the establishment of human contact; we miss the contact-directed expressions found in normal people, and, at the same time, we are struck by the desperate attempts undertaken by the schizophrenic to re-establish contact. Strictly speaking, the latter are voluntary, and deemed to fail. Nobody knows how long a schizophrenic, in his ever-increasing solitude, continues to yearn for contact. I am sure that people who have become unreachable continue to send out distress signals to us, and sometimes, with a lot of patience, some of it can be heard and understood. A typical example of this disturbance in the mutuality of movements is the impossibility of approaching the schizophrenia-sufferer playfully. K. H. Bouman tries, during his ward-rounds, in uncertain cases, to see whether the patient can be engaged in a playful relation.[28] If the patient is schizophrenic this is virtually impossible; in order to play one has to be tuned to each other.

Not only do the movements lose their intentionality and mutuality, so does our most important communication instrument, language. Even when a formal speech disorder cannot yet be demonstrated, the melody, the intonation, everything that aims to draw attention, to seduce or to fend off, is changed. Speech becomes monotonous. The schizophrenic actually speaks out what usually, in contact-directed speech, remains hidden.

Our own interior monologues are full of derailments, bizarreries, thought-disorder, stereotypies, perseverations, etc., often even neologisms. Nevertheless, I do not mean to assume similarity between our internal speech 'for private use' and schizophrenic language (C. Schneider makes important remarks about this issue in his book on schizophrenia[29]); this needs further study. Schizophrenic language shows us the same as schizophrenic movement-disorders; expressions of persons who are outside the community. The absence of spontaneous, communication-directed language is striking; only partly do we become aware of failed attempts toward communication. The schizophrenic scream is like the tormented lamentation of a roaring animal in the desert.[30] If the patient communicates or depicts the changes in his internal life, a great deal of it remains, as a matter of course, beyond our comprehension. We cannot be sure, in the present state of knowledge, how far this difficulty of describing his own mental state is due to formal thought disorder, and to what extent this is a direct consequence of the fact that a schizophrenic mental state simply cannot be condensed into ordinary words. In conclusion, apart from the impossibility of empathy and the disturbed instinctual rapport, changes of motor behaviour and speech contribute to the praecoxfeeling. What about the changes of affect? Often these are thought to be the main source of the praecoxfeeling. The affect of

---

28 K. H. Bouman (born 1874), Professor of Neurology and Psychiatry in Amsterdam one of Rümke's teachers [**Translator's note**]

29 C. Schneiders, Die schizophrenen Symptomverbände. Berlin: Springer Verlag, 1942. [**Original note**]

30 Isaiah 40, 3. 'The voice of him that crieth in the wilderness.' *The Holy Bible* (London: The British and Foreign Bible Society, 1972). [**Original note**]

schizophrenics is only disturbed to the extent that it is related to the rapprochement-instinct; the same goes for the sexual libido. Vera Strasser said: 'the "Austausch-Affektivitat"' (affective exchange) is damaged.[31] The disturbances of empathy and sympathy are evident and they can be described as 'stiffness of affect'. On the other hand, emotions that accompany other instincts appear to be entirely adequate. The lack of exchange of affect is surely conducive to the praecoxfeeling.

A diagnosis of schizophrenia along these lines will only be correct if these phenomena are really present and if they are recognized by means of a praecoxfeeling. If schizophrenia is diagnosed in the absence of these phenomena a mistake will be made. This highlights the intricate relation between the theory of schizophrenia and the clinical diagnostic process.

What causes the decrease in the rapprochement-instinct? I am convinced, on the basis of my clinical practice and my psychological analysis of schizophrenics, that the drying-out of an energy-source is fundamental.

This reduction in energy does not affect all the aspects of the psychic life equally ... ; it affects chiefly, possibly even exclusively, the instinctive life ... It reveals itself in the rapprochement-instinct, and often in the sexual instinct as well; object cathexes are diminished and the libido as a whole shows evidence of disorganization and disintegration. It is a certain fact that in many schizophrenia sufferers sexual disturbances can be demonstrated, often even before the onset of the illness and sometimes even from the earliest stages of development ... The clinical course of schizophrenia illustrates in many ways how energy is progressively lost – the loss of freshness.

*****

If insufficiencies in the instinctive basis are accepted as the fundamental problem in the illness, then schizophrenia should never be diagnosed if there are no actual indications that the instinctive layers are affected. I am therefore used to assigning all patients in whom such evidence is lacking to other categories.

*****

---

[31] Vera Strasser or Vera Strasser-Eppelbaum, psychiatrist in Zürich at the beginning of this century. [**Translator's note**]

Now I should indicate some of the mistakes which can be made if the diagnosis is made on the basis of praecoxfeeling; since the issue of differential diagnostics is beyond the scope of our study, I will merely point out some typical errors.

If one has rich and highly developed empathic capacities at one's disposal, it may sometimes be possible to establish a mutual contact with understanding of the patient's verbal and psychomotor expressions. One may feel that the possibilities of contact have remained within normal limits although in fact they have deteriorated to a subnormal level. If the doctor does not distinguish carefully enough his own reactions, confusion may arise between, on the one hand, the relation which in fact exists and, on the other, his own attempts to establish rapport; a pseudo-rapport may be mistaken for a real one. Faulty diagnoses will be made in both cases.

A praecoxfeeling will arise inappropriately if the doctor himself is inhibited in his rapprochement. This, however, is not the genuine praecoxfeeling but the usual feeling of unease which inevitably arises when one is confronted with people one does not understand. One's own feelings of sympathy not uncommonly cause an unjustified rejection of the diagnosis of schizophrenia. Making this diagnosis is easy if one is disinterested and neutral in one's meeting with the patient, like for instance during a first interview. If one has known the patient for some time and feelings of sympathy have arisen, then one finds it less easy to diagnose the illness, either because unconsciously one shrinks from its devastating implications, or because one overestimates the quality of the rapport which has established itself along with increasing mutual sympathy. If, on the other hand, one dislikes the patient, it will be difficult to set up a relation anyway, so that the diagnosis may be made when it is in fact unjustified.

In this study I have tried to work out how I diagnose schizophrenia. My reader may have noticed that I have not mentioned the so-called schizophrenic thought-contents. Although these may sometimes indicate the diagnosis, they can never in themselves justify it. I am convinced that the diagnosis is made – and should be made – not on the basis of the thought-content, but on the basis of the formal changes in the patient's psychological dynamics which induce a specific experience in the investigator.

Chapter

17

Affective disorder

Binswanger, L. (1964), 'On the manic mode of being-in-the-world'

From (1964) *Phenomenology: Pure and Applied*. Edited by E. Straus, translated by E. Eng. Pittsburgh, PA: Duquesne University Press: 127. Originally presented as a lecture at the first Lexington Conference, Kentucky, USA (1964).

Editors' commentary

In this text Binswanger gives us his idea of the vocation of the psychiatrist and highlights similarities and differences with the physician in physical medicine. He uses the example of a psychiatric interview with a person with mania and describes how it must begin with putting oneself (as psychiatrist) into a relation with the manic person. It is in the face-to-face or person-to-person relation with the manic mode of being-in-the-world that the psychiatrist obtains their orientation. Symptom description and diagnostics, for Binswanger, come later: they presuppose a knowledge of the manic mode of being-in-the-world; however, they lie on a pathway to knowledge of the organism and to therapeutics which Binswanger sees as shared with the physician. Binswanger gives us an existential sketch of the manic mode of being-in-the world. The mode is an over-swing into the festive joy of existence. Existence, he says also has its problematic side – in the form of death – and Binswanger says the manic mode is inherently in tension with this problematic side which we may see symptomatically as mixed affective states or as swings into depression.

In my choice of theme, "the manic mode of being-in-the-world," for today's lecture, I am making a direct linkage to clinical instruction. At the same time I wish to familiarize you with the methodic assumptions and structure of psychiatry.

The young medical student, when he is called upon for the first time to examine a patient here in the psychiatric lecture hall, I am sure will be surprised by the words chosen by the clinical instructor. While the internist or surgeon says, "examine the patient," the psychiatrist says, "try to establish a relationship with the patient." The difference between psychiatry and the rest of medicine could be derived simply from the phrasing of this instruction. But the way in which they agree could also be derived, because – to anticipate a bit – the instruction to put himself in relation with the patient also includes the instruction to examine him! However, in examining the bodily sick person, you use your senses – observing, palpating, percussing, smelling him – while you examine the mental patient by putting *yourself*, as personality, into a relation *with him*, as personality. Here the patient is first of all very different from an *object* of investigation; he is not a direct object of perceiving and judging, but *partner* in a relation with a fellow man, a communication relationship. In short, he functions in the former instance as an organism from the very beginning, in the latter as a fellow man. But we ought not to go too far with this type of examination. In the rest of medicine, you also *question* the patient and expect an answer from him, not seeing him *only* as an organism. In psychiatry again the physical examination is essential, and here, too, a concern for the organism, as the eventual objective of every medical investigation, remains in constant view. What distinguishes somatic medicine and psychiatry in the last analysis has nothing to do with the *goal*, but with the way to this goal. When we say that in psychiatry this way is different, longer, and more involved than in the rest of medicine, we mean two things: First, whoever chooses this way must have as a *physician*, especial ability or talent in relating himself to a sick fellow man; second, as an *investigator*, he must be clear about the scientific methods and problems whose control and mastery he needs on this way. Above all, he must comprehend the enormously simplifying and condensing process of transformation or reduction that psychiatric thinking and acting must go through in moving from its point of departure, *viz.*, from establishing relations with a sick fellow man towards its goal, i.e., to determine pathological processes in an organism.

I cannot hope to show you this process of transformation within an hour's time. I will confine myself to a study of the point of departure, to the examination understood as an entering into a relation with the sick fellow human and to the resulting view of his kind of life form; and, secondly, to a particular sick fellow man, the manic person with flight of ideas.

Like the rest of medicine, psychiatry proceeds solely and entirely on the basis of experiencing. However, what you *experience* here at the patient's side are, as I have mentioned, not changes in, or of, the organism, but changes in regard to communication, i.e., putting yourself in relation and remaining in relation with the patient. Usually you experience these changes as hindrances, complications, or impediments in the course of communication, whether affective, intellectual or purely linguistic. So you will understand the statement made that psychiatric symptoms must be considered as disturbances of communication, or in other words, of mutual understanding; that they actually *are* facts of comprehension. But you ought not to limit this term mutual understanding to understanding through words. You must take into account the whole sphere of possibilities in communication with fellow men, the many different ways of everyday social acquaintance or social intercourse as well as the so called *existential* and the so called *sympathetic* communication. From this it follows that you can only expect to make a psychiatric examination correctly when you devote yourself to the sick fellow human confronting you with your entire *being* and complete *love*.[1] Only then do you have a right to expect that the sick fellow human will open himself to you, affording you a glimpse into the most secret linkages between his immediate experiencing and his illness.

Now, what is the situation in regard to understanding or communication with the manic human being, with flight of ideas? At first it seems that here we do not encounter difficulty in communication, but rather increased ease and speed in making contact.

You have no difficulty at all entering into relation with these patients. They answer you easily and quickly, even breaking in, giving you undivided attention, admiring your mustache or your dress, your intelligence or your manners, overwhelming you with questions about their life, their past, their family promising you heaven knows what next, telling you circumstantially, without being asked, the most intimate details of their life and circle of friends, all the while grasping your hands, inspecting and feeling your ring, your ear, etc. But this heightened facility in communication is only apparent; it remains superficial. If a second or third party appears, the patient loses you from sight just as quickly as he first laid eyes on you, to turn his attention to the newcomer. So now you find that you haven't "come near" to the patient and that you will have to make every conceivable effort if you wish to get beyond the most superficial conversation and learn something coherent. Simultaneously, you quickly get the impression that the patient is also not close to himself, but lives, as it were, away from himself. And, as I've said, nothing is able to hold his interest. Of course, he fills up his house and his room with a thousand and one things, is always with others, uses up many persons, throws his money, so to speak, down the drain, while being obliged again and again to get, discover, stir up, or try something new. His striking "curiosity" is simply a special case of his over-all tireless craving for novelty. In contrast to the really occupied person who always "has" time, the manic fritters his time away and so does not really occupy himself. His so-called hyperactivity which, in the onset of illness, is often still a stimulus for outstanding achievement, projects, scientific or artistic works of every kind, gradually turns into an aimless, meaningless, empty busy-ness. What we call the seriousness of living turns into a game. The patient "takes everything lightly," doesn't see obstacles and difficulties anywhere, or only those he is convinced he can overcome by a snap of his fingers. He misjudges the heaviness of things that no longer stand out in relief, but become light, soft, yielding, mobile, in a word, evanescent or volatile. Hence, one can also say that he mistakes things; even the entire atmosphere in which things are "suspended" is rosy. What appears to us as gray, gloomy, dried up, even lifeless, appears to him as colorful, bright, blooming and bursting with life; I shall return later to this point. Everywhere there is soaring life, light, sun, prosperity; all space resounds with music. He sees, to use a folk

---

[1] Binswanger is using 'love' here in its philosophical sense. E.g. the sense of love in Plato's *Symposium* in which love for another is the means of ascent to contemplation of truth and beauty. [Editors' note]

saying, "heaven filled with bass fiddles." What is true for the world of things around him also holds for his world of fellow men. No one is "up to him"; he believes himself ready to deal with everyone, everyone is near to him, in everyone he sees his friend and fan. Nor with himself does he have any difficulties; everything is easy for him; he can do everything; there are no problems; no sooner thought than said and done. Nowhere do you find distance, nowhere delay or wait. Everything is "handy" for the patient, is at once "handled" and "played away." So he is continually on the move. He does not sit, but stands; he doesn't walk, but hops, dances, or jumps.

From all these particular experiences with the patient it once more becomes evident to you that reaching an understanding with him is not after all as easy as you first thought. You must expend great effort to fix, collect, and review your experiences with him. Here, too, you will then conclude that this patient lives in a world different from yours, a world unfamiliar to you, which strikes you as more or less new and strange. And if one of you should also say that you have experienced something like this after sudden good fortune, especially in love, or during a stay in the mountains, while flying or in alcoholic intoxication, at the beginning of narcosis, in a state of great exhaustion or of hyperthyroidism, while falling asleep or dreaming, then you are only taking the problem back one more step to yourself. For in this situation it is not a matter of being able or unable to put ourselves in the position of the respective patient, a very vague subjective thing, but a matter of understanding and describing *the world* in which such a patient lives (and perhaps we too under certain conditions), an understanding of the world which cannot be attained with purely scientific means, in a purely scientific way. In my view psychiatric inquiry has no more urgent task than to reach an understanding and description of the patients' worlds and of their modes of being-in-the-world. Only then do we *know* what separates them from us (and, in the above instance, what separates us from ourselves), why we must strive to understand them (or ourselves) and how far this understanding is, ultimately, possible.

You can see this same volatility with loss of contour and focus of the world, the same hovering, skipping or jumping within it, when we turn from the world around and at hand to the verbal expressions and idea worlds of these patients.

Since the manic patient is not scrupulous in his speech, we have difficulties here too in understanding him. Instead of a hypotactic sentence construction, organized with independent and dependent clauses, there is parataxis or the mere stringing together of clauses in which it is left to the hearer or reader to discover a logical connection between the separate clauses. The verb or activity word that actually animates and vitalizes the spoken or written representation increasingly recedes, and, where it yet survives, functions almost entirely in the present tense, less often in the past, and more and more rarely in the future.

Once more this shows with all desirable clarity how these patients live almost entirely in the present and to some degree still in the past, but no longer into the future. Where everything and everyone is "handy" and "present," where distance is missing, there is no future either, but everything is played off "in the present," in the mere here and now. This also throws a light on the self of such patients. A self that does not live into the future, that moves around in a merely playful way in the here and now, and, at best, still lives only from the past, is but momentarily "attuned," not steadily advancing, developing or maturing, is not, to borrow a word, an existential self. As a consequence, every existential communication, every understanding from human being to human being, is impossible; the mere contact or association with them is altered. The sick cannot be taken "at their word" which always implies a promissory note drawn on the future; and they let themselves be impressed and influenced all the more easily if one knows how to take them, lightly, just as they go on living, as airy and insubstantial as the world they live in. But there is one thing they will not tolerate: contradiction and restriction of their freedom of movement. In their world there are naturally neither restrictions nor interferences. When they actually encounter them, they are infuriated, become irritable, crude, assaultive, and, in manic excitement, even extremely dangerous.

But to return to language: With the withdrawal of the verb, the name or noun secures the upper hand, more or less decorated with adjectives, so that the final result is the so-called manic "telegram style." Even this style, from which meaning can still be made out, proceeds to fall apart; words are no longer used in accord with their meanings, but simply strung together on the basis of their sounds. We find the so-called "clang associations," rhymes, puns, and word completions, all of which show up very clearly in the word association experiment. Finally, the words are then taken apart into their syllables and letters. At this point there are innumerable interjections like oh, ah, so, etc. Instead of thought making use of word meanings, we find a playful preoccupation with sounds of words and even phonemes. In line with the continuing association with other persons, the steady addressing, aggressing, questioning, asking, ordering, the pronouns thou and you (*Du* and *Sie*) play an important role; yet even the *Du* never expresses true intimacy, for a loving communication is just *as little* possible here as an existential communication.

If we now take up the topic of *thinking*, we realize that because of the close relation of talking to thinking, and of thinking to talking, the ground has already been prepared. Psychopathology is correct in speaking of the manic pressure to *talk*, not to think. The patients verbalize a great amount, but in terms of thought express very little. If they also report a racing of their thoughts, that doesn't at all mean they think a great deal – which implies deliberate and painstaking consideration, composition, and typing together of various themes of thought – but only that much comes to, or rather, overcomes them. And, once more, they have neither the time nor necessary earnestness to think over or through any of these ideas. The logical units of meaning, the thoughts, are volatile or fleeting without contour or clarity. They flow into one another, or are loosely and brokenly suspended in the space of thought. Correspondingly, thought is not continuous, but occurs "by leaps and bounds" or, as psychopathology says, in a *flight of ideas*. And here you have a perfect illustration of the way in which our idea of the presenting symptom is dependent on the kind and degree of difficulty we have in reaching an understanding. If you have relatively slight difficulty in bridging the gaps of these patients' thought in your own thinking, then we speak of an "ordered flight of ideas"; but if it is hard or even impossible for you to do so, then we speak of a disordered or incoherent flight of ideas (Wernicke) or of confusion with flight of ideas (Kraepelin). But at the present time, it is no longer enough for us to view the fragmentary or tattered sentences, words, and thoughts of such patients simply as a disordered heap of broken bits, just a picture of breakdown. Rather, it is our task to discover the new principle by which this disorder may be understood. This principle, however, is no longer to be found within

the verbal disclosure, the meaningful expression, or even thought itself, but only in the *entire form of life*, in the pervasively up-in-the-air, leaping, skipping life style of these patients, as you will certainly have noticed.

Where we speak of form of life and life style, we are speaking of the characteristic way in which a human being or a group of human beings, a people, a class, a caste, but every bit as much, a group of similarly ill human beings, are *in the world*. And it is according to the how of their being in the world that the how of their selves, or as we mistakenly say, their "I," shapes itself. Self and world are not to be separated here, but are merely polar delimiting concepts within the *one* being-in-the-world.

You will realize still better why I said we, in order to understand, must consider the over-all life style of patients in order to understand their thinking as flight of ideas, if I show you verbalizations of manic persons we came across which are perfectly correct from a linguistic and grammatical viewpoint, but which must, nevertheless, be labeled as ordered flight of ideas.

A patient writes as follows to a distant relative: "Would one of your seven sons have the great kindness to be my mother's constant companion? Unfortunately, I no longer can, and am very sad about it." Apart from the slight formal peculiarities, which we will pass over, these sentences could have been written by a healthy person. That they show marked flight of ideas becomes apparent only when we compare their content of meaning with the actual situation of mother and daughter. First of all, the daughter was completely unable to be a companion to her mother because of her frequent and prolonged periods of manic-depressive psychosis; secondly, the mother is 80 years old and has had a constant companion for some time; thirdly a male companion, and especially a young one, is completely out of the question. We establish the presence of flight of ideas in this request only when we make pains to investigate the verbal-cognitive theme in relation to the over-all theme of the situation to which it alludes, or, as we very briefly say, to "reality." Then we establish that the patient does connect up with reality, but that she constructs an – from our viewpoint – absurd connection in thought between the mother and the seven remote nephews. Thereby, she vaults – as seen from without – with an invincible optimism over all of the obstacles that stand in the way of carrying out her thought. We only understand this connection of thoughts in returning to the life style of the patient, to the way and manner of her being in the world.

Of course, we are already familiar with this way and manner; it is the optimistically playful form of life, the misjudging of the gravity and seriousness of problems, *no less than that of things*, the misperceiving on the contours and limits of thoughts, *no less than those of things*. It is a particular kind of "unfocused" thinking we meet with here, lack of focus, however, that does not originate from intellectual disability, but rather from the optimistically playful life style, of which the play of thought represents but a single feature. "Thought" here means not merely a theme, but an earnest thematic elaboration of facts on an appropriate level of being. With regard to the thinking of our patient, we likewise see that serious matters have been treated playfully, just as we found for his contact with things, human beings and language. Here not only the thinking is flighty, but the entire form of life. Thus, you will understand why I regard it as an error to try to localize "flight of ideas" as a psychopathological sub-system in the brain or brain stem. The same applies to the compulsion to talk and be constantly busy; what one can project on to the brain is only the metamorphosis of the life style as such, the manic disturbance of mood as a whole. What can be projected on to the brain in such an instance is only the transformation of the life style as such, the manic disturbance of mood as a whole.

When we characterize the life form, the kind of being-in-the-world of the manic as flighty play, we are making a judgment that has a touch of the moral about it. But it is our task in psychiatry to avoid the moral value judgments with which we all too often label and classify the behavior and conduct of our patients, and, therefore, not only to understand but also to describe their behavior in terms of their existence or being-in-the-world. Existence, however, seen from where the manic patient is, is not frivolous play, but a continuous celebration. This is why he becomes so irritated when the examiner or doctor, who is completely unable to enter the picture in the role of a fellow celebrant and communicate festively with him, disturbs his revelry. To *celebrate*, however, implies to transcend unreflectively or in pure joy in existence the problematical aspects of life, even to the climax of vertigo.

Once we have discerned the essence of the manic life form in the festive joy of existence, we can also understand the intrinsic connection between *manic* and *depressive* life forms. We already know from

everyday life that, running through the festive vertigo in existence, this lordly unbridled to-do, singing, dancing, jumping, skipping, there is a streak of the "demonic." This same streak also reveals itself particularly clearly in the unrestrained festivities with masks at the time of carnival whose linkages with the cult of the dead are well-known. Where life holds its festivities, death is always at hand. The higher, more quickly and wildly life mounts up, the closer it is to death.

What we describe as manic-depressive disorder is merely a pathological formation and intensification of this universal principle of life and death, the entanglement of death in life and of life in death found everywhere. Therefore, it is not surprising that even the great founder of modern psychiatry Griesinger ... emphasized "that often enough melancholy looks through, like a dark background, the most unbridled arrogance of the manic phase." The truth of these words can be easily demonstrated today. You need only listen closely to the descriptions of nature by these persons especially in the form of poems, you need only study their dreams or Rorschach protocols in order to realize that wherever you encounter the phenomena of *mounting* life – the blooming, flourishing, gleaming, resounding, the jubilantly soaring lark and the eagle lifting itself drunken with sun into the ether – you will never fail to find the phenomena of *deciduous* life – the withering, decaying, moribund, deformed or disorganized, the gray, gloomy, hateful, dirty, stinking, the worm crawling in the ground, the death's head, the skeleton, the frigid mask or deformed visage, the discarded shards or scraps of paper lying around, etc. Likewise you will find – much to your surprise – in the language protocols of even the most confused patients with flight of ideas, in the hurly-burly of their outcries, greetings, questions, and commands, a depressive theme which breaks through the tumult again and again in a surprisingly well-ordered verbal form and here, too, of deepest life historical significance.

Inasmuch as the antinomy of life and death, immanent in life itself, finds its most striking expression in manic-depressive disorder, we could describe, in this sense, the manic-depressive person as the *antinomic* man par excellence. This is the person you have been charged to set yourself in relation with, with your entire being.

*****

Thus far, however, we have characterized the manic moment of festive joy in existence in negative terms, i.e., in opposition to the problems of existence and reflection. If we wish to characterize it positively, then we must describe it as a qualmless affirmation of existence, as an attunement of existence in which "all problems have evaporated." Such carefree assuredness uncontradicted by life experience is termed in the everyday language which we have used so much, *optimism*, actually crazy optimism, or briefly, insanity. Instead of further illustrations, I would like to read some words from Goethe that clarify this meaning:

"I never thought that something was to be attained; I always thought I already had it. They could have put a crown on my head and I'd have thought it completely understandable. And yet, just because of this I was human like any other person. But only because I tried to work at what I had grasped beyond my powers, and because I tried to deserve what I had undeservedly gotten, only because of this was I different from an actual madman."

That the manic already "has" everything, that it seems unnecessary for him to attain anything because he already has his hands on everything, is simply another way of saying everything is "handy" for him, as if he had only to stretch out his hand to have a crown on his head. Working through is so very much a part of the make-up of our existence that madness raises its head where it is missing.

What I have termed 'know-all optimism' is only one particular trait of optimism. Manic 'know-all optimism' like the 'know-all optimism' of the dream, of 'high altitude silliness', of the fever state, of intoxication, etc., enables one to believe that he already knows everything he encounters, that no height is too difficult, no journey too great, no problem eventually insoluble, as we saw in the request for the mother's companion, and as we often experience it in the dream. In the same way, dream and mania misapprehend the gravity of the problems of knowledge. They are 'knowledge' without a working through of what is to be known. The dreamer and the manic 'grasp' a swarm of themes 'beyond their powers', brushing their surface to be sure, but without reaching into the depths. In opposition to this unimpeded optimistic, all-abounding manner of thought, which superficially apprehends every germ of an idea as soon as it comes to consciousness, there is once more the depressive life and thought form of deciduous life, which revolves fundamentally about one problem only, the problem of death. However, the depressive form of life is just as incapable of working out that problem through thought alone, but can only violently realize it in suicide. So the extreme falling asunder into nothing save festive joy of existence and nothing save problems of existence leads in one direction to madness, in the other, without timely intervention, to death.

I have guided you along the way of psychiatric examination of mania, starting with the factual obstacles in reaching an understanding with patients to their being-in-the-world and their having of the world, as it emerges from the ground of those difficulties. This *first* stage of the examination is, with mania as also with endogenous depression, especially simple and easy. Here we can generally do without the patients' inner life histories and are able to limit ourselves to what we learn in direct communication with them. That is the principal reason why I chose mania in particular for the topic of my lecture. If we were concerned with schizophrenia, matters would be much more complicated. Then communication extending over months and sometimes years is necessary in order to understand the gradual or sudden changes of such patient's being-in-the-world. For while the manic, like the depressive lives purely according to his mood and in this regard, *ahistorically*, the history of a schizophrenic's illness cannot be understood without the most exact knowledge of his outer and especially inner *life history*. That proficiency in psychoanalytic interpretation of life historical connections is indispensable for understanding the life history, hardly needs mentioning.

The *second* stage in the course of the psychiatric examination is the *diagnostic* reduction of being-in-the-world and, occasionally, of its life historical changes into symptoms, or characteristics of illness. The manic triad: hyperactivity, flight of ideas, elated mood, is the result of this "diagnostic reduction process." Here the patient has ceased to be a partner in a communicating relationship; whenever we discuss symptoms of illness and diagnoses he is already seen as a *case*, i.e., as an individual belonging to a particular clinical variety or species, a particular clinical genus or class. Just as a plant is "specified" by the botanist in terms of certain characteristics on the basis of a botanical system, so the patient is specified here in terms of certain characteristics in accordance with the system of psychiatric pathology. To make you familiar and intimate with this system is the highest goal of psychiatric clinical instruction. For we are here concerned with the backbone of psychiatry as medical science.

And now to the *third* stage of psychiatric examination. Wherever we mention symptoms of illness and its diagnosis, we are already speaking of the *organism*. Diagnostic judgments in the medical sense, whether referring to psychic or somatic conditions, are wholly biological judgments of purpose or value, measured according to the norm of integration of an organism's achievements and functions. In the present instance, this is shown by our conception of the manic triad as expressive of an organismic hyperfunction more particularly of the nervous system. In contrast, however, to somatic medicine we are concerned in psychiatry with a biological doubling of the organism as psychic and somatic organism. I feel entitled to speak of a psychic organism because we can, if necessary, so far objectify psychic life (which, as pure "subjectivity," by its very nature, does not allow objectification), so reduce psychic life to the categories of natural science that we may finally speak here also of processes, functions, mechanisms, etc., all of which would be impossible without the idea of psychic organism. However, once we have turned being-in-the-world into a biological object, then all the pseudo-problems raise their heads, problems we are familiar with under the headings of psycho-physical parallelism, interaction or identity, which have led and still lead to arguments as useless as they are hopeless.

Now concerning the manic triad, we are speaking of a hyperfunction of the psychic organism, whose more detailed examination we leave to *psychopathology*. Only from this examination do we turn to the *fourth* stage of psychiatric examination, to the question of the "localization" of psychic functions and disturbances of function in the somatic organism. The special problems, the unavoidable difficulties and limits of such a localization, cannot be further pursued here. You have probably already noticed that here it is a matter of reducing the third stage, psychopathology, to the pathophysiology and pathological anatomy of the psychoses.

My intention was, as I emphasized at the beginning, to make clear to you how long and complicated a path the psychiatric examination has to follow until it reaches the point where it enters into the general medical procedure of examination and research, into questions of etiology and the courses of illness, of heredity, eugenics and causal therapy. You will only become a psychiatrist in the full sense of the word

when you realize that the psychiatric task in its entirety must not be restricted to one of the single stages or positions on this path, when you skip none of the particular stages as unimportant or incidental, but are always on the way from one position to another, feeling yourself right *at home* in this "on the way." For it is in this being on the way that the actual method of psychiatry reveals itself to you, as well as the *actual being* of the psychiatrist.

Schneider, K. (1920), 'The stratification of emotional life and the structure of depressive states'

From (1920) Die Schichtung des emotionalen Lebens und der Aufbau der Depressionszustände. *Zeitschrift für die gesamte Neurologie und Psychiatrie* 59. Translated by A. Stringaris (Institute of Psychiatry) (2010).

Editors' commentary

In this article from 1920, Kurt Schneider, who later developed the first rank symptoms of schizophrenia, sets out to establish a typology of depression. His attempt is based on the notion of a stratification of emotional life taken directly from Max Scheler's then famous work on ethics (Formalism in Ethics and Non-Formal Ethics of Values), *which is extensively quoted here. Schneider's distinction between endogenous and reactive depressive states has led to a lot of research and debate since. As such, the text may be considered as being at the origins of a rarely trodden pathway linking philosophy to clinical phenomena and empirical science. To the best of our knowledge, this is the first time this text has been translated into English.*

In the second part of his great work *Formalism in Ethics and Non-Formal Ethics of Values*, Max Scheler has provided a phenomenological account of emotional life, which seems to me to be of particular importance in examining certain pathopsychologic conditions. Since this book will rarely find its way to the hands of psychiatrists or of psychiatric libraries, it seems justified to refer more extensively to this fundamentally psychological chapter of his book. The ethical and metaphysical applications of this book will not be referred to here, so as to not miss its psychologically relevant aspects.

There is a stratification, a layering, in emotional life. As an example, our language distinguishes between bliss and a sense of well-being making clear that the two don't just differ in their intensity: there is rather a sharply demarcated difference of the very feelings involved. What points to this special kind of difference is the fact that these different types of feelings can "co-exist in one and the same act or moment of consciousness". This becomes particularly clear when such co-existing feelings possess different valences, one with positive and one with negative characteristics. A person can, as a martyr would, be blissful and at the same time suffer bodily pain, one can also feel "serene" amidst a great misfortune, in the sense of a "serenitas animi" but not "joyful", and one can, when despairing, enjoy a glass of wine. In such cases, it is not a succession of states of feelings that is taking place, as they are all present at the same time, and it doesn't even come to a mixture of different feelings that would add up to a total sum of feelings. Such feelings don't differ merely in their quality, they differ in their "depth". Apart from the sensible feelings, which by virtue of their [respective] localisation remain separable, feelings belonging to the same layer can blend with each other, but not so the feelings from different layers. Only secondarily do feelings from different layers also impact upon other contents of consciousness.

Emotional "depth" is in its essence linked to four well characterised levels "which conform to the structure of our entire human existence". One has to distinguish between: 1. sensible feelings (feelings of sensation, according to C. Stumpf) 2. feelings of the lived body (as states) and feelings of life, vital feelings, (as functions) 3. purely psychic feelings (pure ego feelings) 4. spiritual feelings (personality feelings). All feelings possess an experiential relatedness to the ego and this separates it from other contents, such as perceiving of events and imagining. However, this general Ego reference is fundamentally different in its essence for each of these four types of feeling.

Sensible feelings are localised in particular parts of the body, although they can – as in the case of lust or pain – expand and affect more remote parts of the body. Though they cannot be separated from the contents of sensation, they are nevertheless not just a property, an "overtone" of perception, but rather, from the outset, a new quality. Sensible feelings are never without an object, they are always present as a state; sensible feelings are never a function or an act devoid of "intention". It can certainly become the object of, for example, enjoyment or suffering. Sensible feelings are without any personal reference and they are ego-related only in a doubly indirect way.

They are not attached directly on the ego, in the way psychic feelings are, nor on the body, as true bodily feelings, which by virtue of the fact that we can say "my body" are related to the ego of the soul. They are merely given as states of a part of the body and in this way related to the ego in a doubly indirect way. Sensible feelings are an exclusively current state of affairs, they cannot be remembered or imagined through feeling. We cannot go through a process of "re-experiencing" a sensible feeling, nor can we experience the sensible feeling of others or with others, and we cannot experience a sensible feeling before we have actually felt it. A sensible feeling can only re-surface in an attenuated form; the stimulating object must then also be present. It is without continuity of meaning,[2] occurs as a discrete point in time, does not last, it does not signify anything from the past or the future. Of all the feelings, the sensible feeling is least disturbed through focusing attention on it, quite the contrary. Vital feelings (as we shall be calling the second layer of feelings), that serve to guide our living activities in a meaningful way, are disturbed in their normal process by diverting attention to them and only thrive in a certain darkness. One can be set free from the sufferings of the soul through focusing, analysing, objectifying. The more any feelings resemble sensible feelings, the more they can be "had or not had", can be produced at will, are subject to volition. Every pain can, in principle, be anaesthetised. Pure psychic feelings (those least admixed with vital feelings) are the least manipulable and hardest to produce at will. Spiritual feelings evade any form of volition, are spontaneous, springing from the depths of the person itself, and therefore they are least reactive, like bliss and despair. They cannot be intended, precisely because they are not reactive and they cannot be set as a goal.

Vital feelings, although they don't possess a particular location in the body, take part in what is the expansive character of the body. It is not "I" who feels comfortable, in the same way I feel sad or in despair, rather "I" can only feel "myself" in this way. The "myself" represents my "lived body". The bodily feeling is a uniform act. The fact that sensible feelings can

---

[2] This is the same that, since Jaspers, we call "meaningful connections". The juxtapositions verstehen vs erklären (connections that "make sense" vs causal) connections may be more accurate, however, the Jasperian expression is clearer in the context of psychiatry. [**Original note**]

exist next to it shows that it cannot be composed out by the fusion of such feelings; if this were the case they would have been used up. Besides, the valences of vital compared to sensible feelings can be different: One can, whilst experiencing the strongest feelings of lust, feel feeble and miserable. Vital feelings always have an intentional and functional character. Sensible feelings can be used as signs, as indicators of certain states and processes when investigating an object. By contrast, in vital feelings we feel life itself, in this feeling there is something given to us, the "rise" and the "fall", "health" and "disease", "danger" etc. Vital feelings are part of "experiencing the feelings of others" or "experiencing feelings with others". In vital feelings we have the "remembering of feelings" not just "feelings of remembering". Vital feelings can also indicate direct threats or gains, states which are beyond the reach of the powers of imagination and comprehension. Vital feelings function as a notation for the ever-changing states in the process of life. Vital feelings are particularly valuable because they arise before the experience of actual harms or gains that can affect the process of life from within or from outside the lived body. By contrast, sensible feelings are only concomitant, they are simultaneous. Vital feelings anticipate the value of a given stimulus as well as its onset: anxiety, fear, disgust, appetite, vital sympathy and antipathy. Vital feelings can operate from a distance in both a spatial and temporal sense (they are feelings-from-a-distance) – by contrast sensible feelings require actual contact (they are feelings-by-contact).

Psychic (soul) feelings are by their origin ego-qualities, without the need for mediation by bodily states. Psychic feelings are not at the slightest expansive. The changing shades of the various bodily and vital feelings do not affect the peculiarity of soul feelings. "Deceptions leading to confusion" can occur between the constituents from different layers. Psychic feelings are motivated. According to Scheler, "A man whose psychic feelings aren't motivated and whose continuity of feelings suffers from ongoing breakdowns merely due to changes in bodily produced emotions, would be as incomprehensible as someone who is severely intellectually impaired."

In spiritual feelings – bliss, despair, peace of mind, serenity – all ego-related states are as if extinguished. Spiritual feelings infiltrate all the important contents of life. They are not reactive feelings, they are not responding to extra-personal value considerations and to their motives. "If we can still identify 'something' for the sake of which we believe ourselves to be blissful or despaired, then we are certainly not blissful or despaired." We can of course be deprived of spiritual feelings through the presence of other feelings "through a motivated chain of meanings" that occur at the end of such a sequence of experiences, but when the spiritual feelings are there, they detach themselves from such a chain of motivation and fulfil the entirety of our existence and "world". We can only then "be" either blissful or despaired, not feel bliss and despair, let alone feel "ourselves" in that way. These feelings are either not experienced at all or they seize possession of the entirety of our being. These are the metaphysical and religious self-feelings par excellence.

Following this overview of Schelerian phenomenology of emotional life, I turn to how it applies to psychiatry, in particular to how it applies to depressive states. The focus on depression should not be taken to imply that Schelerian phenomenology may not be fruitfully applied to other pathopsychologic conditions – I am thinking particularly of affective disturbances in schizophrenia. An important lesson from Scheler's distinctions is that the co-occurrence of positively and negatively valenced feelings from different layers, even when these feelings concern one and the same object, should not lead us to assume that we are dealing with affective ambivalence.

We shall be viewing depressive conditions based on the two well-characterized extreme manifestations, the purely unmotivated "endogenous" and the purely reactive depression. These types are so familiar through everyday clinical experience that case presentations are unnecessary. It is immediately evident that a disturbance of vital feelings plays a much greater role in endogenous depression. We know that disturbances of feelings of the lived body and vital feelings can come to dominate the clinical picture of endogenous depression and that such feelings precede sadness and can persist well after sadness has gone. They are often hard to tease apart from sensible mis-feelings, which are localized in the head. That such conditions often change according to endogenous rules is well known. I am reminded in particular of the typical diurnal variations and also of biological symptoms, such as the changes in weight and menstruation. Matters are different in reactive depression. It is not as if disturbances of vital feelings or of sensible mis-feelings are totally absent in reactive depression; however, they are much rarer and, most importantly: they are exclusively secondary symptoms. The primary disturbance in reactive depression is the disturbance of psychic feelings.

How, then, do these psychic feelings behave in endogenous depression? They do seem disturbed in most cases and in a very striking way. Nevertheless, it is easy to show that the "sadness" of endogenous depression is different to that of reactive depression. Let us look first at the symptom of anxiety, where this distinction of types is clearer and well recognized. All of us know from our patients about this empty anxiety that lacks in content and that is prominently a bodily feeling, often an organ feeling. Whearaes the German language does not have words to distinguish between different forms of anxiety,[3] the French make a distinction between "angoisse" and "anxiété". It is similar with "sadness" and this is again shown by experience. Not only in ourselves do we experience the difference between an unmotivated mood change and a reactive sadness, our endogenousely depressive patients are also able of distinguishing between them. Anyone who has ever, for example, had a patient whose relative died knows that the reactive sadness experienced by the patient is different from the endogenous sadness. This is most evident in remission, when the endogenously depressed is again capable of registering such experiences. Educated patients know of the difference between "normal" sadness and the ever-protracted, albeit subtle, feeling of endogenous sadness. These two types of sadness cannot be summed together to a total feeling, they can co-exist in one and the same act of consciousness, since they stem from different emotional layers and they only share their name. We have heard already that feelings of one layer may rub off on another layer. Therefore it is not surprising to observe that psychic feelings of sadness may arise secondarily (as a consequence) of endogenous depression. It is also understandable that patients will seek to find a motivation, a meaning for their vital depression, they invent the words to the melody, as it were and this is not an uncommon pathway leading to delusional ideas.

By understanding that endogenous depression is a primary depression in the layer of vital feelings, we are also able to grasp those not so rare forms which are confined to the disturbance of other vital feelings. In such cases there is not even a dull vital sadness, let alone a secondary disturbance of psychic feelings. Such forms are often labelled along with other conditions as "hysterical melancholia" or "neurasthenic melancholia" (Friedmann). These considerations can even explain why in some manic depressive patients there is a disturbance of vital feelings even outside of their "depression", often even as an ongoing condition (Kraepelin). Even the symptom of the "feeling of being empty of feelings" can now be seen in a different light. It is namely possible that the disturbance of the vital feelings is so severe that psychic feelings cannot actually manifest themselves, in a similar way to how people can come to be dominated by strong feelings of pain. Finally, it should be mentioned that we should only expect the "feeling ill", in its vital essence, to occur only where vital feelings are affected. The reactively depressed, who is not suffering from vital mis-feelings, will feel "ill" only in a figurative way.

In this context it would be an important task to use this framework to examine the phenomenology of involutional melancholy and to establish whether it shows differences from periodic depression, which seems unlikely to me. To draw the analogies for the manic and reactively manic conditions, would be beyond the scope of our outline here. I shall only briefly refer to mixed states. This is to prevent the misunderstanding that I am talking about mixtures of feelings with different valences stemming from the same layer – this would apply to schizophrenia. In mixed states, feeling states may either arise one after the other in quick succession or – and these are the only true mixed states – a feeling state is associated with an oppositely valenced motor response. In mania, vital feelings rub off more easily on to psychic feelings than in depression, the conditions are otherwise analogous.

This characterisation of the types of endogenous and reactive depression should not be taken as a statement about their relationship with each other. It is perfectly conceivable that a vital depression is elicited by a sad event – we do also see in hysteria disturbances of sensible and vital feelings elicited in similar ways, without being able to understand the mechanisms at work. Furthermore, we have seen already that what may originally have been a purely reactive depression – which in contrast to the psychically caused vital depression is characterised by its meaningful connections with the actual experience – can, as a consequence, rub off on

---

[3] Because there is no sharp distinction made between "anxiety (Angst)" and "fear (Furcht)": although we wouldn't use "fear" instead of "anxiety", we would commonly use "anxiety" instead of using "fear". [**Original note**]

to vital feelings. A "vitalisation" of such originally reactive depressions doesn't seem uncommon and it can, as evidenced by wartime soldiers, even go so far as for the depression to persist by "vital rules", even in the absence of what had originally elicited the "suffering". It is similar in the field of anxiety with regards to certain phobias and obsessional states.

I have intentionally avoided discussing the pathopsychology of spiritual feelings, and I am not sure about their fundamental distinction from psychic feelings. Without a doubt, it would be of great interest to examine whether anything similar to spiritual feelings are experienced in psychotic conditions (which would seem unlikely according to how Scheler described their essence) and to point out any differences that may exist between states that seem very similar from the outside: the schizophrenic experience of "being endowed with heavenly grace" and of "ecstasy", and of true person feelings.

Straus, E. (1928), 'The experience of time in endogenous depression and in the psychopathic[4] depressive state'

From (1928) Das Zeiterleben in der endogenen Depression und in der psychopathischen Verstimmung. *Monatsschrift für Psychiatrie und Neurologie* 68: 640. Translated by M. Symonds and N. Kern.

Editors' commentary

This text, like the one that follows (by Viktor von Gebsattel), was written in 1928. Both follow on from Kurt Schneider's 1920 article (please refer to p. 203). Like Schneider, both attempt a phenomenological understanding of endogenous depression and its distinction from 'psychopathic' or 'reactive' depression. The distinction remains a problem in psychopathology to this day. Schneider, looking at the problem from the perspective of layers of emotional life, concluded that it is the vital strata of emotions which are disturbed in endogenous depression and the psychic strata in 'reactive' depression. Straus and von Gebsattel come at the problem from the perspective of temporality and try to argue that the experience of time is disturbed in endogeneous depressive states but not in

'psychopathic' ones. Temporality has been explored by phenomenologists (especially Scheler and Heidegger) as the basis of anxiety, guilt and the immanence of our own death – all phenomena we see amplified in depressive states. Straus and von Gebsattel draw, in part, upon Scheler's ideas on temporality. Von Gebsattel makes use of a case where a young woman with depression occurring within a manic-depressive illness is able to express an alteration in her experience of time with consequent compulsive acts and a heightened experience of being on a path toward death. The texts are interesting and they succeed in drawing attention to the deeper phenomenological structures underpinning depressive states but they do not conclusively resolve the distinctions.

On good days and weeks, when we are being productive, having ideas, able to accomplish our work, or on which events occur that are of significance to us, or we are exposed to an abundance of new impressions – on a journey, for example – we are scarcely conscious of the experience of time passing by, suddenly we become aware that it is already lunchtime or night time, and yet nonetheless evening and morning, the weekend and the start of the week appear widely spaced, the time span that has been traversed seems to be spread out over a long period. By contrast, on bad days, when production comes to a standstill, when we are entirely at the mercy of the repetitive monotony of our everyday work, what we notice is how sluggishly time is dragging by. Everyone can remember tedious school hours, long train journeys, spent checking their watch over and over again at intervals that seemed to take an age to live through, only to discover to their disappointment that the hand of the watch had hardly moved at all. At the same time, when the person looks back on these bad days, evening and morning, the end and beginning of the weeks seem to be closely crowded together, the time span traversed seems short.

The contrast between how lived and remembered time is estimated, something that can be adduced from any number and variety of examples, signals an objective contrast: namely that between the immanent lived experience and the transuent experience[5]

---

[4] By 'psychopathic' Straus means 'reactive' or 'neurotic' contrasting it with endogenous. The term has no resemblance to psychopathy in its contemporary English meaning. [**Editors' note**]

[5] The contrast between 'immanent' and 'transuent' causation was an abstract distinction popular amongst neo-Kantian philosophers. 'Immanent causation' stood for causation within the same entity and 'transuent causation' between entities. We are unclear how Straus is applying this contrast to the experience of time. [**Editors' note**]

of time (Hönigswald), between subjective time and universal time. Measured on the clock, good and bad days, good and bad weeks and years are exactly the same length. Physical, objective time flows, by definition, homogenously, evenly, it has no defining points, no early and late, no today, tomorrow and yesterday, no fast and slow progression. All those characteristics of time as it is experienced, as being fulfilled or unfulfilled, as being structured or unstructured, as flowing quickly or sluggishly, as dragging or flying by, all these are extraneous to objective time. For that reason, physical time is not a suitable means, or at least it is not a sufficient means on its own, of describing the temporal moment of experiences. When we use time as a reference, experiences are only registered as external events, but their fundamental inner property is not represented. Only behavioural psychology employs the sort of principles that would entitle it to make do with objective time as a measurement.

There is no doubt that homogenous objective time is a purely methodical construction, devised for the purpose of measuring and making mathematical sense of natural events.[6]

However, the development of all the sciences has been dominated for so long by physics and the epistemological approaches that accord with its premises that only very recently has due attention been paid once again to the unique character of historical, biological and the immanent lived experience of time. And even now, this understanding has still mainly been restricted to the theoretical disciplines, philosophy, philosophy of history, psychology of thought and theoretical physics. It has still had very little influence on empirical psychology, pathopsychology and biology, although it is precisely by way of the structure of time, and only then, that the diversity of phenomena, the very juxtaposition of symptoms in a pathological case, for example, can form a conceptually understandable unit.

It is a singular connection which formal and content-related structures form with one another in the experience of time. The experience of time thus becomes a means of solving all the problems related to the dependence of the contents of experience on formal processes and functions. Problems that have equal theoretical and practical importance for psychiatry are particularly suitable. The following is an initial attempt to understand, via the experience of time in endogenous depression, the relationship between some accessory psychotic symptoms and the biological cardinal symptom of the illness, and further, to gain through this examination of the experience of time a new differential diagnostic criterion that can be used to a certain extent to distinguish between endogenous and psychopathic[7] depressive states. Before we do this, however, we must explore in more detail the general observations begun above about the experience of time.

It hardly needs to be emphasised that we should not yet understand the transuent experience of time in the same way as objective time, as measured in physics. For even this transuent time accessible to experience still has distinguishable points, a now, today, yesterday, etc. It is the experience of transuent time that we share with other people, and also with the objects of the external world. And whilst it is this that enables a spatio-temporal system of counting and measuring and whilst it can thus be related quite easily to objective time, it is not, however, identical with it.

The immanent lived experience of subjective time, which grows alongside the development of the inner personal history, is not measurable and countable in the same way as universal time. The particularity of how it is experienced will be elaborated in more detail in the account below.

*****

As psychophysical persons, we belong to both types of time, but whilst transuent time is measured according to the duration or the change in the things around us, the measure of immanent lived experience of time is the evolvement of the personality; looking forwards, the experience of anticipated action and its effect, looking backwards, the steps of inner personal

---

[6] I have looked in more detail at the problem of time, at the relationship of the physical to historical and biological time, and at the connection with biological potencies in my essay on "The Problem of Individuality". Reference should therefore be made to what is stated there, and to the literature cited therein. Of more recent works, from a methodological approach Hönigswald's psychology of thought should also be mentioned, and from a phenomenological and ontological approach in particular Scheler's essay on Idealism and Realism. [Original note]

[7] Straus is using 'psychopathic' here in the sense of 'reactive' or 'neurotic'. [Editors' note]

development taken in transuent time. Transuent time passes, whilst subjective time proceeds, grows with the history of the person. The measure of subjective time is thus not an identifiably numerical collection of external stimulatory effects. The number of stimuli, both internal and external, can be the same on good and bad days or the quantity of stimuli on the good days can be exceeded by those on the bad days; the internal experience of time is not defined in this way. External incidents and occurrences only become meaningful events when they have been arranged within the individual life story.[8] Even though the internal life story develops through such events, its own course is still founded in a development along a path towards a particular objective point of time, and it is this that gives it the status of an event. By being arranged within the life story, a value factor is added to external events that are in themselves indifferent to values. Subjective time is therefore historically directed, whereas transuent time is not characterised in this way.

The individual historical development is entirely dependent on biological potencies and the biological history of the individual, from the transition from what is potentially possible to its actualisation. This correlation finds direct expression in the experience of time, insofar as the future is experienced as potential action and its effect. This experience of potential action and its effect, which is grounded in the biological powers, is directed towards the life story. The sense of potential action and its effect enables the individual to anticipate the evolution of the personality in the future enabled by the actualisation of the biological potencies.[9] The structure of the individual experience of time, which is dependent on biological events, in turn conditions and limits the structure of the possible content of experience, so linking biological and psychical events together.

In the example of boredom it would therefore be more correct to describe the situation not as one where a person is hindered in his attempt to give time a content of his own choosing, but rather to give

greater emphasis to the opposition between subjective time and universal time. For boredom only manifests itself when the impossibility of giving transuent time a content is experienced at the same time as the individual potential action and its effects, the drive towards development (cf. Pilker's concept of the drive to be awake). If this need is absent, when the person is fatigued or depressed, then the same external conditions lead to the occurrence of completely different experiences. So, for example, the atmosphere at the end of the working day is such that the internal sense of lingering time can be enjoyed whilst there is a steady progression of transuent time. The pleasure can even be heightened if the contrast is intensified between the sense of peacefulness within and the events taking place externally. One only needs to remember that familiar image of the farmer or workman when he has knocked off work for the day. It is only when he is watching the external events that he really begins to appreciate his own peace and quiet. However, stopping like this is clearly only experienced as a pause between having done something and being about to do something else, and so does not lack the relationship to the future. Every festival, every celebration has this character of a pause associated with it, and only remains a happy experience for as long as it can retain this character.

*****

Certain euphoric and depressive moods are very closely linked to the harmony and the contrast between subjective and universal time, and to the manner in which subjective time rushes ahead of or drags behind universal time. Both the experience of time and these vital dispositions are rooted in the same biological event.[10] It is only for these types of affect that the James-Lange theory of emotions has any justifiable basis. Only through the experience of time and its connection to individual personal history do other experiential contents and functions become indirectly dependent on the biological event. We will attempt to demonstrate how in endogenous depression, delusions, compulsive thinking and the inhibition of certain affects are determined by the basic vital disorder through the experience of time.

---

[8] Note the etymological origin of the German word "Ereignis" and its relation to "eigen", corresponding to the English word "own". [Original note]

[9] The experience of potential action and its effect is not linked to the intactness of the motor apparati, neither of the pyramidal tract nor of the extrapyramidal motor system. [Original note]

[10] Cf. the work of K. Schnieder, The stratification of emotional life and the structure of the depressive states. [Original note].

First of all, however, it should be pointed out again that healthy experience, as has been illustrated in the examples used above, is directed towards the future. Of course, we should not take that to mean that conscious thought normally extends perpetually towards the future. We are talking here about the evolution of time, not about the experience of structuring time, of organising temporal points, the disruption of which process plays a role in organic dementia. As long as the biological development remains undisturbed and thus the possibility of personal development still exists, the future as an anticipated function is also assumed. This fact can be proven in any number of empirical cases; it finds its general expression in the fact that the concept of personal immortality concerns people almost exclusively in the form of a question related to the individual future, whilst the theoretically equal question relating to the individual past is virtually disregarded. Euphoric moods only manifest when they are directed towards the future.[11] Every alteration that the experience of the future sustains, either externally or internally, has a simultaneous effect on the present experience and even on transforming the past, which on no account can be thought of as a rigid entity lying behind us. Past experiences, too, are only illuminated in the light of the future event. The past only carries us and supports us when the way into the future lies open. The past cannot comfort us, or it can only comfort us if the future is not entirely cut off.

The vital inhibition in endogenous depression also initially only influences the experience of the future, by means of the alteration of the potential action and its effect. But as the accumulating internal time slows down, stalls and finally comes to a stop, the structure of what is in the past also changes. As soon as the internal life story undergoes stasis, the sense and prevailing meaning of events along the stretch of life that has already been traversed is altered as well. This alteration is not only related to the content of what has happened, lending a new emotional tone to past events; it is also a formal alteration, insofar as the experience of being determined by the past and of how it is resolved undergoes a profound change,

which has a bearing on everything in the past, consolidating memory falsifications and fabrications. Of these alterations, that of being determined by the past is related to depressive delusion, that of being able to resolve it to the symptoms of compulsion. In its influence on the experience of time, the vital inhibition, the cardinal symptom of endogenous depression, plays a decisive part in the construction of psychotic symptoms, whereby a step-by-step gradation of the restriction of the future experience correlates with the fluctuating intensity of the inhibition, and in turn, the manifestation of certain symptoms corresponds to these steps in the modification of the experience of time.

If the intensity of the inhibition is only slight, and subjective time does not come to a complete standstill, but simply slows down, then in the first instance it is the potential effectivity that suffers in a characteristic manner. The nature of the relationship between non-complex compulsive symptoms, such as the compulsion to control, obsessive thought processes, and *folie du doute*, and this disturbance of the experience of time requires an initial explanation.

Normally, we do not only turn towards the new once the objective demands and systematic connections of earlier experiences have been completely resolved, but rather we deal with what has happened in the past, we turn the transuent past into immanent past, by turning to the future. This normal process of resolution can be demonstrated in individual lives, but equally in the succession of historical epochs. In the history of science, too, problems are very rarely concluded definitively and systematically, but instead they become obsolete questions pertaining to the older generation and shunted out of existence by new questions being addressed and considered. That is why old problems can sometimes suddenly come to life again. In the same way, in the life of the individual, the same form of resolving the past means that it can never be fully brought to a close and can therefore continue to have an effect in the future. Only in this manner can the continuity of the life history be sustained. The experiences of regret and conversion can be understood in this way. This opposition between resolving events objectively and autobiographically is characteristic of the process of volition, too. Thus there is always a residual element of what has not been resolved objectively which is transported and carried over into the future. What has been fully resolved loses its connection with what is in the future, drops out of the life history because it has no

---

[11] The ecstatic feeling of happiness, which should not be confused with the vital euphoric emotions, is experienced as a release from the temporal event. The temporal structure of emotions as indicated here has until now rarely been considered, although it constitutes a fundamental element of its objective formation.
[Original note]

ongoing effect upon it, and henceforth belongs only to the shell, not the body, of the life history.

This form of resolving what has happened by stepping on into the future has the further consequence that in healthy experience we do not experience ourselves as being determined completely and utterly by the past. The condition of being entirely determined by the past is something that will be explored in more depth later in our discussion of depressive delusion. At this point, we should simply emphasise that we are concerned with the experience of determination, but not with the question or problem of objective determination. The manner in which we experience ourselves as being determined by the past must be discussed primarily and independently of any theoretical assumptions about objective determination, psychical causality and the problem of free will.

When depression brings internal time to a standstill, there is no longer the possibility of resolving experiences in the way described above, by stepping on into the future. Inner experience has reached an impasse, and the depressive can no longer turn the transuent past into an immanent one. The demands for conclusion that emanate from things cannot be fulfilled in the future-less experience of the depressive.

If we consider the behaviour of the healthy person in relation to a crucially important letter, we can see that it is not so very different from that of the obsessive-compulsive, who is constantly checking that his letter is correctly stamped, addressed and sealed. In a case such as this one, the healthy person also makes draft copies, improves, alters and revises them, delays the decision, finally makes up his mind and, even after making a decision he is happy with, is often beset with reservations that allow him no peace of mind until he has finally surrendered what is to come to the future. We say a letter has crucial importance, however, when it anticipates many future possibilities, when it definitively determines a certain path into the future. This restriction of future freedom inhibits the decision. The accumulation of the determining force of the past over the future proceeds in these cases from certain content matters. The depressive obsessive-compulsive, on the other hand, when confronted by the formal alteration of the experience of time, the obstruction of the path into the future that is not bound to a particular content matter, is constantly thrown back towards the starting point with every action he takes. He can never bring himself to make important decisions; and when it comes to small

things, whilst there is an initial motion towards an action, a fruitless attempt at resolution, this always leads back to the beginning. It is significant in this case that sick people's doubt is directed towards the manner in which they resolve something, and not towards the various objective possibilities between which the healthy person vacillates whilst making a decision. The compulsion to control thus displays itself as a symptom of the basic depressive disorder, it is just one dependent element within the totality of the alteration of the personality. The non-complex compulsive processes named here are founded in the opposition between subjective time and universal time that is specific to depressive experience. Even more clearly than in the case of the compulsion to control, obsessive thought processes demonstrate that thought is not inhibited in the first instance as a function, but rather in its character as an action. In obsessive thought, too, the past cannot be concluded or laid to rest; the same thing has to be thought over and over, often any banal things, in other cases metaphysical questions displaced from temporal events, because thinking further ahead, thinking as a process of dealing with and constituting the future, is prevented.[12]

---

[12] The fact that all thinking is an activity of the thinker is something that receives too little consideration. When it is considered, however, it tends to be associated with the fallacy that therefore what is said can also only be interpreted pragmatically. Because thinking is an action, the attention can turn arbitrarily towards certain subjects. It has long been known that the thought disorders of manic-depressive illness cannot only be derived from formal alterations in thinking, especially since Liepmann's work on the flight of ideas. But neither do leading ideas and determining tendencies lead a special existence. Their dynamic does not derive from their logical structure, but from their psychological meaning, from the place that they occupy in the framework of the thinking person. The same formal characteristics of thinking could therefore bring about quite different results, depending on which alterations in the whole structure of the personality they encounter. In one case, for example, a constant flitting of ideas from one subject to another, in the other a restless brooding that goes nowhere. I cannot elaborate any further on the difficulties that we run up against in analysing the mixed states of the manic-depressive condition. Kraepelin's interpretation, deriving from independent variations of elementary functions, is no longer compatible with our modern understanding of how the personality is constructed. [Original note]

For the purposes of description, we do make a distinction between compulsive ideas, compulsive impulses and compulsive acts. However, it is already apparent here, and will be emphasised even more clearly in the following discussion, that all compulsive symptoms are compulsive acts that have the character of actions, even if precisely because of the disorder contained within each compulsive experience they do not come to have an external effect. A sick person who feels tortured by compulsive blasphemous thoughts does not just suffer under the thoughts alone, but also under the idea that he is having to adopt these thoughts as his own, and so having to blaspheme God in an internal act. Through this active character, compulsion and time are forced into an internal relationship, which is also genetically significant, even crucial, for the one group of compulsive actions, as we have just observed.

Of course, by no means all compulsive symptoms of depression, such as the compulsive experience of a mother who feels the desire to murder her children,[13] can be thought to derive from the temporal structure of depressive experience. However, there is a further group of compulsive symptoms, encountered in severe inhibitions, that seem to me to be closely related to the experience of time: the compulsion to count, the compulsion to turn one's attention to any external or internal rhythmic processes. Here the ontological relationship between number and time becomes an experience. In the case of these compulsive symptoms already discussed,[14] what occurs is partly to do with an attempt to drive stalling time onwards (one patient states, for example, that time only advances at all when she is doing her crochet work), and partly to do with finding a way of giving substance to the void of external time as it slips past.

*****

We are accustomed in psychiatry to use psychological facts to diagnose and label biological functional disorders, apart from in the group of illnesses related to neuroses. By doing so, the particularity of the biological conceptualisation is sometimes blurred, and characteristics are ascribed to concepts in biological psychiatry that they could only have as psychological concepts. The concept of inhibition is one of these terms that is also commonly used in a half biological, half psychological sense. This teleological approach encourages negative, judgemental terms to start penetrating into biology. As the history of biological theories shows, in so doing we run the risk of transgressing a boundary, i.e. of psychologising biological processes. But only in an experience where the happenings datable to a particular point in time are classified in terms of a comprehensive connection to immanent time, only in an experience of this kind does the non-happening have the form of a gap, an absence, an inhibition, only then can doing and not-doing take on the sense of resolution and non-resolution. It becomes apparent here that the body-soul problem, insofar as it is solvable i.e. insofar as it is a problem at all, can only be solved in relation to the experience of time.

The more strongly the inhibition is felt, and the more the tempo of internal time slows down, the more clearly the determining violence of the past is experienced. The more firmly the future is closed off to the depressive, the more strongly he feels overcome by and tied to the past. The malady that he experiences is decided, indeed determined irrevocably and unalterably, by the past. In the case of the depressive delusion of smallness, the ideas of guilt, ideas of impoverishment, it is characteristic that the effect of the patient's guilt on himself, his immediate family, and the whole of humanity is already entirely contingent on the past. It may well only be expected to make an appearance at a later point in time, which as such belongs to transuent time, but its appearance itself is categorically predefined by acts that cannot be rectified. What happens or will happen is determined by the past. That is also true of hypochondriacal delusion. The onset of terrible illnesses or the advent of their devastating consequences can still be pending, but the actual onset itself has already become inevitable through what has happened in the past. The depressive no longer fears the onset of illnesses like the psychopathic hypochondriac does. (Fear is of course always related to the future event, to something not conclusively determined, whilst anxiety is related to current existence. Fear is based on the possibility of the realisation of an adverse possibility;

---

[13] It is more likely that those types of compulsive symptoms have their basis in depersonalisation. [Original note]

[14] Wundt has already indicated the connection between the perception of time and the perception of rhythm, as embodied by walking, breathing, the pulse. Bücher has investigated the way that monotonous physical labour is facilitated by rhythmisation. [Original note]

but the chance of favourable possibilities still exists. In order to realise these, the fearful person tries to find help.) The psychopathic hypochondriac solicits consolation and support from the doctor, whilst the depressive refuses this, since his fate is already determined. The incorrigibility and unshakeableness of the delusion within the depressive finds its objective equivalent in the knowledge that he has been definitively determined by the past, and abandoned by it to destruction.

Depressive delusions do not have the same underlying experiential material as that of the healthy person, where a delusional meaning is only experienced under the effect of particular emotions; in the case of the depressive the material presenting itself to be processed has itself already been modified under the influence of the altered experience of time. In it, the lines that the depressive delusion follows are already, as it were, marked out in advance.[15]

During the depressive stupor even transuent time eventually seems to come to a standstill, as far as we can conclude from external impressions. At this deepest level of inhibition, it appears that the sick person's experience is that of time absolutely failing to extend and that as a result the person fails to understand events in his vicinity and to understand the temporal order of these processes, as can be seen in objective catemneses. In the case of the stupor arising from schizophrenic inhibition, the same disturbances of the experience of time do not occur.

There remains for us now to consider the connection between the breakdown of certain affective experiences and the experience of time. I have already indicated at the beginning that the moment of time is objectively of great importance in differentiating and classifying the emotions. The well known phenomenon whereby the depressive is capable of grieving for a loss that he has suffered just so little as he experiences joy over some happy circumstance, has suggested the possible explanation that as well as other functions the affective receptiveness is also inhibited. It is still astounding, all the same, that this hindrance affects the emotions of both joy and grief. K. Schneider has tried to understand this striking phenomenon with the aid of the Schelerian theory of the stratification of emotional life. According to this, the depressive and euphoric moods belong to a deeper level than joy and grief; it is possible that the vital emotional disturbances become so intense that emotional feelings are not actually able to emerge at all, in a similar manner to the way in which strong pains could completely govern a person.

With respect to the difficulties adherent in interpreting the feeling of loss of feeling, it may be helpful to consider that joy and grief are compatible only with a certain experience of time. For all grief over a loss involves the internal sense of lack beginning at the moment of loss and extending into the future, and this corresponds to joy, which involves an enrichment starting at the moment of gain and related to the future. Thus joy presupposes the capacity for enrichment, grief the possibility of a lack with respect to the future relationship to the world around. However, when the vital inhibition is such that the experience of the future is completely extinguished and, as it were, a temporal vacuum is created, joy and grief lack any possibility of being realised.

We do not therefore need to assume a specific inhibition of these affective functions beside the vital inhibition, but rather can deduce that the loss of emotions discussed here via the experience of time derives from this underlying basic disorder.

In the psychogenic depressive moods the alteration of the experience of time characteristic of endogenous depression does not occur. The psychopathically disturbed person is not cut off from the future, but threatened in the future. His mood therefore belongs to a completely different dimension, to the relationship between the self and fate, and the particular symptoms therefore differ accordingly from those of real depression. Psychogenic depression is governed by the tension heightened for whatever reason between the self and fate. This tension remains the substance of the experience and determines all further reactions and course of events. The picture is configured differently depending on whether the conflict is solved or persists, whether the sick person succumbs to apathy and resignation in response to his feeling of impotence in the face of the external forces, or whether he seeks to obtain assistance and

---

[15] The variety of forms that paranoid delusions take shows that here it is a case of particular characteristics of depressive delusion, but not of delusion in general. Manic delusions, unlike depressive delusions, are more changeable and less serious, they relate to a present or future aggrandisement of the own self, or to an achievement still forthcoming, or to a piece of good fortune, whose occurrence does not need to be based in the past. [Original note]

relief indirectly via further psychogenic reactions. In all the aspects that we are able to observe in such cases, we can recognise that there is no alteration of the experience of time dependent on the vital inhibition.[16]

The future is threatening and full of dark clouds, but the future is also assumed; the flow of time does not come to a standstill. Only the form in which the future presents itself is refused, avoided, or indirectly opposed. In the fears, complaints, the open or hidden accusations against others, the anger frequently escalated to the point of enjoyment, the suicide attempts, the despondency, the person's behaviour remains a reaction to what is going to happen in the future, and it changes as soon as a propitious turn for the better dissolves the tension that has set in.

The psychogenic depressive mood is therefore not only linked to other psychophysical strata, but is also linked to them in a different way. Through its underlying psychopathic constitution, the limits of the individual's relationship to the environment and the possible forms of reaction to it are indeed predetermined, but the psychogenic mood does not originate from a pathological variation of the psychophysical functions, but rather is a reaction to a variation in the environment.

The statements that endogenously depressed patients make to us about their experience of time, either spontaneously or when questioned, are manifold. Sick people report that time runs dry, seems in their anxiety to have come to a stop. Or again, that the passage of time in general has slowed down, or that time only seems to move forward when a steady mechanical activity is taking place. These statements do not contradict our explanations, yet by themselves they would not be enough to deduce them inductively. However, sick people can really not be expected to be able to make substantive statements about such a general feature of experiences such as time. Experience that can be conceptualised is as a rule addressed to that which is quite specific to the individual moment. It is not the basic forms, but only their salient alterations that become perceptible. Even language works in opposition to this pragmatic tendency and tends to inhibit rather than facilitate

attempts to apprehend the general elements of experience in a conscious manner. It is therefore important that the relationship derived from the psychological analysis of symptoms between the intensity of the inhibition and the appearance of certain psychotic phenomena be examined clinically, if the methods employed here are ever to be rendered fruitful.[17]

Gebsattel, V. von (1928), 'Compulsive thought relating to time in melancholia'

From (1954) Zeitbezogenes Zwangsdenken in der Melancholie. In *Prolegomena einer medizinischen Anthropologie.* Berlin: Springer. Translated by M. Symons and N. Kern (2010). First published as (1928) Zeitbezogenes Zwangsdenken in der Melancholie: Versuch einer konstrucktiv-genetische Betrachtung der Melancholiesymptome. *Der Nervenarzt* 5(1).

Editors' commentary

See commentary above, p. 207.

We will take as a starting point of our investigation the complex of symptoms of compulsive thought relating to time in a case of endogenous melancholia. The patient is a 20-year-old girl, who fell sick with an endogenous depression as a result of caring for her similarly melancholic mother. The girl displayed symptoms of severe weight loss, insomnia, loss of appetite, agitation, and despondency. On the whole her disorder followed the pattern of the so-called manic-depressive mixed state, as can roughly be seen from the following testimonies of the patient. It should be said that the patient, who began treatment with me in the tenth month of her disorder, was fully cured after a total of 14 months, about 2 months ago. Without dwelling on the typical details of her illness, we should immediately single out the particular disorder of her experience of time, which for a long time was central to her awareness of her illness.

---

[16] The fact that it is not possible to talk of an inhibition even in the most extreme cases of psychogenic depression is something that J. Lange also emphasised; cf. also Bonhoeffer. [Original note]

[17] (Note on the proof correction.) Only after completion of this work did I become aware of two essays by E. Minkoswki ... which also deal with the meaning of the experience of time for psychotic phenomena. There are in particular many points of consensus between my work and the essay published in the *Journal de psychologie* in 1923, "Étude psychologique et analyse phénoménologique", fewer with the work published in the *Journal of Complete Neurology and Psychiatry*, 82, 1923, [11] on "Bleuler's schizoid-ness and syntony and the experience of time". [Original note]

The sick girl made the following statements in relation to this:

"The whole day I have a feeling of anxiety, which is related to time. I am constantly thinking that time is flying past. As I am speaking to you, with every word I'm thinking 'past', 'past', 'past'. It is an unbearable state to be in and produces a feeling of being harried. I'm always harried. It starts as soon as I wake up and it is linked to noise. When I hear a bird chirping, it makes me think 'That lasted a second'. Water dripping is unbearable and it drives me mad, because I always have to think: Now another second has gone past, now another. The same when I hear a clock ticking. I've let my watch run down and hidden it. But watches on other wristbands disturb me as well, they really drive me mad. I can't go on the train, because the thought that I have to be at the station at 2.05 is just as unbearable, it makes me anxious, in the same way as the thought that I need 20 minutes to get to X. If I imagine my wedding, I can't bear the thought, because I have to imagine that the ceremony in the church will last an hour. When my sister E. writes: I arrive next Sunday at 8.09, I can't understand it. I can't understand how people can make plans and make sense of such dates and can still stay calm. It makes me feel alienated from other people, as if I didn't belong, as if I were completely different. When people talk, I can't understand them, well, my mind understands them, but actually I don't understand how they can talk so simply and calmly and not be constantly thinking: now I am talking, so that's lasting for this and this amount of time, then I'll do this, then that, and all that will take 60 years, then I'll die, and then others will come along, who will also live roughly the same length of time and will eat and sleep like me, and then others will come again, and so it will go on, without any sense, for thousands of years."

"And also when I see people moving, each time they move, for example when someone is crossing over the lawn, each step they take I am thinking: one second, and another second – and that makes me horribly agitated and fills me with anxiety. I have these thoughts constantly. Even when I don't expressly think them, I have the feeling of them inside. I often think that I am not sick but that I have perceived something that everyone else hasn't perceived; that I've just formed such an unhappy view of the world that the others don't share, but which is actually quite logical; I have no idea how it's possible to think in any other way."

"These thoughts and feelings are linked to anxiety. It seems strange to have to think like this. And then it seems strange to me that I will never be able to stop thinking like this. It is completely impossible to imagine that someone would ever be able to think in a different way once this has started. The worrying thing is that this state is getting worse. It is getting worse because the periods of time that I have to think about are getting shorter and shorter, which makes me more and more agitated, so this state can only lead in the end to the asylum. The state began with my not being able to divide up my day at home. But now the periods of time that I have to think in – that lasted an hour, that lasted a minute, that lasted a second – are getting shorter and shorter. And when I do my needlework, every stitch, every time I stick the needle in, makes me think of time. The state is linked to sound, and to perceptions, and it is closely linked to thoughts of suicide, because the whole thing is strange and unbearable."

Another time she said:

"When I am talking to you, then the word 'talking' goes, then the word 'goes'. First it's words that go like this, and then letters. It all goes, bit by bit, step by step. This disturbance with time started in a flash once, in the summer, when I noticed a cyclist moving his legs and it made me think for the first time: 'up, down, a second, another second'. Often there's no external cause for these thoughts, then I just have to think that I'm going up the stairs at home or here: one step, and another step, one second, another second, and so on."

"In my opinion this can never stop. Every single movement makes me think: now I'm doing this, now that, for example hanging clothes in the wardrobe, dressing, undressing and so on. It is terrible thinking like this, it's a type of killing (?), that's why it is related to thinking about suicide."

She explains what is "terrible" with a sketch:

[A → death]

This line signifies her allotted lifespan. She is placed at a point A along this path, the final point of the path is death.

"Everything I do makes the line that separates me from death shorter. That's why I am anxious of everything I do, but also of thinking. When someone says, for example, that he's looking forward to spring, to the flowers in the garden, and so on, I can't understand that, because I always have to think that when spring has come then the line has got a bit shorter again, death has come a bit nearer again. How can one look forward to that? That doesn't mean that I'm frightened of death, not at all, I actually think of it as being something rather pleasant, but the thought that everything is going by and that life is getting shorter and shorter makes me anxious. And when I am crocheting, too, the emphasis isn't on the fact that the cover I'm crocheting is getting bigger, but on the fact that as the cover gets bigger the lifeline is getting shorter and shorter. I find that terrible. That is why I always want to take my life, to escape from this thought, even though I do really like life."

Another time she said:

"I am terribly anxious." – Of what? – "Of one minute passing by and then another and death coming closer and closer. I am anxious about the journey to Switzerland. The others are looking forward to it and thinking about all the things they'll do, for example, that they will do such and such a thing on the first day, such and such a thing on the third day, and so on. I am just skipping over the 3 weeks of holiday and all I can think is that after three weeks I will be lying in bed again and nothing will have changed except that I will be 3 weeks nearer to death. The whole thing is so pointless, the journey as well. This pointlessness is so agonising: everything just keeps passing by and passing by and doesn't make you happy and just carries on passing by until death comes. Don't you understand that once a person has started thinking like this they can never stop?"

"I think my illness has its roots in my anxiety about growing old. I always used to sit around at home, and time was passing, and nothing became of me, and that disturbed me. When my sister married, I started working out: in one year, in two, in three years it's my turn. It's my turn, just like it's all the other women's turn. That seems so pointless to me. And it's the same with speaking in a group: now it's his turn, now this person's, now mine. I speak just because it's my turn, and that's so pointless. – I do feel happy sometimes, for example, when someone gives me a present and when someone is nice to me, but there's always something terrible about everything, because everything actually just doesn't matter. At times that feeling was so strong that I couldn't do anything at all, couldn't get up out of bed, couldn't get myself dressed, because nothing matters anyway. Also playing games, for example ping-pong or tennis, I can do it, but only if I force myself to, I have to force myself, actually I can't do it, and it's still pointless, actually I always have to think: now I'm hitting the ball, now the other person, now I'm bending down – what's the point of all of it. I have to force myself terribly just to live at all. The awful thing about it is that I can control myself so well that the others don't notice anything, I can even laugh and have a good time. If I was mad and going around shouting and screaming, I wouldn't suffer so much. I have to force myself to do everything, everything needs overcoming, only a quarter of me joins in, no, not even a quarter."

*****

We see a patient who is compulsively, constantly preoccupied with time. More precisely, she suffers from the sensation of time elapsing, from the constant impression of its passing by. Thus she is aware of something that at least to this degree does not normally enter into anyone's consciousness. Our thinking about time can focus on time passing, but this focus does not occur as a primary experience, but rather is controlled by a particular problematic of life and has as a prerequisite an estrangement of the person from the immediacy of life of the totally naïve, unreflected feeling of existence. However, to the extent to which this focus has an effect, the impression can arise that the lifeline allotted to the individual is being reduced through every act, through his whole affective, motor, volitive behaviour, a fact for which Balzac invented a grandiose symbol in the Peau de Chagrin. Here the lifespan is pictured spatially, in the form of the stretched expanse of leather, which, shrinking and disappearing with every wish granted, gives a graphic image of the inexorable disappearance of the life time. A spatial symbol therefore illustrates the time, corresponding to the fact that we can only hypostatise the in itself non-objective entity of time by means of spatial schemata. If we remember that our patient also hypostatises the passing of time and the disappearance of the life time allotted to her in the form of a successively crumbling line, then we can straight away, at the very outset of our investigation, notice that the time our patient speaks of is not the time in which we normally and permanently live, but that it involves here an unusually objectivised time, that is, a particular formulation of the essence of time, whose occurrence requires its own explanation.

In order to see clearly here, one has to hypostatise in two different ways: firstly, that normally time is not experienced as something passing by but as something to come, a fact that Max Scheler expressed in this manner: "our primary experience of time is directed towards what we call the future. This univocal directedness towards the future is essential to the form of existence of life."[18] Secondly, time is not normally experienced as the medium by which the process of our dwindling, our decay, a diminishing and disappearing of our personality occurs, but rather, conversely, as the medium for an increase, a development, a "growth of our personality" (E. Straus). However, these two moments, that we are primarily orientated towards the future, and the other moment, that we stretch out into this future, grow into it

---

[18] This is taken from Max Scheler, 'Idealism and realism' (Scheler 1973e, p. 341). [Editors' note]

and thereby experience an increasing fulfilment of self-realisation, an increase in self-development and self-enhancement, these stand in just as comprehensible and necessary relation to each other as the other two moments: the experience of diminishing, of lessening or disappearing of our personality and the passing or elapsing of time.

Normally however, we do not become aware of this objectively ascertainable experience of time passing and elapsing, because the momentum and drive with which the unfolding life of the personality, with its projects and plans, carries this into the future tends to obscure completely the element of time passing. Only when this development and course of the personality comes to a standstill for whatever reason, be it because a problematic of the feeling of existence halts the active drive related to the future and makes it into something conscious, or be it because the vital inhibition of melancholia paralyses and constrains it, only then can the temporal determination of experience, thus altered, now become something conscious, even perhaps become a permanent state.

In the case of our patient, the changed temporal determination of experience becomes just such a permanent state. Every time she hears dripping water, the clock ticking, a bird chirping, every time she hears a word, sees a movement, every time she sticks the needle into her sewing, she is forced to think: "one second, another second", and "past, past". She registers how things go past, and in a compulsive manner.

What is striking is that such things are registered at all. The ticking of a clock, the individual movements of a person, words, etc., these things are not generally noticed at all ... There is a disorder that requires explanation in the very fact that more or less irrelevant elements of situations, which relative to the distribution of emphasis in normal thought behaviour are random and incidental, receive more attention. We are familiar with such attention disorders from other situations. So a tired person will tend to register irrelevant things, street signs, for example, house numbers etc., whose observation is determined more by the more passive relationship between the here and now than the more active relationship between the here and then.

*****

Let us reiterate then: it is the passing of time that forces itself upon someone in the first instance, and the individual contents themselves by which the passing of time is experienced have no other meaning than as stations along the pressing impression of time passing. The contents are interchangeable; what is crucial about them is that through them the experience of time takes on a concrete and thereby perceptible, even identifiable character. Thus in fact it is not primarily contents that impose themselves on one, but rather an imposing sense of time passing, and the contents are selected according to aspects of their suitability for the manifest representation of time passing. They are simply crests of waves that make visible and emphatic the inexorable stream of time. The passing of time is only given structure and perceptible content through the individual acts of perception. The basic experience of the patient is therefore the passing of time, and this temporal determination of her life constitution has the effect that contents come to her attention that illuminate this process.

We know the effect of the patient's disposition on the passing of time. It is clearly this, that the orientation towards the future of the personality disrupts the approach to the coming time. The normal temporal structure of experience is disturbed by melancholia. This normal temporal structure of experience – the personality's orientation towards the future – is altered by the endogenous inhibition. The personality's progression, the urge for self-realisation, its course towards what is to come and developmental momentum, this is all brought to a halt. It is condemned to come to a standstill in areas where normally no standstill occurs. The future is shut off to it ... Melancholics complain about nothing as much as they complain about ... a decline in their mental faculties, an increasing reduction of their ability, their domain, their worth, a growing loss of strength and health – even in cases where such a decline and deterioration cannot be objectively detected, that is: the inhibition of the process of becoming is experienced as a decline in one respect or another. Expressed in temporal terms, the inhibition of growing time appears as a passing of time and has to appear as such.

A precondition for this "passing of time" is that personality's urge for becoming is inhibited but not actually destroyed ... We can express the condition of melancholia in the following way: the sick person would in fact like to live, function, act, love, develop, progress, and that is why his inability to do so, his own self-consciousness, is so keenly sensed ...

It is therefore not the destruction of the urge for becoming in the personality but its inhibition that forms the background to our patient's compulsion to register. It should be remembered that this inhibition reaches into deeper layers than the psychically grounded inhibition of aspiration.

*****

The patient said: "Everything I do feels as if I wasn't actually doing it; only a small part of me is involved in doing it; it is always as if I was staying behind, as if I wasn't entering into what I was doing, as if something inside me wasn't changing along with everything else." This stopping of the personality in the middle of what it is doing is what causes its futile inauthenticity, which is what the patient complains about. The action does retain its objective meaning, but its sense of becoming is lost, and this in turn condemns it to pointlessness. "A terrible feeling always accompanies me, and this never changes however much life around me changes." In short, the experience immanent in time stays still despite the activity. If the patient surrendered herself completely to her condition, then she would do nothing at all anymore. It requires a battle against the tendency to do nothing. She has to overcome her instinct all the time, force herself to do everything, always exert herself: she is not carried forwards by an internal course of action, that which otherwise carries everything we do and accounts for all its ease and also for its meaning, the victorious, joyful and meaningful nature of everything we do. Indeed, from time to time the inhibition wins out and the patient remains in bed, does not dress, refuses food, etc.

*****

Let us recall the diagram that the patient sketched and which was concerned with death. She states that a constant anxiety accompanies everything she does, everything she says, even everything she thinks. This anxiety is actually fear of death. When she crochets the emphasis is not on seeing the cover grow but on the fact that with every stitch the lifespan allotted to her is shrinking. With everything that she does the lifeline shortens, and so death comes closer to her. That is terrible for her, she says. Everything passes and passes and gives her no pleasure and passes until death stands before her. She cannot understand how people can make plans or speak about the future, about spring, for example, and be pleased, because everyone must know that death is creeping closer with every event. She even pursues this futile process of time elapsing even further, beyond death. For then more people come, and they also live to 70 and then die, and so it goes on pointlessly, for thousands of years. Looking into the future is for her simply looking at death ... Each individual step in life does not have the significance of any meaning, or any fulfilment like it does for us, but instead it means absolutely nothing, only the nearing of death. Indeed, I believe we should say that in this constant experience of time passing by, death itself, as the embodiment of passing time, as its absolute and final form, is included. For us, however, it is problematic that death is experienced as the embodiment of passing time. For seen in this way death must provoke feelings of anxiety, horror and terror.

In order to understand this fear of death, however, we have to make a distinction. We must make a distinction between death that is immanent to life, and death that is transcendent to life.

As healthy people, too, we stand in a permanent relation to death just as we stand in a permanent relation to time. This relation is however not a conscious relation. As long as we are living our life actively and productively, we do not actually think about death. But we still live it. Death is immanent to our whole life. Our whole life is lived under the motto "Die and become". Becoming is always intrinsically a partial dying. We always give up some points of life to go onwards. A created work is always a completed piece of life. In a love that has been fulfilled we bury a piece of life that will never return. In the transition from childhood to youth and then to manhood, we leave stages of life behind us and deliver them, as it were, to death (Feuerbach: Death and Immortality).

What is peculiar about this death immanent to life, however, is that we do not approach it, but that it follows on behind us. It grows as our life unfolds. Life is actually constructed around death and unfolds through a death that is immanent to its individual forms, which eventually absorbs these forms again when they have been brought to a close. ... Death that is transcendent to life differs from this death that is immanent to life, in that it is a power that seems to come towards life from the outside in order to bring it to a conclusion from outside. This death is an imagined death, a subjectively posited death, the caricature of death immanent to life. It is an invented product, just like imagined, objective time.

Tellenbach, H. (1982), 'Melancholy as endocosmogenic psychosis'

From (1982) *Phenomenology and Psychiatry*. Edited by A. J. J. De Koning and F. A. Jenner, translated by A. J. J. Koning and B. Swingler. Academic Press: London.

Editors' commentary

In this text Tellenbach draws on concepts from Heidegger and ancient philosophy to discuss the phenomenology of severe depression. He regards severe depression as a psychosis in the sense that it is a transformation of experience as a whole. He wants to understand this phenomenology as arising out of a person's liability to becoming severely depressed ('endo-') and specific environmental happenings which may come to envelope that person ('cosmo-'). Tellenbach proposes that melancholic people typically select melancholic environments due to 'hereditary factors', what in current terms may be described as a gene–environment correlation. The text is unique in combining a whole-person with a life-course approach to melancholy.

... For a century there has been talk of "endogenous psychoses" in psychiatry, but what do these concepts really mean? Is it not grotesque that we have been speaking about "psychoses" without knowing scientifically what we actually mean? The first worker to attempt to give a satisfactory definition of psychosis, meeting with reasonable criteria, was Binswanger (1960). Admittedly, he had to arrive at this definition from the heights of the transcendental phenomenology of Husserl. When Husserl said: "The real world only is, in so far as the constantly prescribed presumption that the experience will constantly continue in the same constitutive style", it enabled Binswanger to characterize psychoses as modes of being in which this constitutive coherence of experimental continuity is questioned – and with it the feasibility of the course of life in the normal way (Binswanger, 1960, p. 15). This definition of psychotic hits the decisive point, namely the break in the constitutive style of experience. When we speak of melancholy below, we have in mind the psychotic melancholia – the melancholy that meets with the criteria of Binswanger. That is why we want to avoid using the word "depression", which has become as ubiquitous as it is unhelpful.

But what about the meaning of "endogenous"? We cannot go into the historical development of the concept here and we only want to refer to three meanings of the word. First, endogénité for French psychiatry (Magnon, Falret, Baillarger), and Endogenität for German psychiatry (Frauser, Bumke, Tiling, Gaupp and, quite originally, Kretschmer), was a convergence of premorbidly given disharmonies of the personality, an unfolding of typical temperaments in "their" psychoses. Secondly, for the early psychoanalysts, especially for Abraham (1916), Endogenität was at last identical with "an Endogenität (1/86) of the oral and anal zone, varying in degree and from child to child". In the neo-classical" phase of psychoanalysis, especially according to Klein (1960), Endogenität is first of all a success or failure of infantile processes of introjection. Thirdly, endogenous is for somatic psychiatry something "cryptogenous", that is, a still unknown genetically determined organic brain disease. For somatic psychiatry endogenous psychoses are physically based mental disturbances which are "not yet" understood. The biological psychiatrists stick to this despite the constantly repeated and obvious clinical fact that the manifestations of endogenous psychoses can be so obviously influenced by pathogenic situations.

*****

However impressive the analytical art of interpretation is, it fails to make very central features of melancholy understandable, for example the so-called "vital disturbances" and the difference of disturbed days and symptom-free days (when everything seems fine) when the pathodynamics obviously suddenly stop. Here it becomes clear that the analytical explanation cannot show the "origin" of psychotic–melancholic symptoms. It is just not true that melancholy has these psychodynamic modifications as its basis. It is rather that these psychodynamics (like the somatic findings) become possible because of a modification in an original being before his differentiation into Soma and Psyche, has taken place. The totality of the modification in melancholy can neither be explained by psychoanalytical illumination of motives nor by somatic research into causes. In order to come closer to the phenomena of this modification, we need a positive conceptual theory of this presomatic and prepsychial original region of Endogenität.

On our way to this concept we next ask ourselves: which phenomena characterize melancholy as one of those psychoses, which psychiatry distinguishes from other psychic disturbances under the heading of "endogenous". This question presupposes a radical distinction between symptom and phenomenon. We always relate symptoms to an event which has a causal basis. With symptoms that exhibit themselves, we experience that there is something present that does not show itself immediately, but rather announces or betrays an illness or disturbance. In this sense psychological symptoms invite diagnostic conclusions about something somatic or unconscious. We take what the melancholic shows us as a phenomenon. We are questioning in a realm prior to the distinction between psychological and somatic. We question the phenomena in their ways of modification of existence (Dasein) in melancholy. We question which existential determination of existence (Dasein) in melancholy has been modified (it will be Heidegger's (1977) "thrownness") and whether the appearance of these modifications can be shown to exist in all phenomena of melancholy. As long as we are exclusively dependent on that which is phenotypically derived from perception and conception, we can only found a positive concept of Endogenous on that which is apparent.

Among the phenomena in which Endogenicity manifests itself in melancholy, the alteration of rhythm is pronounced: in disturbances of the sleep – wake rhythm; in so-called diurnal variations; in the influences of the changing seasons, times of predilection for the manifestation of melancholy; in the constancy of the monthly cycle; in the disturbance of the regular behaviour of digestive and sexual appetite; the phase-like character of melancholy; in the periodicity of the cycle; in the frequently fluctuating moods and drives, as already described by Kraepelin. And lastly in the abolition of rhythm in the structure of existence, for instance in the permanence of sleeplessness, the permanence of being ill-humoured, the permanence of anxiety, in the monotony of being agitated and in the stereotyped movements (lamenting, hand-rubbing, etc.), and especially in the basic phenomena ranging from inhibition to stupor.

As phenomenal characterization of Endogenicity we also include the modification of the whole of being-human, which allows us in typical cases to make the diagnosis beyond the bounds of race, language and culture (we refer here to typical transubjective conformity of behaviour and expression). It is often something that can be already experienced in a kind of atmospheric sensing or through an intuition

of the whole, even when manifest symptoms are not present. As distinct from conformity of symptoms, that always refer to definite fields of disturbance and are therefore particular changes, the individual facets and phenomena of melancholy always contain the whole. In other words: in all phenomena constitutive of an endogenous modification, the same origin shows itself.

Further characterizations of the endogenous modifications show themselves in the appearance of psychoses in salient points of maturation: adolescence, critical age, senescence. Maturation itself is the cardinal phenomenon of a normal "Positive" endogenous modification. This is similar to the "generative events" which so often accompany endogenous modifications, ranging from states of ill-feeling around the menstrual cycle to the psychoses that occur in connection with pregnancy, childbirth and menopause. Another feature of the endogenous is the reversibility of melancholy, which, as distinct from the reversibility of organic psychosyndromes, is dependent on so many differentiated conditions. On the other hand, it can also be of such a "situation-indifferent" spontaneity that deep states of melancholy can remit in a short time, in which the beginning of the remission can occasionally be determined to the minute.

All these phenomena indicate that there is an "atmosphere" from which self-determination is absent; it is in a region of the personality-structure which is beyond volition; it is a basis that one cannot choose but into which one is thrown, but which one nevertheless (and this is most decisive to understanding endogenous psychoses) has to take in one's existence – in the same way as one has to take one's steps of maturing existentially. One is thrown – also in the sense of heredity – into one's race, sex, physical constitution, talents: into all that which one is "by the mercy of nature", or what one can possibly be according to what has been given to us as a possibility by nature.

To those who can fall ill with a melancholy, there is included the possibility of a development of a specific typicality of the personality, a specifically structured (premelancholic) primary personality. One can find a representation of this melancholic type in Melancholie (Tellenbach, 1976), to which reality the development of a monopolar melancholy is necessarily connected. (This has been objectified statistically by the research of Zerssen et al. (1969).) Its decisive characteristics consist of a being-pinned-down to orderliness, high demands to individual production, a painful concern with avoiding guilt . . . and lastly an inclination towards a sympathetic, even symbiotic mode of communication. It is these decisive characteristics that make the melancholic type appear in a special high-ranked social aspect. He is pinned down to, and fixed in these forms of, realization of his existence. In fact it is even better to typify the positive aspect of this characteristic as a double negation. The melancholic wants never under any circumstances to be disorderly, unscrupulous, non-performing (lazy), independent, unreliable, etc. One always senses a certain concern in him to get off this path of positive qualities: it ranges from inhibition (not-being-able-to-perform, to-have-let-everything-get-into-disorder, to neglect oneself, etc.) to imprisonment of mind and body in a stupor; it is a being-overpowered by guilt in the delusion of sin; it ranges from inner distance from fellow men to depersonalization; it is a never-ending debit. Against this background the melancholic type appears in the quality of his social aspect as "too normal" a type, while the precariousness of this type consists of the being-pinned-down to this form of normality, i.e. to this "pathological normality".

We must state explicitly that the element of the endogenous can only be considered within the context of the world. The sleep–wake rhythm corresponds to the revolution of the earth, to which it adapts itself constantly – as we experience in adjustments after transatlantic flights. Sex refers to heterosexual sex; digestion refers to food and drink; the natural variations in drive and mood correspond to the different atmospheric character of times of the day and the year. Experimental research into animal-biological rhythm speaks of "Zeitgebers" that correlate with periodicities. According to Aschoff (1954) these are not only meterological timekeepers (such as light, local time, temperature) but also ecological–sociological timekeepers, such as the appearance of prey (the leaping of the salmon towards insects), the olfactory effect of oestrogen cycles on male rats, feeding times, the regularity of noises etc. According to Aschoff (1970), this interlocking is relevant for human beings with respect to the "totality of the periodic expressions of life in its civilizing environment in so far as he becomes aware of them. The reflection on the connection between these environmental processes and original natural rhythms suffices to uphold this time-keeping function." Although a shift-worker has the possibility of acting against environmental periodicity, he is still connected with the original rhythm.

One can see how endogenous predispositions correlate with worldly ones, and it is easy to show that these correlations are typified by vital meaningful characterizations (Kunz, 1966). For human beings, light is colourfulness and brightness which illuminates the world; darkness is primarily an affective atmosphere. The other sex is implicitly stimulating, or rather it stimulates procreation. Morning and evening, day and night are ultimately not just astronomical–calendrical determinations, they are situations of vital meaningfulness (one only has to think of Michaelangelo's sculptures), just as spring and autumn are situations of becoming and "unbecoming" that are especially significant to older people. In all these situations, the endogenous possibilities and wordly intentions are always attuned to each other in such a way that one has to speak of endocosmogenic relationships.

When we proceed from the human environmental possibilities, that which correlates with the determination of vital meaningfulness can be very distinct. For instance, a jealous person sees in the approach of another man towards his wife the specific meaning of the threatening loss, while such an approach can be a matter of indifference or even an honour to the man who is not jealous (Tellenbach, 1967). . . . What we call Typus melancholicus, is characterized by a certain sensitivity and susceptibility to situations which convey beyond awareness – vital expressive meanings. It is therefore possible that situations (moving home, pregnancy, childbirth, promotion, marriage of a son or daughter, retirement, etc.) can take on a pernicious meaning for the melancholic type of person. There is an influence emanating from such situations that is not obvious to other people; an influence in the nature of disorder, guilt, stagnation and a "not-measuring-up-to" the demands made on oneself. This type has to set himself these demands and will exist in contradiction with himself, because of his inability to measure up to these requirements (we characterize this as "remanence").

With regard to the interlocking of endogenous predispositions with vital meaningful contents and the pronounced influence of the situation, we wish to speak here of a Heraclitian distinction. That is not just of the cosmos as "koinos kosmos", i.e. of nature, law, the objectivity of spirit and nature, but also of "idios kosmos", man's own world in which he enfolds himself and which is also determined by the life which one has lived. In this perspective, melancholy always exhibits itself as endocosmogenic psychosis, no matter how different the importance of "endogenous" and "cosmogenous" may be in the individual case. When particular situations correspond to a great extent with specific endogenous possibilities in such a way that they become incompatible with these potentialities, then the system of melancholies follows a sequence of pathogenic situations. One only has to look at the diagnoses of female patients, who have been in the clinic as in-patients through 10 to 15 phases, where the precursors to the diagnosis of "melancholy" changed throughout their lives, from puerperal melancholy to a melancholy related to moving home, to a climacteric and senescent melancholy, and even to a cerebral–sclerotic melancholy. One would not want to state that it is within the power of these situations themselves to evoke a melancholy through real causal connections. It is much more within the power of the pathogenic situations to bring the melancholic patient to the limit of his possibilities, which is the result of a specific one-sided development of the personality. Exhaustion, childbirth, pregnancy, retirement, moving home, cerebral sclerosis, critical age, are first of all situations, and the question is to what extent they can become pathogenic. We cannot go into details here concerning the similarities of these situations which are pathogenic (which we called "includence" and "remanence" in our phenomenological analysis) and have to refer to *Melancholie* (Tellenbach, 1976).

This situational aspect, however, should not be looked at as too static. What furthers our knowledge of the relationships of typical structure and pathogenic situation is the demonstration of the dynamic interrelation between endon and cosmos. In doing so, it becomes clear that only those pathogenic aspects of a situation are decisive – those which address and demand something from the melancholic – when he is pinned down and is also incapable of adaption. When the peace of this rigid order is disturbed, there is always the possibility of the situation becoming pathogenic. It is therefore always something within the person that can turn a primarily quite irreplaceable and even relatively enjoyable situation, into something pathogenic. One can see here how such a "situation" is something that can be induced by the characteristic qualities of a person. "Producing and unfolding-oneself" within the framework of

fellow-man and environment means to this type constituting this connection as "his" situation. In other words: within the development of the melancholic, the tendency grows to "situate" his fellow-man within his personal world (but also everything that is "at hand", for instance the environment in which he dwells) in a specific way. ("At-hand" refers to "Zuhandensein", a term from Heidegger where the object is understood as "object-to-me" ["handiness"], in its meaningfulness. This is different from the object as "Vorhanden", which is the object for itself, where the objective is thematized. The reader is referred to Heidegger's philosophy for a fuller understanding of these terms.) In this context, to situate means to include the human environment (and also the things which are "at-hand"), in one's own life-design. This is characterized by a tendency to include oneself with one's fellow-man and objects in the neighbourhood ("includence"), and also the concern of being unable to measure up to one's own ideal production ("remanence"). If one of the "fellow-men" withdraws himself from this inclusion (or when leaving the dwelling place, when moving home), then the situation, which has been constituted by the melancholic himself, becomes pathogenic. So it means that the melancholic type has himself already made such circumstances (situations) pathogenic. For instance, a patient has for long created the conditions in such a way that a situation like moving home and/or marriage of a daughter is already pathogenic (after being so accustomed to the house lived in or because of the symbiotic relationship with the daughter). The endogenous modification can result in a melancholy, just as situations that are hardly provocative can trigger off jealousy in jealous people. Such a person comes to situate a situation in such a way that he even develops a delusion of jealousy, in which he exposes himself and his wife to this "Nebenbuhler" (a German word meaning that particular "rival" to whom one is nice and comes close to and therefore different from the "rival-proper" whom one wishes to fight) (Tellenbach, 1974). He has a particular need for closeness to this "Nebenbuhler". Proceeding from the assumption that there is a hereditary predisposition to develop as a melancholic type, it does not follow that a certain environment is needed in which the child's typicality is reinforced and developed. It is rather the type himself who singles out those influences from his environment that make the potential specific possibilities evolve. In most cases it is so that the social validations of the striving towards production and the orderliness are favourable to the development of melancholy. The results of transcultural psychiatry show that the countries with a dominating producer-society show a higher incidence of melancholy (Tellenbach, 1969; Wittkower and Hugel, 1969). In cultures in which syncytial family structures have been superseded by progressive individualization through western influences, psychotic melancholies are occurring more frequently. "When high production and success play an important role in the value-system of a society, when individualization is encouraged with a sense of duty and personal responsibility" (Wittkower and Hugel, 1969), a constellation is given which favours the development of melancholy. But also when growing up outside such structures of the live-world, this type will develop situating his environment more and more in such a way, that in the end, the situations constituted by himself can become pathogenic.

Thus, a conception of monopolar melancholy as endocosmogenic psychosis can be summarized as follows:

Genetically the predisposition is given that the melancholic is being pinned down to a particular way of orderliness and/or avoidance of guilt.

This specific constitution is not like Locke's tabula rasa, on which one can write whatever one wants, but rather is like the constitution as Leibniz understood it, which means that a person will only take up those imprints that are allowed by his own ontic constitution.

In this sense, the hereditary predisposition of the melancholic type corresponds with forces of the co-human environment that are related to this specific predisposition, and bring it to reality. One could say that the table (tabula) mentioned above, performs an active selection, and only those signs are accepted that meet the criteria it is willing to receive.

These forces are often, though not always, met in the attitudes of the family (more often in the mother's attitude than in the father's). In principle, the influence of such specific forces of the family is not necessary. The social structure of the environment, of the "cosmos", in the sense of a high endorsement of production and orderliness, suffices to favour the realization of these specific possibilities.

In his development the melancholic structured personality tends to situate the co-human environment (and the objects "at-hand") in a certain way, that is, they constitute their situation so that it can lead to constellations characterized by the phenomena "includence" and "remanence". If the situation leads to a formation that comes into self-contradiction with the personality, then a pathogenic situation has arisen, out of which the endocosmogenic modification into melancholy occurs.

Chapter

18

Obsessive compulsive disorder

Straus, E. (1938), 'The pathology of compulsion'

From (1966) *The Selected Papers of Erwin Straus: Phenomenological Psychology.* Translated by E. Eng. New York: Basic Books. Originally published as (1938) Ein Beitrag zur Pathologie der Zwangserscheinungen. *Monatsschrift für Psychiatrie und Neurologie* **98**(1): 61–101.

Editors' commentary

This text by Straus on the pathology of compulsion (what we would now call 'obsessive compulsive disorder') is a twin publication with von Gebsattel's on 'The world of the compulsive' (next text). Both were written in 1938 and published in the same journal.

Straus is clear that his inquiry is neither physiological nor psychological but rather 'existential' or 'anthropological'. He wants to understand compulsive symptoms as arising neither out of brain processes (though he is generally sympathetic to such approaches) nor out of psychological processes (Freud's insights, he claims, are the wrong way around in this disorder). Rather, his aim is to understand compulsive symptoms as arising out of what he calls the human being's 'sympathetic relations to the world'. The disturbance at this tier of the human person he regards as an 'existential' disturbance.

According to Straus, it is the 'ease' with which the healthy person is carried by life (in their thinking, feeling and acting) that is unavailable to the compulsive. In eliciting this phenomenon of 'ease', Straus draws upon descriptive case histories but also upon art, philosophy, ethnography and mythology. It is a rich, if unfinished, picture and we think it illuminates some of the current debates on how to understand obsessive compulsive disorder. One can be critical in places. The nihilism Straus expresses about treatment seems unduly pessimistic in the light of current evidence. The metaphysical position Straus adopts is at times both dogmatic and vague. Are the sympathetic relations with the world (the 'physiognomic realm') unavailable to the patient in toto, with their compulsive symptoms being an expression of some form of solipsism or autism? Or, is it that participation in the 'physiognomic realm' is hindered only by the unavailability of one aspect of that realm (what Straus calls 'ease') with compulsions being a defence, or guarding, against the remaining and dominating aspects ('decay', death, formlessness, etc.)? Though Straus may be unclear here, he stimulates a mode of thinking about the psychopathology of compulsion which remains as relevant to our era as to his.

We are but following conventional usage when we term the, compulsion sickness "compulsion neurosis," just as, until recently, paralysis agitans and chorea minor were still classed under the heading of motor neuroses even though their organic bases were already determined or considered probable. I tend to the view that the phenomena of compulsion do not originate in the circumstances of the sick person's life history. At the same time, I believe that it is only an existential analysis that will enable us to penetrate more deeply into its pathology.

*****

The compulsive's warding off has diverse shadings – shadings of terror, dread, repulsion, and disgust. From all these shadings of parrying I shall take only one – disgust. But I shall not be able to adhere to this limitation too strictly, since disgust is modified in the individual instance by dread, terror, and repulsion.

*****

For the sake of brevity, let us begin with this: Disgust is the defense against invasion by decay. In using this definition, it must be kept in mind that I am referring to decay as a hidden characteristic and, thus, one that can express itself in many different ways.

In a study of disgust published some years ago, Gustav Kafka (1929) asserted that disgust is directed toward all outgrowths of the organic. This interpretation of the phenomenon comes so close to being correct that it is doubly misleading. First of all, it is factually incorrect. We aren't disgusted by ivory tusks, antlers, bits of coral, pearls, or snail shells – all organic products – nor, probably, by mummies, dried sea horses, and skeletons. The dried starfish, like deer's antlers, are beyond the process of decay; both have assumed fixed forms. They are petrified, dead, but not decaying. Kafka's view is also incorrect in a still deeper sense, for he is looking for manifest characteristics instead of hidden ones with their manifold changing expressions. Of course, organic outgrowths often have the character of decay but not necessarily so. A purely physiognomic dissolution of organic form is at times sufficient to evoke disgust in us for sheer life and not merely for its outgrowths. Even a "swarm," which obscures organic form or in which it seems to dissolve, can produce a feeling of disgust that we are spared when seeing a single individual of the same species. On the other hand, inanimate nature, taken in a strictly scientific sense, can exhibit the physiognomic characters of generation and decay. The "winking lake," the wide-open ocean, and the carefree stream all invite us in – quite different from the stagnating pond, even when, objectively speaking, we must grant that it is "clean." In the first instance, we plunge in, becoming one with the lightness, joy, wide openness, and play of the waves; in the second instance, we are repelled by its murkiness and lifelessness. In other words, while eager longing and the defense against disgust are both entirely sensual, the expressive characters exciting the longing and the aversion are neither rigidly determinate nor simply given by nature. The expressive characters are also partly shaped by tradition, in ecstasy and longing no less than in disgust and defense. Some centuries are enamored of fleshiness while others look for slenderness; there are ages that award the palm to the mature, and others in which the juvenile takes the prize.

*****

Expressive characters are many and various; in addition, things themselves change their expressive character from one situation to another. Something that is disgusting in one situation may lose that character in another. The athlete's profusion of sweat may be sensed as expressive of vital strength and activity.

Then it provokes a very different feeling than does the fever perspiration of a patient or the odor of a sweating throng. Taken as a thing, a hair is still a hair whether on another's curly head, on a coat collar, in a soup, or used as material, such as horsehair. I need not descend to details to show how the same thing – hair – changes its expressive character entirely with these changes of situation. Combed-out hair disgusts us, but, in some historical periods, a true cult of snipped locks has existed. Cut hair is every bit as much an outgrowth of the organic as combed-out hair or horsehair. One last example: Faust demands that Mephistopheles bring him a cloth from Gretchen's breast as a love-token. Used clothing, our own as well as others', disgusts us, but, for Faust, the cloth is not a piece of underclothing; for him, it is part of the beloved, saturated with her scent and essence. A cloth from Gretchen's linen chest would not have served equally well. The antithesis between clean and used does not coincide with that of pure and impure. The expressive character that something reveals does not depend only on its qualities as a thing and on the particular situation; it is just as much a matter of whose eyes alight on it.

*****

The Flemish painters – Rubens, Jordaens, and others – saw the world with eyes different from the Nazarenes or Pre-Raphaelites who came later. Rubens is indefatigable in portraying the live world in all its luxuriant fullness. If the milk spurts from a woman's breast in the midst of drunken festive processions or a curly-locked urchin gives free play to his inner prompting,[1] then all of this can only aid the painter to represent the brimming, and brimming over, abundance of life.

---

[1] For the child, many things are still free from the often very considerable disgust felt when met in grown, especially aged, persons. Disgust remains a stranger to the child as long as he is unacquainted with death and decay. In the child, we can still accept much that will later provoke disgust because it is an integral feature of his burgeoning life. The "Manneken-Pis" in Brussels has survived decades without challenge. Of course, another circumstance also plays a part. His display is no offense to human dignity because the child has not yet gained dignity; in him, nature is without odium. Indignation does not pave the way for disgust. The innocent eye allows us to discover the fullness of life in the goings-on of the Brussels "Manneken," too. [**Original note**]

This particular sense of life has undergone a pervasive change since the days of the Dutch painters.

*****

Rubens' paintings of fauns and nymphs are a perfect example of how, even in its details, the physiognomy of the world always depends on the observer and how quickly what is appealing can become disgusting without any actual change in the thing itself. Some persons are irritated rather than delighted by a painting of Rubens. Its lushness they see only as corpulence; its abundance, only as bulkiness; its burgeoning, only as swollenness. For them, the living metamorphoses into the decaying.

*****

In this sphere, the norm cannot be exactly determined, and yet it is clear when the limits, in either direction, have been violated ... There is such a thing as a pathology of sympathetic relationships, and ... the phenomena of compulsion fall within it.

*****

Just as in Aristotle's view (*De Anima* 424a 2–10), sensation is intermediate between the extremes of what can be sensed (white and black, for example) but must contain both potentially without actually being either, so the healthy person is also potentially between the two value extremes; he can turn in this direction or in that. The sick person, however, has been displaced toward one pole. His center has shifted to such an extent that he finds himself completely surrounded by decay. Thus, he is no longer able to discriminate; he is without insight.

For the compulsive patient, the world is filled with the decaying. Wherever he looks, he sees only decay; wherever he goes, he meets only with decay. All his activity is expended in warding off the decayable that presses in on him from every side and at every instant; and so these patients are never finished washing and scrubbing their own body.

The following case history will illustrate this more clearly.

A twenty-five-year-old woman, Mrs. F. L., who had suffered from compulsions for several years, reported that her illness had appeared suddenly at the time of her first pregnancy, when she was twenty-one. She still recalled the day and the particular circumstances. Her mother had asked her to come along to the cemetery to visit her father's grave. She had cried and hadn't wanted to go (although in previous years she had frequently visited the cemetery); she had become frightened: there was such a smell there; there were vapors from what the buried persons there had died of. She hadn't wanted to give the reason for her refusal; finally, she had overcome her distaste and gone along. On the way, however, she was terribly frightened, and, at the cemetery, she had to be "on guard" continually, lest she breathe normally and inhale some of the vapors.

Her examination was made more difficult by the fact that the patient made strong warding-off movements almost continually; struck herself in the face; wiped her cheeks and neck; screamed; made clicking, gurgling noises; and threw herself around in bed, first pulling her pajama tops and then the covers over her head. She only quieted down when the conversation was directed toward rather impersonal topics. Whenever the theme of her compulsion came up, her outbursts started again. The patient termed these uncontrolled movements "showing off" and added that she was no longer able to suppress them. Her back and shoulders were sore all over from rubbing. After the first interview, the patient had to vomit because "everything had been called by its plain name."

Since that visit to the cemetery, the patient continued, it had been one thing after another. At first she had been unable to say or listen to anything about dead people or coffins. She felt disgusted at everything old and grayheaded. Earlier she wouldn't have sent any beggar away, but now she couldn't even look at an old man's hand. When she did so, she had to scream and run away. She felt frightened, but there was something else, something inside her she couldn't describe. She had tried to control herself, but the more she tried the less she was able to. It was as if a strange power directed her, like in hypnosis. She had "lost her grip"; that was how she had gotten sick. The only one who understood her was her husband. Having "lost her grip," she didn't know where "to stay." It simply took hold of her. It was as if she had no life of her own, as if someone were squeezing her together. For the past three years, she had also been having frequent bad dreams. When she awoke, she had told them to her husband, and this had been a big "show off." Afterwards, she demanded that her husband take deep breaths so that she could be sure that someone else could stand to hear such thoughts, and that made her strong again. She was living like a parasite, from others' strength. She had demanded that her husband sleep in the same bed with her so she could cling to him and be protected."

For the past three years, everything had revolved around dust. Her child lived in the next room with her mother, so she had "strange dust." Because of this, she had to reject the child. Her own mother and child were not allowed to enter her room. She suffered greatly because of this; she loved her child and wanted to kiss her, but then it would bring germs into her room.

The patient is no longer able to do her own housework. She stays almost all the time in one room of her two-room house, constantly fighting the dust. It is almost impossible for her to go out, for coffins are sold on one street, someone once killed himself on another street, she once met a cripple on another, and the fourth street runs by the cemetery, etc., etc.

Compulsive thoughts keep coming like ants, like a car going faster and faster without being able to stop. Then she has to fight off her thoughts and doesn't know where "to stay." She screams for something to hold on to, hides in a corner, crawls into the closet or in bed, hides underneath her husband's coat, or tries to call up something beautiful in her imagination; then she has something to hold on to.

During her stay in a sanitarium, she once saw a coffin standing in front of the house and had to run away. She ran all the way home from the suburb to her husband because she had "lost her grip." When her doctor later stood on the spot where the coffin had been and breathed deeply to show her that he was able to bear the thought of the coffin, she was also able to.

The illness, whose numerous symptoms I have only sketched here, ran its course with some ups and downs while becoming progressively worse.

What is unusual about this case is the pervasiveness with which the patient experiences the disturbance of her sympathetic relationships. Remarkable, too, are the simultaneous defensive measures: the rudimentary warding-off movements, the magical participation in her husband's and her doctor's vitality, and the technique of cleansing.

In the psychopathology of compulsion, it has been customary to distinguish compulsive thoughts, compulsive fears, and compulsive impulsions, and this patient, too, employs such terms. Nevertheless, such distinctions do not hit the mark. The patient does not suffer from isolated thoughts, imaginings, impressions, and impulsions. She suffers from having to live in a world filled with evil demons. In the dust with which the patient constantly struggles, the demonic can still be detected. The dust, like a demon, is both ubiquitous and elusive. The struggle against dust is an effort to endow the demonic with the rational form of a thing, rendering it susceptible to being warded off; but the effort is futile.

In the hope of understanding compulsion better, attempts have been made to spot experiences of healthy persons comparable to the symptoms of compulsion – e.g., the inability to get rid of a tune that keeps running through one's head. Actually, as the preceding case history shows, there is no analogy at all between such disturbances and compulsion phenomena.

Finally, there has been a controversy about whether the experience of compulsion is a disturbance of thinking or feeling. But the compulsive patient does not experience a disturbance of a psychological function; rather, with such a disturbance as basic, he lives in a world whose structure is altered from that of the normal world. His world and his being in the world has undergone a fundamental change. Only by taking account of this transformed style of life is it possible to make the compulsive syndrome intelligible. Such a radical disturbance of sympathetic relationships alters the over-all physiognomy of the world, even in the mere reception of it …

Through this analysis of disgust, I have tried to obtain some insight into the structure of the compulsive patient's world. I started from one symptom frequently met with in compulsion sickness. Now it is time to judge whether our attempt has succeeded. If it has, then it ought to be possible also to better understand other typical symptoms not yet discussed – e.g., doubt, pedantry, magical behavior, and miserliness. (See Binswanger, 1933.)

All these symptoms are met with at times even in healthy persons, so they seem to differ from normal behavior in degree only. However, I wish to maintain that the mode of being of the compulsive is essentially different from that of the healthy person. Since the compulsive's symptoms are not merely phenomena incidental to his illness, it must also be possible to demonstrate their essentially compulsive character. This, in turn, requires that the world of the normal person be contrasted with that of the obsessive in an even more radical manner. Such a confrontation promises a reciprocal clarification of the normal and the pathological.

To the norm as integral are opposed the multiple forms of pathology. So it is not enough to simply indicate that there is deviation from the norm; the specific deviation must be shown. The truly characteristic feature of the norm, in its opposition to compulsion, is, it seems to me, ease (*Gelassenheit*).[2]

This we know, that even the most conscientious work will draw critical fire. Unexpected events upset the most beautiful plans of the politician or businessman; the accidents reported in the newspapers day after day show that all the measures taken to prevent them are still inadequate. From this standpoint, compulsive patients, in the last analysis, would be justified in their endless doubting, controlling, and searching for reasons. They are actually right insofar as it is possible to improve precautions by taking new measures or insofar as all reasons can be supplanted by better ones. Yet, we call obsession morbid and consider it a vital disturbance. And justifiably so! If we had to wait for an absolutely reasonable basis, for absolute certainty in our actions, then everything would come to a stop. We live "for the time being," and we know – more or less clearly – that we live in the provisional. However much we strive for conscientiousness, we still put an end to our deliberations. In all action, we give up certainty and entrust ourselves to the future, relying on ourselves, on the circumstances, and on others. Closing a deal in everyday life is always pragmatic.

But we are only able to live while "letting things be" because we feel ourselves joined by a sympathetic tie with other parts of the world and borne along by them. But anyone who – like the compulsive – cannot live in the provisional, as a single part in a sympathetic tie with other parts, is opposed by the world in its totality. And both the methods and aims of life together undergo a radical change.

*****

We know how compulsive patients seek to avoid the necessity of personal responsibility, how they – sworn enemies of improvisation – would even like to regulate everyday life according to a plan elaborated to the last detail. One of my patients was rarely able to fall asleep before daybreak because she passed night after night making schedules in which she tried to include everything that she would have to do as a housewife the following day, down to the tiniest detail. Travel was a nightmare for her. The change from everyday routine, the unpredictable, the little bit of adventure that even tourist bureaus have not been able to eliminate, all interfered with her making plans and spoiled any pleasure she might have had in the trip from the very beginning. As soon as she would try to make a travel decision, the trouble began, for, in such a decision, deliberate choice, curiosity, and mode became relevant – all unmeasurable factors.

Because all action is directed and, therefore, of necessity directed in a one-sided way, the patient is plagued by a wish to undo what has been done. If it were only wicked thoughts that the patient wished undone, then one could consider this tendency as a kind of repentance. But the undoing is to be understood literally. An effort is made to reverse the personal history, to return to the starting point, to literally retrace a path. Time loses its quality as historical time. When a healthy person, on the way home from work, takes the same streets he used in going to work, he has no intention of annulling his earlier way thence. But this is precisely the meaning of the compulsive's urge to retrace a present or past path in the opposite direction.

This compulsion to undo was particularly marked in the following case.

A biologist, Dr. B., had received from his university a stipend for several years of study abroad. He went first to Berlin. After some time, without any warning, he began to suffer from compulsive disturbances. At first, "images" came to him while he was working with the microscope, images he had great difficulty warding off. He never said anything about the theme of these images. With painful effort, he was able to continue his researches for a time. But he experienced increasing interference not only from his struggle against the images but also from his compulsion to count and recheck his preparations many times. Hoping for improvement from a change of surroundings, he discontinued his studies in Germany and went to England. But he was unable to stay there for more than a few months because the professors used words that he could not bear to hear. Later, he was not even able to repeat these words. One could only gather from his remarks that they must have been words like death, dying, and corpse.

---

[2] There are many related words in German suggesting the importance of ease or "looseness" in normal behavior, e.g., *lässig, nachlässig, zuverlässig, sich verlassen auf.* [Original note]

His next stop was France. But, there, the sight of so many men dressed in black frightened him. He quickly realized that their clothes had nothing to do with mourning; nevertheless, the sight of black so disturbed him that he returned to Germany.

When he returned to Berlin, it seemed to him that the porter who carried his trunk had a skin disease, so he had the trunk put in storage. During the subsequent ten months, he was unable to decide whether to claim the trunk, although it contained scientific records and important official documents along with his clothing and underwear. It was impossible for him to resume his studies during his second stay in Berlin. If a "bad thought" came to him on awakening, his entire day was ruined. He was unable to use many of his books because they had been printed in places which were taboo for him. He could no longer visit the library and laboratory because of particular impressions that interfered. As before, these were men in mourning, persons with badges indicating blindness, and mortuaries. On one occasion, he had sat opposite a blind man on the streetcar. Subsequently, he was unable to use this particular line any more, and, soon after that, he was unable to take any streetcar at all. Disturbing impressions came to color anything that stood in even the slightest relation to it.

But, when Dr. B., after a long struggle, finally resolved to go for a walk, he was then gripped by a compulsion to undo. This compulsion was particularly strong on bridges and railroad overpasses. Sometimes he was successful in going on in his original direction after a single return trip over the bridge. This compulsion to undo was not a façade of anxiety in the presence of rejected impressions; Dr. B., rather, sought for definite objectives so that he could retrace a particular path he had taken some time previously. He was particularly bothered by recurrent thoughts about a place he had once passed more than three years before. Several attempts at undoing had failed because new building made a reversal in exact detail impossible. Now, to the need to undo was added the need to restore the way to its original condition. This, more than anything else, was what kept him in Germany. When his money finally ran out and his visa had expired, he was still unable to make the decision to leave. At the same time, he was unable to do what was necessary to extend his stay. His situation became desperate. The day I decided to bring his case to the attention of his consul, he suddenly disappeared. He had been careful to see that all his responsibilities would be attended to. I have never learned what became of him.

The tendency to undo is the distinctive feature of this case; its theme, its defense, its anxiety at the spoken word and its life-space structure are the same as in the earlier cases. The power of the compulsion over the patient is also clear.

*****

So may one call on compulsive patients to give up their system from one day to the next. Only I fear they will not do so, for even the possibility of death will not bring many of them to renounce their ritual. A patient I knew for a long time literally washed herself to death ...

What good can it do in such cases to try to prove to the patient that "he is playing with reality?" Of what use is "breaking up his system" to him? Of what use is the insight that he is "abusing logic?" Most patients know these things anyway, before treatment. The symptoms of compulsion actually stem from the incapacity, following the breakdown of sympathetic relationships, to live in that nonlogically grounded tentativeness and particularity on which man's capacity for action depends.

In every action, we must impose an order on things. This means that a tension must necessarily arise between the private individual order and the general order ... The compulsive patient would like to act according to a constituted general order; he would like to act in accordance with the categorical imperative. But the categorical imperative is a general formula. When we try to apply it to the concrete instance, we are once more thrown back upon ourselves.

*****

A philologist is unable to finish his studies because he is compelled to read every book word for word. He cannot skim a book, cannot read it by paging back and forth, arranging passages from his own viewpoint; rather, he must crawl from word to word so that everything he reads forms an endless chain he can never articulate as a whole.

Another patient had sorted out the individual items of wash in his linen closet according to their importance and age. Among them were two dozen brand new shirts. But he continued to wear only his old and worn ones because the two dozen had to be kept unbroken.

To someone no longer able to guide his daily affairs according to need, wish, mood, and possibility of success, numbers seem to offer certitude. Numbers, of course, are well-defined, exactly determinable individuals, many even, through their particular position in the number series or through their preferred use, are downright individualities. But even this security doesn't last. For the certitude afforded by the full meaning of the single number is soon placed in doubt by the multitude of numbers. When I have resolved not to leave the house before brushing my coat twenty times from top to bottom and twenty times from bottom to top, why should it be just twenty times? Why not thirty or fifty times? Why not two or three times twenty times? And did I do it exactly twenty times? Did I make a mistake? Must I not start over again from the beginning? The guarantee of numbers breaks down, too; the requirements must be raised repeatedly.

The principles of order to which obsessives subordinate themselves consequently become increasingly odd and bizarre. In this connection, I suspect that the following factor is also involved: What is sought as a solution for specific personal difficulties is an impersonal general schema. But none is forthcoming because what is being demanded, in a sphere ruled by mere opinion (*doxa*), is certitude itself (*episteme*). The place of the suprapersonal principle actually intended is now assumed by that which lies at the farthest remove from everything familiar, personal, and intimate: The odd offers itself as a substitute for the impersonal, the extraneous. The end result is that what should lead away from all arbitrariness reveals itself as the very extreme of the arbitrary and unreasonable.

*****

A patient who consulted me described his trouble in a way very relevant here. This forty-two-year-old man said that he had suffered from compulsive apprehensions of criminality for the past nine years. Therapeutic efforts of every kind to reduce his worry that he could mistreat children, murder, or steal had been of no avail. To meet these dangers, the patient has devised a series of precautions. But, at one point in his ritual, he is still completely unsure whether his devices are for preventing a future action or for assuring him that he has not already committed one of the crimes mentioned. The following is a typical example: The patient has stored his rarely used bicycle in a shed, but he keeps the bicycle lamp in his house. When he sees any unfamiliar bicycle parked along the street, the patient is overcome with anxiety lest the lamp he has at home is the one he is going to steal. As a precaution, the patient crosses to the other side of the street long before he comes to the bicycle; but, if there should happen to be bicycles on both sides, all he can do is walk down the center of the dangerous street. "I will certainly get run over some day doing this," the patient said, being quite able to give an account of his temporal confusion without being able to interpret it. Here, we see a compulsive apprehension and a compulsive drive that are indistinguishable with any degree of reliability. The loss of sympathetic contact with his own development removes the patient from a temporal perspective. Future and past then lose their characteristic difference and appear interchangeable. In other words, the compulsive drive is not a genuine drive at all; the compulsive apprehension is not a genuine apprehension. The patient realizes evil in his own nature but as if it were in another. Evil is experienced as possibility through the interruption of contact with one's own development; evil is experienced as nontemporal, potential being never actualized as deed but which also never abjures its power by ultimately repudiating the deed.

Now, we must say a word about doubt as it takes the form of theoretical doubt in compulsion sickness. All questions lead to ultimate questions. Accordingly, answers to every conceivable sort of question can be final only when they are based on the final questions and principles. As healthy persons, we seek, in the principles, to attain a grasp of the totality. But neither are the principles themselves fixed. The healthy person discovers peace in religious devotion to the totality; or he seeks it within a tradition where the historical and changing seems final and unchanging; or he accepts makeshift answers and lives for the day, alternating between satisfaction and resignation. All these paths are closed to the compulsive patient. His doubts never leave him, and they develop into an impotent interrogation of the final meaning of everything. Thus, there is definitely a relationship between religion and compulsion neurosis, but it is just the reverse of the connection assumed by Freud.

The history of human thought bears witness to man's incessant struggle to secure a grasp on the whole, to rise above particularity and tentativeness. But the very same history teaches us that, as long as we are healthy, we remain inexorably confined to both.

*****

The disturbance of sympathetic relationships affects the compulsive patient in his relations with the world as a totality, so that he is no longer able to dwell in the tentative, the particular, and the perspectival. ... We could now conclude ... [b]ut a more thoughtful treatment of the symptoms of compulsion cannot afford to by-pass the problem of the "magical." In taking it up here, I hope to be able to tie the beginning and end of this study more closely together.

*****

[E]verything in the magical world tends strongly in the direction of a magical technique of participation.

Arme Heinrich was to be healed through the sacrifice of a virgin.[3] His cure was considered a purification through magical participation in the purity of a maiden. But the magic healer requires a magic means for his rite; he needs the live heart of a maiden.

*****

"The Pangwe girls use lush flowers and fruits as beauty magic, because they make them just as lush ... If one aims a sharp point at an enemy from near or far, he will waste away and die" (Jaide, 1937)." It is not the point itself that is effective but pointedness, as its inner nature, that results in the effectiveness of the point. The pointedness enters into direct spatial action with the thrust of the spear, but it can be just as effective at a distance. Despite such general efficacy one can make special use of the pointedness by aiming the point in a particular direction. Originally, then, the point acquires its potency from being filled with the "mana" of pointedness; thereby, its effect is no longer confined to any particular place or spatial area. ... The sorcerer can make the pointedness serve him by setting up a sharp object at a certain time, in a certain spot, and pointing in a certain direction. In this way, the strength of the magic, despite its ties to place, hour, and means, is nevertheless able to overcome all spatial distance and limitations...

Magic is a technique in the realm of the physiognomic.

*****

---

[3] "Der Arme Heinrich" is the central figure of the medieval German verse epic by Hartmann von der Aue. [**Original note**]

The so-called primitive interpretation of the world is a first step toward any kind of world interpretation. We encounter it on a primary level in the history of human thought; it is not a protoform in the biological genesis of thinking. Just because magic corresponds to the primitive's interpretation of the world, it comes always to the fore when men, as individuals or as members of a group, are surrounded and overcome by the physiognomic. This is exactly the situation in which the compulsive finds himself. The physiognomy of his world has been altered in its very depth. It is not only the new and increased power of the physiognomic that distinguishes his world from that of the healthy; it is the dominating physiognomy of decay – the radical absence of wholesome forces – that marks this world.

It is perfectly correct to speak here of the physiognomy of the decaying; still, we ought not to overlook that, by contrast to the world of the primitive, this is a decaying more sensed than seen. Moreover, the world of the compulsive is fraught with decay in a monotonous manner; it does not have the physiognomic spectrum and articulation of the primitive world. Because the decaying is more "scented" than seen, the compulsive suffers a violent shock whenever the decaying assumes a definite form. He is no less frightened at the sight of a sick person, a cripple, a corpse, a coffin, or mourning wear than he is at the written, printed, or spoken words referring to these things.

A healthy person also knows such anxieties. Convention dictates that we pass over many things in silence or that we employ a euphemism or circumlocution. The names of things enable us to take hold of them; the unnamed and anonymous does not yet seem to exist for us. The name establishes a new communication – not only naming but also evoking and convoking things; it gives us power over them at the same time that it puts us in their power. The name lifts things from undefined possibility into definite reality. The pathic moment is complemented by the gnostic. What was said goes into the record, is put down in chronicles, becoming valid and real thereby. The spoken word also lifts the decaying from a vague indefiniteness to unassailable certainty.

*****

Against these omnipresent frights, the sick person develops his particular ritual. The details of the ritual may be understood from the life history; incidental features, such as the requirement to knock three times, may be traced back to associative linkages. But the design of the patient's "magic" ritual corresponds, in the first place, to the magic character of the world in which he lives.

The literature contains many references to compulsives' beliefs in the omnipotence of their thoughts...

Isn't it only wicked thoughts that have such power? A compulsive woman, childless and unmarried and whose sister had to be hospitalized, is seized by the idea that if her sister should die, she would get her child to raise. A few days later, this sister actually dies; from then on, the patient was unable to get free of a self-indictment that her own wish could have brought about her sister's death.

Most of us at one time or another have played with such thoughts, but we reject them; we know we are playing a dubious game, and we attribute no more power to such thoughts than to their opposites. For the compulsive, on the contrary, whether he looks at the world or at himself, evil alone appears real to him. The compulsive's feeling of guilt is more a sense of horror about his being evil than about any particular evil deed. He is crushed by his universal feeling of guilt before he has ever begun to act.

Consequently, compulsive patients combat an enemy who is at once an overpowering, omnipresent, and intangible; with inadequate weapons, they join a hopeless battle. Their fate is that of Sisyphus and the Danaïdes ...

In every action into which we have been coerced, assent and refusal, our yes and our no, are joined in a peculiar way. In resolutely opposing an alien power, we reject its demand and affirm our own conduct. If we yield to it, then we acknowledge the extraneous demand and are once more in agreement with our correspondingly altered behavior. If we are coerced by force, our no continues; we are unable to oppose ourselves in such a case since we have suspended action. But the person who has been coerced to act can still make a decision. His opposition, to be sure, reverts to submission; even he who acts under coercion must, in acting, affirm his own doing as well as the other's demand. The conflict, however, remains; he rejects his own conduct and repudiates the other's demand. Avoiding final commitment, he submits to the power of a demand whose right he contests.

Now, in compulsion sickness the conflict is not, of course, with the power and right of an alien demand.

As long as the strength of the compulsive's opposition continues, he straightforwardly resists the power of decay. Only with collapse does his experience become ambivalent. Only when overtaxed does he begin to reflect. But in reflection, the invisibly decaying cannot be comprehended. The standpoint of the compulsive patient is definitely not so "far out" that he would not interpret the world in accord with general opinion. The compulsive still shares with the healthy person the reflected gnostic evaluation of the world. But he understands the modifications of the pathic [i.e., the modifications in sympathetic relations to the world] no better than the healthy person. Consequently, in reflection, his own doing is incomprehensible; it seems absurd to him, as if it were happening under coercion. His own warding off is interpreted as an inner compulsion. So it is that we are wont to say that the compulsive has "insight" into his absurd behavior. Yet, if his insight were perfect, he would long since have given us an interpretation of compulsion and would have spared us the trouble of attempting one.

Gebsattel, V. von (1938), 'The world of the compulsive'

From (1958) *Existence*. Edited by R. May, E. Angel and H. F. Ellenberger, translated by S. Koppel and E. Angel. New York: Basic Books: 170–87. Originally published as (1938) Die Welt des Zwangskranken. *Monatsschrift für Psychiatrie und Neurologie* **99**: 10–74.

Editors' commentary

This piece picks up on similar themes to those discussed by Straus in the previous text but von Gebsattel gives a richer and more detailed case description with some striking turns of phrase to capture the world of the person with severe obsessive compulsive disorder. Despite its vagueness, the text is intriguing, offering another example of an existential anthropological analysis.

I. The Problem

What always fascinates us in encountering the compulsive person is the unpenetrated, perhaps impenetrable, quality of his being different. Seventy years of clinical work and scientific research have not altered this reaction. Kept alive by the contradiction between the intimate closeness of the presence of a fellow man and the strange remoteness of a mode of being completely different from our own, the affect of psychiatric amazement never ceases. This excitement constantly thrusts upon us the question about the world in which the compulsive lives; for our world, in which he is found, does not seem to be his. Actually, the contradiction found in the phenomenon of the compulsive does not distinguish him from others encountered by the psychiatrist; but the lucidity with which the compulsive illuminates his own abnormality, without finding it out, and the consequently increasing paradox of his existence, only heightens, if possible, the acuity of the psychiatric affect and keeps it going with particular emphasis.

The focus of our inquiry is the compulsive person *in toto* and primarily the special way of existing by which he is set into a specific world of being (*Daseinswelt*) different from our own. In this, we wish to go beyond the mere analysis of function, act, and experience, likewise beyond the depth-psychological drive theory of psychoanalysis, and beyond the simple character and constitution theories of compulsivity as stimulated through the compulsive phenomena in post-encephalitis. The results of these types of research form the premise of our method, which we should like to designate as a constructive–synthetic one. The following inquiry aims at a phenomenological–anthropological–structural theory, which will prepare the ground upon which the data obtained by clinical analysis can then take root and attain their proper meaning.

It is the proper psychiatric affect of astonishment, the experience of an encounter with an unexplainable other being, that should enter into the initial posing of our question. For what becomes effective in this encounter is just this unexplainable other being in his human totality. This "being-different" of a fellow human being – which stirs equally our sympathy and our intellectual curiosity – is not exhausted in the difference of his functions, his life history, his character, etc. – in other words, in what one usually calls the symptomatology of the sick person. The latter appeals to our curiosity, interest, or scientific understanding. The wondering has an existential meaning. One wonders not only as a scientist or as a psychiatrist; one wonders much more as a fellow man – i.e., on that level of being which precedes being a scientist or a doctor and which provides the foundation for both.

II.   A Case History

*****

Case H. H.

Patient is seventeen years old; gives an impression of being shy, embarrassed, dejected, introverted, inhibited. Intelligent – ambitious. Had earlier been the leader of his class, learned without an effort. Had to be removed from school (*Gymnasium*) in August 1937 because of total failure – an eventuality which had been in the making of several years.

He complains about his compulsions, everything being compulsion with him; not for one second is he free of his compulsion. Wishes intensely for freedom from his suffering, but does not believe in a cure. Considers his case unique. He has been suffering from compulsions for eight years without knowing what was bothering him; considered himself abnormal. At the time of his first confession, his thought revolved exclusively around the confession, which he never considered valid because in spite of hour-long efforts, he could never arouse a "perfect repentance" in himself. Anxiety about vows tortured him. In the prayer of angelic salutation, he felt he had to visualize each letter; should he fail to accomplish this, it would be a "mortal sin." He had then to vow to himself that he would accomplish it, he had broken a vow, an oath, and must confess he had perjured himself 150 times. In connection with the repetition of penitential prayer, there appeared a counting compulsion. With respect to the sixth commandment, he behaved as follows: One must confess when one has thought or done something unchaste. Actually, no such thing happened, but if a boy in school said something unchaste and he heard it, he did think it, because one cannot hear something without thinking, and he did do it because every thought is an act. Very severe scruples. Later he stopped confessing. At about twelve years, first nocturnal emission, which he took for "bed wetting." The next morning he noted an odor on himself and established that his penis was wet. Since then he observes that his penis drips. Hours on end he would sit on the toilet, waiting for the dripping to stop; he would dry his penis carefully and wrap it in toilet paper to prevent urine getting on his shirt. Should he be disturbed in this, he would stand for one or two hours with his pelvis pulled in, hands propped on the table in front of him, to prevent his shirt from becoming wet before his penis should have become dry. In spite of these measures, an "odor" developed that stuck to his clothes and his coat and controlled him all day long. This is still so today. He is constantly possessed with the thought of smelling bad and, thus, with being conspicuous, which prevents him from talking to and associating with people. He cannot even telephone because of his obtrusive body odor. Even when he is alone this odor disturbs him in everything so that he cannot do anything. He is just about "nailed down" by it. Because of this odor which he considers to be something objective, he is shy and embarrassed.

In general, compulsions rule him in every performance. They begin at once with getting up in the morning. This must proceed according to a ritual that has been laid down exactly. He divides each action, each performance, into the very tiniest single movements. Each movement must be carried out exactly, and to each he must attend carefully. Everything is ordered and laid out in this way – getting up, washing, drying, getting dressed: first this movement, then that one (dividing compulsion plus control compulsion). Often he must stand with arms upraised, clutching his sponge, before he can go further. Then again he must remain standing and think everything through once more, especially if he feels there is something he did not do right, or if he was "lost in thought" (i.e., was not attending closely to his task). This recapitulation appears especially after some disturbance or omission in the completion of his ceremonial. He is often tortured by the impression that what he must do has not been done right, or not precisely enough or consciously enough, and for this reason he is actually never "well washed" or "neatly clothed." He requires many hours for his toilet, never really gets through, and arrives late for everything. And for that reason he has a "guilty conscience." This compulsion for order rules everything, even the way he eats or goes through a door; in the latter act he must never come in contact with anything. If he touches something, he becomes dirty. If his father, in visiting the hospital, hangs his coat over his bathrobe, the coat is soiled with urine and he must take care not to hang his coat next to his father's in the closet at home, otherwise he cannot put it on again. By contact, dirt can be spread over innumerable objects.

A washing compulsion is also present. He can read only when he accidentally comes upon something readable. Should he want to read, he simply does not get to it because he must take each word apart into its single letters. He never has any peace; something always has to be analyzed or inspected, something always has to be recapitulated, or repeated, or washed – and in everything he is disturbed by his own repugnant body odor which is the most tiresome thing of all. He is depressed and without hope and thinks that people like himself, if left to themselves, could starve to death. No sexual life.

III. The Disturbance Aspect in the Compulsion-Syndrome: "The Anankastic Phobia"

Our chronic anankastics confirm thoroughly the twofold nature of the compulsion-syndrome as recognized in psychiatric circles: ... The phobic aspect of the compulsion syndrome with its obtrusive, unshakable quality of possessedness is emphasized by French psychiatrists, who speak of "obsession" and of "obsessional neurosis," whereas German psychiatry underlines rather the factor of "compulsion."...

In contrast to many authors, we side with those investigators who consider the phobic touch of the compulsion syndrome almost indispensable. We recognize, however, that the anankastic phobia must be considered only a symptom of a more basal disturbance, pertaining to the fundamental disturbance in the patient's relation to the world – to the very thing that delivers him to the anxiety-world. But the nature of this disturbance – which precedes the phobic phenomena and is "basal" in relation to them (de Clérambault) – cannot be determined precisely, notwithstanding certain reports by patients, as we shall see.

Examples reveal these anxiety-worlds to us. They appear, for instance, in the form of a phobic odor of one's body.

A Phobic Odor Illusion

In the center of the compulsive illness of H. H. stands ... the being obsessed by an illusory body odor. We have learned that, biographically, this illusory odor originated from the first spontaneous ejaculation and, from there ... implanted itself in the urinary and excretory system. This case stands out as a model for anankastic disturbance of volition. The cleaning process after elimination often takes hours – and in spite of this the penis often remains moist, that is, unclean, and accordingly capable of transferring this uncleanness to clothing in the form of a repulsive odor. We see here a rather considerable impairment in getting things done and bringing them to an end;

there is a complete failure to perform the *acte de terminaison* (Janet). If the process of cleaning the penis with the aid of special procedures does, at last, seemingly succeed, then the clothing odor which soon appears, and which is always the urine odor transformed by the specific properties of certain fabrics, immediately proves the contrary. The cleaning process itself and, indeed, elimination are defiling, and this defilement spreads on the one hand spatially (to clothing) and on the other temporally, in that from one point to the other it extends itself through the whole day. Indeed completely in keeping with the anankastic illusory phobia, there is a complete absorption in the illusory urine odor. Every life situation now has the significance of serving as an occasion for realizing the latent obsession, regardless of whether it concerns meeting people, telephoning, working, reading, playing, eating, thinking, praying, etc. Becoming aware of the repulsive odor is always disturbing by nature. It is tied up with feelings of pain, aversion, shame, and disgust. The reflexive character of the phobic disgust-reaction is unclear. It prevents, in general, every normal act, every normal occupation, every normal experience of rapport with people; it isolates the patient completely and confines him within the obsessive circle of nauseatedly having to smell himself.

Of all the symptoms in H. H.'s compulsion syndrome the odor is the most unpleasant, because it is always present and incombatable; and because of its localization in the center of the self-concept it is particularly painful. To himself and to others he is a "disgusting skunk." Changing clothes from head to foot several times a day or frequent bathing does not bring relief; the impression of smelling bad or at least "funny" lingers on and forces the phobic, intense, cramping preoccupation with himself (*Reflexionskrampf*) which in anankastics, especially in puberty and adolescence, is often precipitated by a feeling of repulsion towards one's own body.

We see that the phobic odor-illusion is intimately bound up with a disturbance in the capacity to bring things to a close – especially with the incapacity to have done with the bodily act of cleaning. The persistence of the odor of the urine is the reverse side of the incapacity to turn to the tasks of the day – e.g., school work – and to move further into daily activities and toward new goals. To the extent to which the incapacity for this decreases, the patient's preoccupation with the odor-illusion increases. Every problem the day brings in is left lying – and on this inhibition the reflexive occurrence of the odor-illusion always rekindles itself, as it were, so that the preoccupation with the illusion forms a homogenous continuum, filling up the time that is passing. Upon this odor H. H. is "nailed," thereby expressing fittingly that the persistence of his body odor is synonymous with being fastened to the past, at the cost of the future, which, in turn, is represented by the tasks that offer themselves. H. H.'s not getting rid of the past pollution is, at closer sight, the pollution itself in its genuine meaning. It appears as a personal emanation loaded with an offensive odor, but it only appears as this phenomenon. Behind this appearance, and making it possible, stands H. H.'s incapacity to let his energies stream into the implementation of a task-oriented self-development and thereby to purify himself from the stagnation of energy. This incapacity is the actual disturbance, perhaps related to the endogenic depressive inhibition; in any case, a choking or blocking of the life course is evidenced in it; therewith is impeded the temporalization of life – "Becoming" is blocked, and the past is fixated. This fixation can be experienced as a pollution which, in man, is expressed in the experience of the anxiety-producing body odor. For it is not at all a question of a real odor or of an actual soiling; rather, odor and soiling are symbols of a life deprived of one of the possibilities of purification – i.e., of its orientation toward future. Thus, we recognize that the compulsive patient does what he does not mean to do; what he does mean, he cannot do. The lack of freedom which manifests itself in compulsive behavior belongs to the essence of his situation.

IV. The Defensive Side of the Compulsion-Syndrome and the Nature of Compulsion

The case of H. H. is instructive still in another respect. Like many anankastics, he suffers from a disturbance in the capacity to act, which is revealed especially as an impediment to beginning something new and completing something. H. H. cannot finish anything because the inner life-historical articulation is missing from his outer action, and therewith the experience of completion. A splitting of action and occurrence is present; this takes on grotesque forms when H. H. stands in the room with his coat on and explains that he cannot go out, for he does not know whether he has really put his coat on. We see that an action can be completely executed, in the sense that it has served to implement a purpose, without being completed – or indeed, having occurred at all – in terms of its life-historical meaning. Although it is done, it is as if it had not been done. The person, as a living being moving ahead in time, does not enter into the objective performance of his action, and therefrom arises – after the completion of the action – doubt as to the reality of its occurrence. At least one more explicit action is needed – e.g., stamping one's foot, or swallowing, or clicking one's tongue, something – such as a command, a "fiat," in the sense [William] James uses it – to give the impression that what was done was really done.

From the case history of H. H. we know that he met this disturbance in his capacity to act with a method that in France has been called *la manie de précision*, in other words, with a compulsion for exactness. His ceremonial consists in dividing every action into parts, into smaller and smaller movement particles, which are precisely determined according to their content, precisely marked off from one another, and precisely laid down in terms of sequence. One can speak of a "dividual" (*saccadierten*)[4] form of action. Thus, the morning toilet consists in a fixed number of single movements, precisely separated from, and following upon, one another. In order to keep to the schedule, it is necessary to put in a control-compulsion and to check, with alert attention, all the movements and their sequence. Mistakes that slip in undo the effect of the act, and hence immediately a repetition compulsion sets in – he must begin again from the beginning – or suffices to carry out the repetition in mental form – by way of recapitulation compulsion. Every imperfection that slips in is, in addition, experienced by the patient as guilt-laden and is punished, so to speak, by an intensification of the illusion of his body odor.

The intensification of the body odor illusion (which justifies H. H. in his feeling in being a "disgusting skunk"), running parallel with a failure in exactness, makes clear that the inexactness not only is considered as an impairment of the action but is experienced also as a soiling. One may recall that everyday language also

draws a relation between "clean" and "exact": whoever shoots precisely, shoots "cleanly"; precise handiwork is described as "clean work." We call a piece of work "not clean" when it is not carried out with precision, and can thus not stand as completed. There is no doubt that H. H., with his "dividual" compulsion for exactness, is out to fight for perfection in his action, which constantly eludes him; for his disturbance consists just in this – the outer completion of the task does not at the same time include the process of Becoming in the person, his unfolding in time, and an act of self-realization.

At the same time, H. H. defends himself with his dividual action – although unsuccessfully – against the possibility of pollution, which constantly lies in wait for him in the form of the repulsive and lasting body odor by which he is possessed, half as a hypochondriac, half as a depersonalized patient. It requires only a small outer disturbance or an insignificant failure in his apotropaic (warding off) ceremonial for the pollution to erupt from relative latency to actual fact.

*****

What is not sufficiently noted is the often possible proof that the compulsion phenomena take place against the background of a personality that is potentially intact but condemned to powerlessness in asserting itself. Already in everyday life it is characteristic for the experience of a compulsion that there is a simultaneous "yes" and "no" – a compliant act with an inner refusal, or a refusal to act combined with inner compliance (if – e.g., I feel compelled to sign a statement which I reject). In the case of psychopathological compulsion, both compulsion and being compelled originate in the ego-sphere: the ego is the *object* of the overwhelming force, but it is also the *principle* of the overwhelming force. The ego challenges the actions that spring from the very same ego. The challenging party and the challenged party are both of an ego nature, are both ego-spheres that do not coincide but stand in opposition to each other. This contradiction stems from the fact that in that portion of the personality which is altered in accordance with the compulsion syndrome, the free personality shines through in its disposition and in its idea. On the one hand, the nonsensicalness and strangeness of the anankastic disturbance is thereby increased; on the other hand, the reactive defense against this fundamental disturbance takes on the character of unfree acts, of an encroachment, of a compulsion. From case

---

[4] *Saccadiert* connotes both fragmented and disrupted.
[Translator's note]

to case varying degrees of the shining through of the potentially healthy personality can be found, and it may be observed that with the weakening of this transparency phenomenon the painfully compulsive character of the acts also becomes weaker. Hoffman,[5] in an excellent paper, gathered statements from compulsive patients in love with their compulsions that bear eloquent testimony to this point. The more the compulsive lives in his phobic preoccupation and the nearer this approaches the overvalued idea (though criticism never is *completely* silenced), the more he is absorbed in his compulsion, and the less challenged – i.e., the more unimpeded – remains the latter. But the more the compulsive distances himself from his phobic preoccupation, the stranger and more nonsensical does it seem to him, the more does he experience the necessity for defense as unavoidable, the more does its compulsive character stand out. Ultimately it is always the underlying personality which, potentially shut out, yet still healthy in its disposition, reflects like a mirror the experiencing and acting of the anankastic. This reflecting defines the experience side of the compulsive phenomena – a fact which up till now has not received sufficient attention.

Let us carry out a little further our analysis of a banal compulsive act – as, for instance, a compulsion for precision – by contrasting the compulsive precision with the healthy practice. In this setting it occurs to us that the healthy person reserves the special exertion of his will to perfection for certain activities where "it matters," whereas the greatest part of his activities takes place without being burdened by an explicit intention to be exact, but without lapsing thereby into inexactness. The healthy person trusts himself, along wide stretches of his way, to the automatically realizable "sure hit" in his conduct, without troubling himself about the difference between exact and inexact. Indeed, he allows himself errors and slips without being shocked where these are of no particular consequence. He knows that the human being is not a precision machine, and therefore he allows the irrelevant to come to expression without pinning himself down to any too-definite rule of conduct. For him, the approximate, too, has its right, and the preliminary its significance. Hence, he always lives in an atmosphere of freedom – where things can be so,

but also otherwise, in a certain loose and capricious casualness of action. Harmless informality and variable irrelevance are, after all, important elements of our freedom. To take into account this side of existence does not prevent, but actually heightens, the readiness to precise action where precision is needed.

In contrast to a healthy person, the compulsive makes just this Unimportant and Irrelevant the object of his will to accuracy. A reversal of the normal relief map of what is important thus characterizes the practical world of the anankastic which simultaneously presents itself as a flattened one. Just where the healthy person bustles about freely in his business, cheered on by the irrelevance of the manner in which it is executed, we see the anankastic succumbing to the need for rigidly laid down, stereotyped executions, while the objectively important action drops out. An impoverishment in freedom now imposes itself in the fixating on irrelevant facts or part-acts and their sequence; there are no alterations; variations are forbidden and guilt-producing. Accuracy does not enter for the sake of attaining some purpose that matters, but has become an end in itself and has the characteristic features of the unmotivated, the reflexive, the formal, the sterile and the rigid.

If the compulsive were a depersonalized individual … he would complain that everything he does is incomprehensibly dead, empty, and meaningless, or even that it is not his own action but that of a stranger. The same void, which in the depersonalized patient is simply suffered, is found also in the anankastic: just as little as the other is he able to enter his task as a person who is "becoming" and to fill it with himself. But in his case, the incapacity to become stands in him as a non-Becoming (*Entwerden*), as an orientation toward formlessness which must be warded off but cannot be warded off. Precision is the counterpart of this orientation to formlessness to which his inhibition in Becoming inescapably delivers him. That the formless appears in the image of a possible contamination, we have shown repeatedly. Dirt is a lack of order ("matter in the wrong place"); it is lack of form (excrement, for example, as matter) which unforms itself (*enstaltend*) and causes "disformation" (*Enstaltung*). The necessity of defense by means of formal order and precise action would not work if there were not constantly at work an orientation of the personality toward the formless, and it would not be *experienced* as compulsion if the possibility of something like a healthy performance of life did not form the background for the defense.

[5] Herman Hoffman, 'Der "Gesundheitswille" der Zwangsneurotiker,' *Zeitschrift für die gesamte Neurologie und Psychiatrie*, 110(1), (1927). [**Original note**]

Just a few words about the repetition compulsion which is found in every compulsive illness. Here, too, we may remember that the life of the healthy is unthinkable without repetition; his is, to be sure, not comparable with the anankastic repetition. For, in the strict sense of the term, the action of the healthy person, his daily toilet, breakfast, going out, etc., is already something other than repetition because it never appears detached from the orientation toward the future that controls the personality in its respective action ... It is just the absence of this relationship in the anankastic, however, and the resulting ineffectiveness and spiritlessness of his action that lead to the genuine anankastic repetition. This accomplishes what it does accomplish only through its purely volitional character – it brings the action to a kind of sham completion.

How should this performance of repetition be understood? Where do we find analogies for such unusual courses of events? We know this kind of repetition in the liturgic realm where formulas of prayer take on, through repetition, a meaning of conjuration. A kind of conjuring effectiveness also qualifies the anankastic repetition, even though it is not a spontaneous and fundamentally meaningful act: it conjures up a kind of completion which purely practically it cannot achieve at all. It achieves this in the way magical acts achieve effectiveness ... The repetition does not bring about the real completion of the action, but a kind of sentimental belief that it has been completed

*****

V. The Compulsive Patient and his World

1. Our previous considerations converge in the insight that it must be possible to interpret the world of the compulsive patient (which according to Binswanger should always be understood as "his special way of being-in-the-world") from its inner logic.

Already the observation that the world of the compulsive patient appears even to himself to be apart from the *koinos kosmos*[6] of average waking reality – without the latter undergoing any structural destruction as

sometime happens with schizophrenics – brings up a whole series of problems. These must be put aside in favor of the simplifying statement that the arrangement with the everyday world through action and self-realization is omitted by the compulsive and is replaced by another arrangement, proceeding according to other structural principles, with a differently structured existence-world.

In general, it may be said that the world of the compulsive is constituted by forces inimical to form, whose quintessence we have called the "anti-eidos." A peculiar world opens up as soon as we use this kind of approach.

The actions and omissions of the compulsive are determined by encounters with an environment (*Umwelt*) that does not consist of the usual objects of our sympathetic experiencing and our cognitive or practical conduct; rather, their coinage bears the stamp of a "physiognomic" character ... If we accept the reports of certain compulsives that all objects around them take on "meaning," we must recognize that we are dealing here with a breaking through of archaic modes of experience to which there corresponds a "primal world," a world which, as Werner says, is "physiognomically given."

... Indeed, the broad sphere of physiognomic settings which constitute the world of children and primitives appears, in the specific anankastic world-structure, limited and restricted to a definite sector. Only that which is inimical to form, which moves towards "un-form" or is apt to bring it about, enters as a deciding factor into the anankastic world ... Thus the physiognomic is here given as an energy – symbolizing "un-form" – that threatens and repels. Effective threat and repulsion are the physiognomic criteria of the anankastic counterworld – as when, for example, objects of daily use which had not been unpacked according to predetermined rituals and, therefore, are affected with the stigma of pollution, are also charged with the potency of the polluting magic force. Thus the physiognomic construction of the anankastic counterworld also turns out to be a reduced structure.

To talk of the "revival of primal forms of reality" is actually a convenient way of covering up important facts, particularly the fact that physiognomic features are interspersed in our real world anyway. In our environment there is no object which, besides its categorical forming, does not have an expression, that is not somehow animated or tuned and can, therefore,

---

[6] Refers to the celebrated aphorism of Heraclitus: "When men dream, each has his own world (*idios kosmos*); when they are awake, they have a common world (*koinos kosmos*)." [**Translator's note**]

speak to us in a fundamental way. It is only that these physiognomic structures become almost completely hidden from us through the categorical rational ones. Only in the poetic atmosphere does the silent language of things come to life again, not because in such an atmosphere a person begins to phantasy, but because in the higher sympathetic receptivity of the poet the real language of things actually arrives at expression . . .

What about the transcendence-character of the anankastic world – if we understand "transcendence" in the Husserlian sense? . . .

To this the following may be said: Fundamentally, the encounters of the anankastic, his collisions with the powers of disformation (*Enstaltung*), do not take place in a vacuum. Even if they do not invariably adhere to real objects, the physiognomic features that determine his actions do impinge upon him as though very much from the outside. In his own experience, it is the world of things which in its taboo-like meanings takes its shape toward him . . . The intentional transcending of the anankastic takes place within the immanence of his own possessedness and surroundedness by the powers of the "anti-eidos." We speak of this particular situation and nothing else when we say that world-deprivation (*Entweltlichung*) is one of the chief characteristics of the anankastic object-sphere. Just this reductive character in the construction of the anankastic world differentiates it from the equally physiognomic–dynamic world of the primitive . . . There is certainly some connection between the physiognomic impoverishment of the anankastic world and the exclusive receptivity of the patient to those contents that symbolize the loss of "eidos" of existence, such as dirt, destructive fire, contaminating bestiality, images of putrefaction, etc. Both belong essentially together . . .

Let us return to our thesis that the physiognomic is here given as the force symbolizing "un-form" which threatens and repels. Above all our thesis illustrates that the compulsive patient lives in a world different from ours. This differentness of his world and the differentness of his existence in it are two sides of one and the same fact which requires interpretation. What entered our awareness from this other kind of world is a sum of negations. What struck us above all was that the friendly, inviting powers of existence step back in favor of the hostile, repulsive ones. Everything that normally draws the individual into the world and invites him to fuse with

it is condemned to a peculiar kind of ineffectiveness. Even taking nourishment is for H. H., according to his statement, a continuing torture because the inviting appeal of food that effects its incorporation does not engage him – rather is he threatened by the exclusive possibility of contamination through it. So it is with all the features of the world which call for connection and union with it and thus make possible the extension of one's own existence, the moving into the world and being active in it, penetrating into it – conquest, joy, activity, spreading out. Indeed, it can also be plainly shown that the world of the anankastic is characterized by the omission of the harmless, the obvious, and the natural. What is called by Scheler the "ecstatic possession of the world-contents" and by E. Straus "sympathetic communication" is here impeded. Threat and repulsion are all that remain. A world without mercy and without grace of Fate (*Schicksals-Huld*) opens up, or rather, shuts up before the anankastic. Its characteristics are narrowness, natureless monotony, and rigid, rule-ridden unchangeability – all of which are most essential alterations of the mode of moral, spatial, and temporal being-in-the-world. We must forego further interpretation of this.

*****

We have already expressed ourselves about the time-structure of this behavior, without exhausting its analysis. What may still be mentioned in a preliminary way is the peculiar mixture of dawdling and rushing that marks the temporal structure of anankastic behavior . . .

. . . It is not merely the slowing down or hampering of inner time that differentiates the compulsive from other categories of patients, in whom the fundamental disturbance is likewise to be sought in the realm of Becoming (as in melancholics and depersonalized patients with syndromes of emptiness). What distinguishes the compulsive is his way of handling the disturbance of inner temporal events. . . . [S]een quite naïvely, the fact is that the compulsive does act. True, anankastic activity is itself – as we could show – an expression of the disturbance in the capacity to act; nevertheless, the compulsive patient is forever in action. From early till late we see him in constant tension, ceaselessly at work to have it out with the enemy who, as H. H. says, is "forever at his heels," regardless of whether this encounter consists more in intellectual or in practical defenses.

Let us anticipate and name this "enemy" immediately; it is nothing else but the pseudo-magic counterworld of the anankastic, the quintessence of the forces that symbolize "un-form," which we have recognized as his world. From everywhere this world pursues him; from outside and from inside it breaks in upon him. Threat and repulsion (taboo) are its agents ... [T]his orientation can appear only in images like excrement or dirt, poison or fire, ugliness, unchastity, "corpsiness" (*Leichenhaftigkeit*) – in short, in such images as are suitable to refer to the form-destroying potencies of existence. The demon of this environment (Umwelt), or counterworld we have called the "anti-eidos," in order to define the quintessence of all form-destroying potencies of the existence in one term. In the ubiquity of contaminating dirt, or in the urine-odor of H. H., the form-destroying potencies of existence in all the repulsive features of the anankastic world-image attain actual realization. Only this makes us understand the desperate and everlasting defense of the compulsive. His contest with the world has no other content than the battle with the form-destroying powers of existence, a battle that has the character of a powerless and fruitless undertaking ...

... Of the various types of patients who are impaired in their Becoming, the anankastic represents that one for whom the inhibition in Becoming means a loss of form. That the impairment in Becoming can, on principle, be experienced in this way appears to us meaningful. For only in the process of Becoming does the form of life complete itself and the "eidos" of the person become realized ... [T]he impairment in Becoming can be experienced as a dissolution of form. The compulsive, in any case, does experience it so. Every interval of passing time, then, is experienced as a threat of increasing the possible losses of form in the chained person and deepens the worry of those who have become deeply struck ... [T]he image of dirt or of death afflicts him with constant contamination. The whole world shrinks to this one repulsive physiognomy which can crop up in almost any content and which plagues him with its threat as it forces him into a defense with its repulsion-producing energy. But only because the compulsive is threatened with the loss of his own form, of his own eidos, can the symbol of the form-destroying forces gain mastery over his imagination and determine his actions ... All individual compulsive acts can be explained on the basis of the fundamental disposition of the anankastic which we have here presented.

19

Other topics

Scheler, M. (1913), 'The psychology of so-called compensation hysteria and the real battle against illness'

From (1984) *Journal of Phenomenological Psychology* **15** (2). Translated by E. S. J. Vacek. Originally published in 1913, now found in vol. 3 of Max Scheler's *Collected Works* (Bonn: Bouvier). These section headings within the text have been supplied by the translator. Likewise, many of Scheler's paragraphs, which sometimes run to almost five hundred words in length, have been broken down into smaller paragraphs. Scheler's bibliographical references and those of his editor, Maria Scheler, have been included as footnotes.

Editors' commentary

In this text from 1913, Max Scheler enters a debate that continues to arouse sentiment until this day: does compensation generate illness and lead to moral decline?

The text is remarkable in several ways. Firstly, some of Scheler's complex ideas are applied to issues of wide practical concern. Secondly, the arguments make important links between individual psychologic causation and large-scale public health and policy matters. Thirdly, Scheler posits psychological mechanisms – such as the role of attention focus in the generation of somatic symptoms – that seem to anticipate contemporary psychological theories.

Scheler agrees that statutory compensation may produce 'compensation hysteria'; however, he states boldly that compensation hysteria should be completely distinguished from what he sees as the rare phenomenon of malingering. He claims that compensation hysteria is independent of cognitive representations of the potential material benefits. Instead, he argues that the prospect of compensation is given to consciousness as an emotional colouring. It is this 'feelingful presence' of compensation that changes what is the person's usual automatic striving for health. In doing this, Scheler views the phenomenon of compensation

hysteria through its relations to emotions and their importance for moral judgements.

In order to fully understand the enormous, large-scale social phenomena of our time, we need to go beyond the research method which is commonly used in these issues. Such research employs statistics and tries to find objective causes through statistical results and correlations. This method needs to be supplemented with an investigation into the psychological origins and the elementary psychological laws that are highlighted in these phenomena. This shift of method is important, for example, in understanding the origins of the presently alarming decline in the birth-rate, a topic which we cannot take up in this essay. It is also important for understanding ... those pathological phenomena that have sometimes been given the name "traumatic neurosis" and sometimes the expression "compensation hysteria."

*****

I.   First Law: Effect of Prospect

Here we may only glance at those psychological laws that are manifest in that large-scale social phenomenon called compensation hysteria.

A.   Distinct from Pretense

Compensation hysteria should be completely distinguished from all forms of either clear or semi-conscious pretense of sickness or its prolongation, as well as from all forms of half or wholly conscious, willful occasioning of accidental injury; it thus should also be distinguished from the so-called "compensation addiction" that is only an intensification of these phenomena. Whenever a more or less clear representation, expectation, or hope for some compensation leads to such sham practices and artificial counterfeits for the natural expression of the state of health, or leads to self-harming practices or to a willful slackening of the requisite "caution" which would otherwise be exercised (e.g., when near machines), then it is a question of the misuse of the statute, not a question of the effect of the statute on psychic health. Since every statute can be misused, such a misuse (even if very extensive) is not a significant objection against the particular statute. Cases of this sort are confined for the most part to the morally lowest segment of those insured. An exception to this moral judgment occasionally occurs when a specifically hysterical impulse for revenge, namely the impulse to make a social observer suffer by harming oneself (counting on a sympathetic participation on his part), acts as the cause of the behavior, something that certainly is very rare. (This impulse became a "custom" in the practice of suicide among the Chinese and Japanese.)

On the boundaries of such cases, however, there still remains one form of "pretense" that we can call automatic pretense in contrast to willful pretense. In automatic pretense the influx of the impulse to pretense occurs independently of the conscious will, and this influx is itself already the sign of a psychic ailment. Thus in a hysterical patient the first impulse towards becoming helpless and breaking down is probably thoroughly automatic; nevertheless, this process shows a certain regularity "on the basis of" (however, not according to a "calculation of") the respective "circumstances," so that, for example, the patient will fall down on a carpet but not on a marble floor. In such cases, the behavior is determined by the meaning and the value which changing "circumstances" possess for the individual's interests. One can demonstrate the presence of this mixture of automatic compulsion an situational determination by an abundance of symptoms known to us from cases of hysteria, such as hysterical blindness, constriction of the field of vision, deafness, lameness, etc., as well as the automatic formation of false representations. Although these representations are not willfully substituted for the truth as in the case of a "lie," they should be distinguished from "errors" and "illusions" by the fact that they remain really "in the interests" of the one sick.

Now it is in accord with this particular law of automatic pretense that the process which ultimately terminates in the pattern of sickness called traumatic neurosis doubtlessly originates. For it is not just the "representation" or the "expectation" of the prospective compensation that causes the (similarly named) pathogenic processes of intensifier "self-observation"

and hypochondriac behavior, rather – and this will for the present seem miraculous – it is the very "prospect" of compensation which does this. Moreover it is not necessary that this fact must also be given to conscious awareness in the form of a present representation, expectation, to say nothing of any calculation. Whenever it is the representation, expectation, or any "counting upon" the compensation that causes the behavior, then we still have pretense in the usual sense.

B. No Explicit Representation

Now the untutored will probably ask, how, without such representation or expectation, can the payment of compensation in the future come to have any influence at all over psychological behavior? Do we not have here a totally mysterious assumption? Could the mere existence of a law that links a provision for compensation to certain intrusive cases of sickness or accident have an effect on the insured if he does not even know of the existence of the law and does not envisage these provisions? In these questions, the true and the false are peculiarly mixed. To be sure, if, for example, an "uncle in America," long said to be dead, dies and leaves me a million Marks, this fact can for a moment, before I grasp it, have no psychic influence on me. By the same token, the one insured must "somehow" also "know" of the existing legislation and live under its "influence" on his psychic behavior. But here it is precisely a question of the nature of this "knowing" and "influence."

For a long time now we in psychology have been rather well aware of the phenomena and laws which we are discussing here. William James, the late, outstanding American psychologist, recounted in his Psychology the following observation about himself. James was accustomed on certain afternoons of the week to offer a required series of lectures in "formal logic," lectures that he used to deliver very reluctantly because his own interests were at cross-purposes with formal logic. He made the observation that already early in the morning he was peculiarly ill-tempered, "nervous," averse to any task. He paced about in his room, moved this or that to and fro, gathered bits of paper, etc. All this happened, however, without in any way thinking about or "imagining" his afternoon lecture. Naturally, if someone had asked him, he would have known that he had to give this lecture; the lecture would also have certainly "occurred" to him if he had, for example, been reminded of it through some association. Still, in order for him to act out this "psychic influence," there was no need for a representation of the lecture.

Who has not had something similar happen to him a thousand times? We often say, for example, one man has a "future," another no "future." And we know how good "prospects" cast a bright and cheery tint over our soul, how they color all our experiences; and we know how bad prospects cast everything within us into darkness. However, there is definitely no need to represent this "prospect" of ours. The mere fact that it "is a prospect" for us already colors, brightens or darkens the present passage and content of our experience.

Quite obviously we have an example of this phenomenon in the case of "cost-hypnotic suggestion." If in the hypnotic state some task is suggested to a particular party, for example, to perform a certain deed at a certain time, the person in the waking state "knows" nothing about this task.[1] But then it happens that a peculiar unrest makes itself felt, specially colored with the content and meaning of the task. This unrest is evinced prior to the time when the person experiences an impulse to do the particular deed and then carries it out. Here again the one under suggestion clearly does not imagine the deed. He "comes to know" it only as he performs it.

Now, in the normal range of psychological processes, an "interest" in something can take the place of the hypnotizer and his suggested command, "you do this and that." This interest is not a matter of "taking an interest in something," which is a conscious, spiritual act; rather it refers to "having an interest in something," a state that the one "having" the interest does not need to know anything about (no more than the one hypnotized knows, in his waking state, that he has been given a task). Yet such a man automatically behaves differently than he would if he did not have this interest. And if this interest in gaining something (for example, a compensation payment) is connected to the realization of a certain condition, then an automatic "tendency" to bring about just this condition will also arise. And it will do so without the slightest trace of a representation of that condition and without a trace of an act of the will to create the condition.

There is an organic life-instinct and (in extreme age before "natural" death, according to Metschnikoff) also an inversion of this instinct into a natural, organic death-instinct. Neither of these have anything to do with a "will" to live or a "will" towards death (such as, for example, someone has who is suicidal and in fact does not disavow life, but rather rejects only his present conditions). In parallel fashion, there is also an analogous organic instinct for sickness and health, and possibly for an accident or for the avoidance of accident; again both are completely independent of any conscious attempt to possess good health or to be or to look sick (or become sick). In fact, they are so independent that, for example, an old man, in whom everything is pressing toward death and who would greet death as a release, can still "will" life in order, for example, further to pursue a task which deeply stirs him, or in order to fulfill a duty; and the reverse is also true.

If, for example, all forms of health insurance prolong the length of time for convalescence, then the prospect of compensation clearly has an effect which is completely independent of any representation of this prospect. This prospect influences the automatic striving for health, precisely in the sense of a lessening of the strength of this striving. And all the while, this dwindling striving may be concurrent with consciously wishing to get well as soon as possible and with strictly following all the directions of the doctor. Doctors, speaking from their experience, usually say to their patients that, without the cooperation of the sick person's "will to get well," all their instructions may be in vain; what they mean by the words "will to get well" is clearly this automatic striving for health which is totally intractable to conscious will and choice. Therefore, it would be completely mistaken to say that the prolonged time for convalescence is due to the fact that the patient "wills" to be sick longer and thus may perhaps either disregard or less than strictly follow the doctor's instructions. Naturally, the legal statute can also be abused in this fashion. In itself, however, the whole phenomenon has nothing to do with such misuse.

C. Effect of a Prospective Gain

One can now also pose the theoretical question: how then can the mere "prospect" of a benefit have such an antecedent efficacy when that benefit is not at the same time represented and "taken into account?" The answer arises from a lawfulness that I have

---

[1] It is presupposed that this ignorance was suggested to him. [Original note]

explained elsewhere[2]. This lawfulness consists in the fact that for us the practical "significance," "importance" and the "value" of past and future as well as present events occurring around us can be "given" to consciousness – whether in perception, memory or expectation – originally and prior to the representation and concept or judgment upon that particular event. (We possess a definite power of feeling or, as the case may be, of "prefeeling" or "postfeeling" the valuable qualities of that event.) There is a parallel here with memory.

Whenever we "remember," the phases of formation of the memory process occur as follows: in the first stage of consciousness, the object "meant" is remembered as something that was "happy" or "sad," something "dirty" or "beautiful," similarly as some "sin" or something "good" and "praise-worthy" (as in a "pure" conscience); usually only then does the image or the concept of this item become available for being grafted onto these value-phenomena. Similarly, the practical meanings which lie for us in our future are still present to our consciousness even if we lack any definite representation or reckoning of what is to come. They may be present only as the "breadth" or "constrictedness," as the "greatness" or "triviality" of the scope for our possible experiences and practices. Thus we have the phenomenon that our future seems to "smile" or it sadly "frowns" on us; thus also the peculiar pressure that, as they say, "circumstances" can exert on a man without his being able himself to specify just what exerts this pressure.

The benefits of compensation is one example of such imageless practical meanings which have a color quality that needs no representation of the compensation.

Now, however, it is known that the efficacy of this purely feelingful presence of the events and experiences lying in our past or future or contained in our present environment is richer and more extensive than the efficacy of that small island which, plunged in that larger sea of feelings, is more or less bathed with the light of representations, perceptions and concepts. And, secondly, this feelingful presence possesses an efficacy that is at once both qualitatively different and quantitatively more intensive than that of representations.

It is a qualitatively different kind of efficacy since it is able to influence even the automatic and purely drive-like processes of our experiences. Thus, even though we use the same degree of conscious will-power to avoid an accident and practice the same conscious "caution" against any dangers in our work activities, still, when the prospect of compensation is "working" in the way described, the drive-like impulses, which are present in all work, as well as the diffusion and sequence of these impulses can nonetheless still suffer a deflection in a direction which will release movements causing an accident.

It is also, we said, a stronger efficacy. The strongest effect of a past experience never occurs when it is present to us in the clear, distanced light of memory and when the time of its occurrence is well-located in our life-history. The least powerful memory is the one that is "right there" before us. Memory's strongest effect occurs when the past has so entered, as they say, "into our flesh and blood" that it peculiarly colors all of the other contents of our consciousness with its meaning. Then, for just this reason, the past as a single experience is no longer involved or remembered, since it has itself peculiarly modified the very experiencing, of every single experience.

The efficacy of "tradition" belongs, for example, to this type. In tradition the past experience is not itself specially given to us; rather its value and meaning appears to us as "present," and not as "past" as happens in memory. Conscious, clear memory simply kills the power of tradition and delivers us from its binding, silent authority. The science of history, for example, performs such a deliverance for nations, churches, etc. Thus historical science first situates in the past that which still seems to carry on a shadowy life around us, even seems to be our present life itself.

Now, there is a phenomenon analogous to tradition in the givenness of our future. This future is as little an "expectation" as tradition is a "memory." There is just that living antecedent efficacy of "being a prospect" without "expectation," analogous to the living ensuing efficacy of the past without "memory." And the analogy continues: just as the enduring content, for example, of an earlier suffering appears as "present" or "still always moves our heart" in such a way that the content is related to present things and not, as happens in memory, to "past things," so also an antecedent efficacious content appears to lie not in the future but rather to be "present."

Sickness or an accident, to which compensation has been linked and towards which an automatic

2 Scheler, M. (1973). *Formalism in Ethics and Non-Formal Ethics of Values.* Evanston, IL: Northwestern University Press: pp. 194ff.

striving is drifting, "appears" already present, is already "felt," "already gets itself ready."

D. Based on Prior Illness

All that has been said reflects only the laws under whose rule sickness sets in. This sickness, however, cannot occur unless some kind of earlier sickness or accident, some "trauma," has preceded it. That automatic drive to sickness (or to an accident) which arises through the prospect of compensation is activated and receives, as it were, material or food from an earlier experience's consequent effects upon the totality of a man's organic sensations and organic feelings. Now there is of course some such material, ever changing in its magnitude and temporal proximity, in nearly every man. The more it is sizeable and recent and, further, the more it still stands in some recognized causal relation to the dangerous circumstances that are present in the nature of the particular job, the more probable will be the onset of sickness.

In the process of becoming sick, however, new psychological laws will now set in; and they will be of a different type. When the focus of the drives toward health and sickness has been fixed by the beckoning compensation and changed in direction toward "sickness," the drive-based attention (not, therefore, voluntary attention such as in "noticing," "observing," etc.) now concentrates rather on every possible "sign" or inner "signal" of an already present sickness.

This change takes place according to the same pattern that occurs, for example, in the field of external sense perception. There, under the control of the strong, drive-determined expectations, and along the lines of the direction of these drives, the given sense data are elaborated into false unities of thing and meaning; and in this way "illusions" appear. Or we have the case of what is called hallucination when the "partial perspectives"[3] of a thing, which certainly go beyond the pure sense data, no longer come to consciousness, and the sense data are elaborated in such a way as to fixate merely on the pure matter of sensation. Similarly, the same kind of elaboration occurs here, only now in the data of the organic sensations and organic feelings. The data of factual inner sensations and sensible feelings are illusionarily elaborated

or, in the more difficult cases, hallucinatively elaborated into possible systems of "symptoms" of all sorts of drive-induced sickness-patterns. These elaborations arise prior to that drive-based attention which takes over and is directed toward such systems of "symptoms."

In these symptoms, a particular sickness seems just as much "perceived" as in the case of one who is organically sick, for this perception connects with the after-effects (for the most part really present) of earlier sicknesses. A similar thing takes place here as occurs in hysteria where changing, organically uncaused pain-complexes spring up or suddenly shift to and fro. So thus, finally, there results a mixture of the hypochondriac and the hysterical pattern of sickness, built upon an original trauma.

E. True Sickness

Of course, at this level of the process of becoming ill, the organic sicknesses, which are supposedly experienced in these illusions of inner sensation and feeling, are in fact only "imagined." The particular individual, however, is not in the least thereby "a pretender," since his statements and other expressive movements conform just as faithfully to the truth of the content of his factual imagination as in the case of the one who is truly sick. It is therefore completely senseless to want to judge him morally on this account. Here we do not have a case of a culpable misuse of a legal statute; rather it is the statute itself that necessarily produces the described state.

The adversaries of the statute rather often forget this influence of the statute. When these adversaries inveigh in moralistic tones against an "addiction to compensation" and speak of a "moral decline," they hardly seem to note that they thereby exonerate the statute itself. When, inversely, friends of the statute by contrast view all the pertinent phenomena as merely "incidental misuses of a law that is on the whole beneficent," they too seem blind to the fact that these phenomena have nothing at all to do with any "misuse," but rather the statute itself produces them.

The affected individuals, on the other hand, may not be called healthy merely because these illusory organic sicknesses are only "imagined." Of course they are organically healthy. A person who, in the above way, comes to be convinced that he has a stomach ache in fact does not have a stomach ache. Nevertheless, the fact that he arrives at these fantasies and lasting fixations is already the consequence of his sickness, a

---

[3] For example, the visual object and its respective visual aspect. [**Original note**]

psychic sickness, however, and not an organic one. He is therefore not somehow a psychological *malade imaginaire*, but rather he is psychologically a really or factually sick man whose sickness has as its consequence, among other things, the imagination of organic sicknesses.

For this very reason, his sickness also offers a case for applying the law (and the compensation benefits linked to this condition); thus the same law will be applied whose existence occasioned the sickness in the first place. If, as one might psychologically misconstrue, such a sick man just willed to turn his attention and "observe" his inner sensation-states or if he made false judgments about these states (or "mistakes" about them) because his judgments were led by mere "wishes" to obtain the compensation, then the case would of course be completely different. In this case one could also find moral fault in him and accuse him of abusing the statute. None of these things, however, can ever produce a psychic sickness, and they are in no way applicable to the sickness-pattern of traumatic neurosis.

It is essential that, first, the one afflicted feel an invincible, drive-based compulsion, which is completely independent from willful attention, as it forages about within himself; that, secondly, this shift of the drive-based attention towards his condition is already induced by the previous "appearance" of some sickness; and that, thirdly, this attention is already directed along its path by the drive-based will-to-sickness which is itself conditioned by the mere prospect of compensation. Any possibly voluntary acts of attention, including the sensing of inner organic stimuli, fall subsequently under the rule and in the scope of that new drive-based attitude which itself is already of a pathological nature.

II. Second Law: Effect of Attention

There is yet a second lawfulness in addition to the one already named. This one is certainly even less thoroughly researched. It is known that a continuous focusing of attention, let us repeat, of the drive-based attention, toward the sensations that commonly accompany the automatic life-activities such as breathing, heart-beat, walking (apart from the impulse to get started), speaking, the automatic segments of work-processes, and so on, is able to hamper and disturb the normal flow of these activities. Indirectly, as a result of these functional disturbances, this turning of attention

usually also leads to the pathological patterns of heart-trouble, asthma, stuttering, paralysis, and so on.

In addition a new purpose or intention can result as a reaction to an illusion that arises in the manner described above, the illusion, namely that one of these activities is not rightly functioning, even though in fact functions well. This new intention attempts willfully to help the course of the processes, that is, willfully to direct partial processes that otherwise perform automatically, but it often brings about that disorder which wants to prevent. So, for example, an individual becomes a stutter, when he volitionally intends the expression of his thought, indeed of his present thought, rather than intends his thought itself and those thoughts he will say next. It can also happen here that turning one's own attention to the particular processes is a result of experiencing another's attention turned on them. Thus, even under normal conditions, one feels easily restricted in speech or writing when another looks at one's mouth or the movement of the pen.

Now in our case both sources of this paying attention are present: the illusion that "things are not going well" (stemming from the illusion the "symptoms") and the attention paid by another person. Wherever the compensation benefits are linked to accidents or illnesses that are the results of the work-process, not only will any negatively tinted experience such as, for example, those linked to earlier life-disturbances, immediately connected with these results of the work-process, but all; even the automatic part of the work-process will attract and strongly hold one's attention. As this happens, however, the automatic activities in fact will be disturbed and the real danger of an accident thereby significant increases. Similarly, factual, pathological disturbances, e.g., of heart-activity, will flow from some previously imagined sickness through the middle link of this lawfulness. In addition, now to play the role outside "observer," there is all the attention which those who are professionally obligated and officially entrusted with administering the law daily and even hourly devote to monitoring the work processes which endanger health.

III. Social Psychology

We have now arrived at the last point which this small study wishes to bring up: the whole phenomenon has in addition to its general psychological side also its sociopsychological side which up till now has hardly been appreciated.

A. Justice, Economics, and Compassion

Our great German sociopolitical legislation certainly does not find its justification in the idea of caritas, compassion, or love. Many of the "racial ethicians" make this mistake about its nature. Rather, it is warranted in part, first, by the demands of justice. That is, the whole society and its highest organization, the state, have the duty to take responsibility in their entirety for those damages to the life, etc., of its members which arise from the nature of the dominant, operating forms of industrial work (whose products everyone more or less jointly enjoy).

Secondly, in greater part, it is also justified simply on the purely economic ground that the forces working in the enterprises must themselves be taken care of, if the gross national product is to grow to its peak . . .

This factual "justification" of legislation is decidedly not identical with its psychological effect or with the way its provisions are received by the insured. It is highly questionable to what extent the insured consider the provisions set up for them as warranted in the first sense; (in the second sense, they certainly do not). And it is questionable how much they actually feel its fruits for them as nothing but a mere gesture, frozen into a "statute," of social compassion on the part of the ruling classes toward "working people."[4] . . .

B. Social Pity

*****

If anyone feels that he is looked at with pity, especially in such a way that it is not his deeper and individual self – which here plays no role – that shapes the course of the pity, but rather his existence as a specimen of a class, then the results can be twofold. Either his class pride and his class self-confidence is strong enough so that motivated by shame, he rejects this pity and the welfare-benefits induced by it; or the pity felt strengthens and deepens his susceptibility for suffering from disorders of a particular kind, however

much the welfare-benefits deriving from this pity may bring relief from this present disorder.

Thus, for example, a child who has hurt himself cries all the more loudly the more we commiserate with him. And although we might little by little remove the painful sensations as well as their causes, his suffering of these ebbing sensations in spite of their diminished intensity becomes greater and swings so to speak out beyond its original cause, namely, the blow and the accompanying painful sensations. He will focus on some small part of the hurt. If the compassion continues, these small parts coalesce with one another at any sort of provocation and finally lead to a kind of yearning for suffering. The stimulation of this yearning is dependent on a pitying observer, and it leads to actual sufferings that would not exist without the pitying observer.

We also have here one of the roots of certain hysterical symptoms. The patient's deeply saddened and tearful countenance turns to a serene brightness and a perfect peace of soul as soon as the doctor or any other person leaves the room and watches the patient, say, through a peephole. However, even in this case, the patient definitely is not "pretending" or "play-acting." He cannot he compared with someone who merely puts on a staged expression of suffering or who verbally alleges that he is suffering, that is, in cases where the expression and the experience are designedly disproportionate to one another. Rather he really suffers; and precisely because his expression and his verbal utterances are natural and appropriate to this suffering, there is missing here that relative transparency of the state of affairs which is present in the artificial split between experience and expression which occurs in cases of pretense. All the same, the duration of this "real suffering" is totally dependent upon the presence of an observer.

Suppose, moreover, as almost always happens, that an interest is linked to the presence of another's pity and that this interest can be promoted by the activity that flows from the pity of an observer. Then the patient's suffering which evokes the pity once again will increase without any special "representation" or "expectation" of any advantage to his interest. This case too, therefore, has nothing at all to do with any "counting" upon another's pity.

Still such counting often does occur. I do not know any more terrifying case of this kind than the one recently reported from Russia (in the Frankfurt newspaper). According to this report, near a large city

---

[4] Of course there is no consideration whatsoever given here to the party's political views, according to which the main body of all German workers would certainly reject this "conception." Rather it is a matter of the feelingful "conception" which can fully contradict the party-views. [Original note]

there was a home for the maimed. Children from the poorest classes were adopted by the home's operator, they were deliberately maimed, for example, blinded, in order then to transfer them to the Russian beggar-army for a certain remuneration and for evoking on their behalf "charitable gifts." This case, of course, manifests a criminal and willful exploitation of pity, a production of pain and malady for the goal of reaping the profits from the pity induced by them.

The same kind of processes can, without any trace of moral guilt and in full independence from will and "counting," occur through one of the possible forms of the automatic efficacy of pity itself. In morally legitimate compassion, authentic sharing, if it is true, is so "beneficient" that "sorrow shared is sorrow halved." This happens only insofar as, first, there is no transference or contagion of feeling in the pitying and thus also none of that "multiplication of suffering" which Friedrich Nietzsche quite wrongly attributed even to authentic pity.[5] Further, this happens only insofar as the intention of the one receiving pity is directed solely and exclusively toward the act of psychic participation itself, but not, whether consciously or in the form of that antecedent efficacy of the mere "prospect," toward the profits which can accrue to him due, to the other's experience of pity. If the latter is the case, then the suffering which evokes another's pity also becomes automatically an "interest" of the one afflicted. But then his suffering must in the long run increase, in spite of the relief he thereby obtains from his particular maladies. For, then, his threshold of suffering (under the same sensations and external conditions) is increasingly lowered, and finally a yearning for suffering is born, with the result that the conditions for suffering are directly sought and his caution in the face of danger correspondingly purely automatically diminishes.

If now – to be sure, contrary to its true meaning – the legislation and its provisions are comprehended and experienced by those affected as a put-down, as a concretion of social pity, then all these psychological laws we have discussed immediately enter into the picture of this large-scale social psychological phenomenon. This is so because the lawfully established and therefore strictly regulated profits combine with that quantum of society's pity towards the insured

which the provisions represent. Then the insurance law functions sociopsychologically, with the fullness of its machinery, bureaucracy, and so on, simply as an ensemble of pity-filled acts of attention directed toward the insured and toward those work-processes in which certain health dangers or accident risks are present. The law's action then is no different than the case where a child hurts himself and an observer, filled with pity, takes notice of the child. Because of the form of the law and the associated stability of it influence, the repeated pattern of the "swing" of suffering "out beyond" its original cause must finally produce in those affected all of the above mentioned symptoms of individual hysteria.

C. Spread of Suffering

We should also give thought to a second sociopsychological impulse which increases, although only quantitatively, the phenomena in question. We are thinking of the mutual psychic contagiousness of suffering which arises not only as a response to factual suffering and pathological disorders (when these are perceived by another) but also as a consequence of the pathological psychic attitude which, as we have seen, leads to an "imagined" organic sickness. These "attitudes" possess an uncommonly strong, psychic contagiousness.

This contagion is so much the stronger the more all those in any way prone to it tend, in Charcot's words, to "look out" for themselves; in their case, the psychic process of contagion increases in a geometric progression, since every growth, arising through contagion, in that attitude immediately reinforces again its starting point. This kind of susceptibility to contagion is increased among those affected by the law, to the degree that a person's individual consciousness gives way altogether to the class consciousness of his particular stratum and to the degree that the feeling of a communal fate more and more suppresses the feeling of having one's own distinct fate. In these matters, the process of contagious suffering essentially begins, on the one hand, with the lowest strata, and, on the other hand, with the groups most hereditarily disposed for compensation hysteria. This process then essentially moves, on the one hand, in the direction of higher quality labor and, on the other hand, to hereditarily less disposed groups; and thus, while the process diminishes in these latter strata, it comes to include ever more healthy elements.

My analysis cannot ascertain just how large is the factor of hereditary constitution. Nevertheless, I know

---

[5] See for this the author's book, *The Nature of Sympathy*, 1973, pp. 14–18. [Original note]

that there are those who have already spoken of a "national disease created by a law." They hold that both the economic profits which the law brings to the labor class and the consequences of these profits upon the health and welfare of that class count for less than the demands of public health which are encroached upon by the law. It seems clear to me that these people significantly underestimate the size of constitutional factors which are the preconditions for those previously described pathogenic processes. If the size of these factors were not considerable, then, considering the enduring presence of law, compensation hysteria should have assumed completely different proportions than those which the statistics and the statements of nonpartisan medical observations reveal.

If this is the case, then, from the viewpoint of racial hygiene, the fact that an increase of pathological phenomena has arisen due to the law gives even less cause for fear. This is so since the number of the individuals hereditarily disposed to that psychic illness definitely does not increase. Instead it is decreased since the law activates these hereditary dispositions and thereby negatively affects the existence of these individuals and their potential for propagation. We should therefore consider whether, without the law, these same pathological dispositions would not just have found simply another form of expression, and whether the individual pathological phenomena would not also have appeared, although distributed in other systems of pathological patterns. If this is so, then we may not say that a law has produced a "sickness" but only that a law has produced a new pathological pattern of sickness.

D. Social Justice

Finally, working from what has been said, I would like to draw a social ethical consequence which elsewhere I have more precisely justified:[6] the consequence that the deepest and morally most valuable acts and motives of the human being, namely love and authentic sympathy, ought to be removed from the social sphere and sphere of social evil and moved into the sphere of the individual personal relation of man to man. In their stead, the idea of social justice and that of energy-saving in human work should take ever greater possession of that social sphere. This consequence requires the ruling strata to learn to sufficiently respect the worker in order not to shame him through an ostentatious pity and its resultant "beneficence." Rather the worker must look upon the particular statute as the sort of thing to which in accord with social justice, he has a right. He must always energetically reject everything that might be to him "humanitarianism," "pity," "love" as a member of a class instead of as an individual.

In response to the victory of the humanitarian idea prophesied Herder's Ideas, Goethe, as is well known, wrote that he feared that according to this ideal "everyone" would thereby become "the humane hospital nurse of the others."[7] In a certain sense, this state of affairs arrived since the state as well as the taxes of each one of us jointly bear the burdens of social security against illness, accidents, and so on. The situation can be attributed as much to the mere application of the idea justice to our civilization's forms of labor and business as to that deeper principle of solidarity which was so unintelligible to Goethe's individualistic moral spirit.

But, on two points, Goethe already had rightly sensed the great dangers which subsequent history has brought to maturity (of these, very small and incidental dangers is that group of phenomena discussed here by us). First, the motive of "humanitarianism" – that great mock attitude that has replaced the fundamentally different idea of Christian love[8] – carries within itself the danger of causing the very evil which this attitude one-sidedly fixates or including, in the social sphere, the disorder at which it stares as hypnotized – and to which it might bring relief. Secondly, the extent of the close attention which a people directs to disorder and harm has an upper limit, after which it ceases to be helpful in bringing relief from that disorder. Indeed, it tends to create new disorders. Furthermore, it blinds the nation and humanity to the amount of value and happiness which prescinding from all other sources of happiness – springs forth from a no less noble solidarity in joy and from mutual shared feelings the positive goods of the world.

We gladly want "everyone to be the hospital nurse of the other" – in not "only" this, as Goethe feared. Rather we wish that everyone might also be the one

---

6 Scheler, M. (1973). *The Nature of Sympathy*. Hamden, CT: Shoe String Press.

7 Scheler, M. (1972). *Ressentiment*. New York: Schocken: 121–2. [**Original note**]

8 Scheler, M. (1972). *Ressentiment*. New York: Schocken: ch. 4.

who awakens joy in the other simply through the witness offered to him of his own joy.

Gebsattel, V. von (1963), 'The meaning of medical practice'

From (1995) *Theoretical Medicine* **16**: 41–72. Translated by J. V. M. Welie. Originally appeared in 1963 as *Vom Sinn des ärtzlichen Handelns*. It was reprinted in Gebsattel, V. E. von (1964). *Imago Hominis: Beiträge zu einer personalen Anthropologie*. Schweinfurt: Neues Forum: 58–74.

Editors' commentary

How does a physician approach a patient? Von Gebsattel suggests that he starts with an understanding of how the patient relates to 'his painful condition'. The 'what' of the disease are not diseases, but only diseased human beings. The author argues that a scientific perspective dangerously ignores existential aspects, which are the essence of the disease, at least in the eyes of the patient. He applauds science when its findings provide a 'measuring rod' of the state of the patient's affliction, but not when it is seen as the measuring rod of what it means to be human.

Von Gebsattel then lays out three meaningful stages, in the encounter between physician and patient, as being the base of medical practice. An elementary sympathetic call for help, an alienated stage of true medical thinking, and a personal pastoral stage of spiritual medical partnership. In other words, the encounter between doctor and patient is an encounter with man's deepest existential foundation. For von Gebsattel this is understood through a Christian theological lens and is an example of how religious beliefs influence clinical work. For many readers such reliance on religious preferences for clinical practice will seem unusual.

At the beginning there is the question of the physician to the other person: "Why are you here?" and: "What is wrong with you?" All categories of Aristotelian logic are contained in this most fundamental question. How? Where? When? Whence? Why are you suffering? Hence, it is with questions that the attack on the disease starts. Is the physician pursuing the disease itself, or are his investigations directed towards his opposite, the living fellow-human in pain?

The physician usually does not consider this question – disease and fellow-human are the same in his eyes; now and then he does not even notice that he cannot see the wood for the trees, the living human being for the symptoms. Initially, for the physician the disease is nothing but an aspect of the other being, that is, a segment of the whole and living human being. And if he does not want to be anything more than just a manager of diseases, the physician will not look beyond this segment. But surely the depicted presentation of the question essentially does not differ from the one posed by a veterinarian or a tree surgeon in the encounter with his charges. The only difference lies in the answer, since the veterinarian will not receive an answer *expressis verbis* and only has signs and signals as his guide. Yet the muteness of animals and plants is certainly not merely a disadvantage for the diagnostician. For all too often it is necessary in the encounter with patients to first get rid of a host of absurd imaginations, confused thought processes, and unreliable statements – conscious or subconscious – by the patient about his own condition! But despite all prejudices which the patient entertains while facing himself, the very fact that he does face himself reveals the uniquely human factor in being ill. Blindly is the animal caught in his disease, submerged up to its ears, so to say, in the disease, maybe twisting in the snares of its pains, but unable to go beyond its body which, like the pain, forms an unsurpassable limit. The human being, however, can take distance from his painful condition, and actually does take distance incessantly, at least tentatively. In the relationship to himself he also relates to the disease, confronts it, takes it tragically or easily, surrenders or defends, impatiently or resignedly; briefly, the relationship of a human to himself (*Selbstbezug*) which is always a mediated (*vermittelt*) relationship, accompanies him into his disease, takes from the disease its pure immediateness and goes through the disease back to the individual. Thus, disease turns from a mere incident into *his* affair, to something that he *has*, something that he *handles*.

Since the "What" of the disease is inextricably united with the reactive self-relationship of the patient, that is, since this relationship of the patient to the disease is what forms the entirety of his disease, the interest in the area of the basic concepts underlying medicine has been focused on the issue of the diseased human being as such. "Real in the true sense of the word are not the diseases, but only the diseased human being." This phrase stems from von Weizsäcker, if I am not mistaken. In any case, it can be considered the motto of what is now called general medicine or medical anthropology. In this perspective, disease is understood as one way of being human. Under the flag of "the diseased human being" nowadays sails the reflection of the metabiological and metapsychological, that is, the ethical and religious foundations of medicine.

It should be realized that after the period of romantic medicine in the first half of the nineteenth century – for example, Schelling, Schubert, Ringseits, Ritter, Justinus Keiner – a period which was relatively fruitless for medical practice, medicine, while binding itself closely to the natural sciences, loosened its connection with theology and philosophy. Medicine thereby lost the anthropological theme, which had been its primary theme once before, that is, at the end of the eighteenth and the beginning of the nineteenth century. Meanwhile, this loss of a fundamental notion that surpassed the various sciences, and its cataclysmic consequences remained hidden for a long time: too impressive were the marvelous successes of the biomedical sciences, such as bacteriology, serology, hygiene, pathological anatomy and physiology, as well as the successes of medicine itself, particularly surgery, but also clinical medicine in all its specialties. And even though the increasing somatization and technicalization of medicine threatened to confuse the average practitioner more and more, the effects of this confusion were neutralized for a long time by the representative and creative physicians of the scientific era. Their elevated humanity had made them immune from the deterioration of the medical ethos. It was only during what the sociologist usually calls the "abnormalization of society" that the disarray in the nature of medicine was revealed.

What took place was a very rare exposition: in a world in which the most unusual and most terrible events had happened and in which abnormality had forfeited its psychiatric and psychopathologic qualification, the shift in the attitude of physicians became visible to everybody in particular examples, a shift that was prepared over a long period of time, yet became symptomatic only in specific extreme incidents – I am thinking of "euthanasia" and "involuntary experiments with human subjects." It was von Weizsäcker who said that in Nuremberg the spirit of scientific medicine was brought to trial. What he meant to say is that those responsible for these outrageous deeds and misdeeds were certainly not sick people considerably off-track, nor abnormal individuals, but very much everyday people. Hence, it does not suffice to explain such events by pointing the finger at those responsible on a State or Party level. Rather, these events revealed,

very much like a sociological experiment, that the average representative of scientific-positivistic medicine had no defensive power against the dictatorial invasion of forces foreign to medicine that arrogantly tried to determine the medical practice from the outside.

As mentioned, this was not the result of a pathology of those physicians who were in the power of an equally abnormalized collectivity; the collectivity could exercise those powers only because in the territory of medicine itself the axioms were lost which should have guided medical practice normatively. "What healthy and what sick means in general, is a question about which a physician is the last to rack his brains," Jaspers has once remarked. The newness of the contemporary situation consists in physicians having started to ponder such issues – something that has not happened for a long time. The first medical anthropology was, as far as I know, developed after the World War in Vienna by Oswald Schwarz, a urologist, psychoanalyst, and philosopher in one person, who analyzed the importance of the act as the human "vital category" (Vitalkategorie) in the area of medicine. It was always philosophically-oriented physicians who were stirred in an anthropological direction, such as Binswanger, von Weizsäcker, Kütemeyer, Matusse; or sometimes theologians, if they had as sound a scientific knowledge as did George Siegmund.

In closing itself off from philosophy and theology, science is as unable to conceive of a concept of disease as of a concept of health. This conclusion is verified over and over again in discussions with extremely positivistically-oriented physicians. They claim competence in the evaluation of health and disease, but if one urges one of them to provide more precise definitions and conceptions of value, then he escapes into the plentitude of disorders which he encounters everyday, and it is shown that his general concept of health and disease does not differ from that of the layman. In this context I have to remind the reader of Max Scheler's "natural perspective on the world" (natürliche Weltanschauung). This means that in everyday life the scientist or scholar lives in a prephilosophical world; in a world in which the sun comes up and goes down, which is filled with qualities whose presence he disputes as a scientist, yet that determine his everyday behavior, and which he cannot evade. Similarly, the concepts that regard the value of health and disease are part of the natural perspective on the world: health is simply desirable, disease undesirable, and in everyday life this view is entertained by the physician as well.

Yet, these original conceptions of the value of health and disease change when they become part of the perspective which the expert holds about the world and the human being; for conceptions of value do not exist in the scientist's perspective of the world. Actually, a diseased human being does not exist in the eyes of the scientist, or if he does, only as the object of medicine and its auxiliary sciences. Undoubtedly, the subdiscipline of medicine perceives the subsections, which it has set apart from the whole of the real human being in accordance with its methodology, sharply and clearly, particularly in their pathological appearance. But the disease is not identical with the pathological. What the scientist is not at all interested in are the existential aspects of a human's diseased state, where these aspects actually are the essence of the disease in the eyes of the patient. For the pathological is only of interest to the patient on a second plane. The scientific objectification of the patient contrasts sharply with the latter's very existential way of being, that is, his being a subject, an individual, a man or a woman, a person, the totality of all those aspects; science objectifies something that in fact cannot be objectified. Yet science objectifies the human being, turns him into its object, which science can do only by abstracting from the living reality altogether. The real, true human being, whether healthy or diseased, is necessarily beyond the scope of science. Rational, methodological analysis of its object requires science to be reductive, even if its object is the person. What is more, science cannot be blamed for this procedure, since it is a prerequisite for all scientific knowledge and thus a *conditio sine qua non* of scientific successes and triumphs. As long as its findings are merely the measuring rod of what has afflicted the human being or his organs, this reductive and abstractive approach is not problematic; but it is when these findings become the measuring rod of what it essentially means to be a human being there are problems. In the area of medicine, the scientific attitude threatens to turn the living fellow-person with all his needs, into the mere object of a technological contact and the irreplaceable unique person into a regular "case."

It cannot be maintained, as has often happened, that it was the introduction of psychotherapy into medicine, particularly psychoanalysis and individual psychology *(Individualpsychologie)*, which radically changed the situation. The introduction of psychology certainly was not equally significant as the postulated introduction of the subject or, even more, the person into medicine. On the contrary, Freud's and Jung's ambitions went so far as to also investigate the human soul by means of a scientific method. They talked about the *mechanisms* of depth psychology, about psychic *apparatus and functions*, about affective and impulsive *dynamics*, complex and libido *energies*, and they talked proudly about energetic processes such as the alpha and omega of the psychic reality. Not the encounter with the diseased human being, but the analysis of the diseased mind was the theme. The mind was turned into the object of therapy just like any other corporeal organ of the human being. That it concerned the mind did not change the basic scientific attitude in the least. After all, the mind was, to be precise, but an organ that was overlooked by traditional medicine, just one organ among many, and the analysis of its functions was the continuously debated subject of research. When in traditional medicine corporeal organs were considered the seat of diseases, now also the human mind was available for the localization of other diseases. The newness of the contents, the emphasis on the subconscious, the analysis of impulses, instincts, affects, the talk about psychic entities, all that seemed to be fully consistent with a scientific position.

But despite the efforts psychotherapy undertook in this initial phase to adopt the scientific attitude, to bring its object under this perspective, this venture did not appear to work out very well. For essentially the human being cannot be divided, and the radical division in material apparatus on the one hand, which the so-called organic medicine had to take care of, and on the other hand, the psychic mechanisms of the neurosis were carried on by the psychotherapeutic clinic *ad absurdum*. Long before the name itself was developed, psychosomatic medicine had taken a hold. Concepts surfaced such as "psychogenic causation of organic diseases" (the so-called organic neuroses); in addition to conflict neuroses, the hysteric conversions of psychological ideas in the language of the body were recognized – in the so-called "organ dialectic" *(Organdialektik)*; briefly, the functional connection between the various layers of the personality became more and more evident, and the slogan "mind–body unity" emerged. At the same time it became clear that individuals are able to escape the mental and psychological problems of life by fleeing into seemingly organic diseases, and this forced medical thinking to complement the purely causal approach to processes with a final approach, already pointed towards the meaning of disease in the context of life itself. In addition to the question concerning the cause, the question concerning the purpose was acknowledged, which was the question about the meaning, even if only in a provisional form.

Furthermore, the scope of medical thinking was considerably expanded when internists and neurologists of the standing of Bergmann, von Weizsäcker, Siebeck, and others made it their business to introduce the experiences of psychotherapy (in the narrow sense of the word) into the internal medicine clinic in the form of "biographical medicine." The technique of anamnesis, traditionally the principal instrument for arriving at a diagnosis in the area of psychiatry, upon transformation in the conversation-hour of depth psychology, became the biographical method of the internal medicine clinic. The patient's biographical perspective on his own existence had thus become the very focus of history taking. For man essentially exists in history, and in the sometimes cowardly, sometimes addicted, sometimes obstinate, but always egocentric opposition against the developmental law of personal being, the therapist nowadays recognizes pathologic disorders of a totally new type. In comparison with such centrally and existentially threatening disorders of the personality – I call them "existential neuroses" – biographical and psychosomatic medicine has to deal with disorders that regard the marginal zone of life; examples being: biliary colics that occur in connection with professional degradations; an angina attack which appears recurrently in connection with erotic crises; a tuberculosis which breaks out at dramatic turning points in life; a Basedow [Graves' disease], such as I observed myself, following thirty hours of deathly fear after a fall in a glacier trench.

But what exactly was so clearly revolutionary about the infusion of psychotherapy in the medical thinking of those days? Certainly not, at any rate not primarily, the mere introduction of the psychic reality in medicine or in some other newly discovered psychopathological science, for example of the unconscious, or the affect dreams of pregenital sexuality, or of the archetypical world. Neither was it the piecing together of these new discoveries into a depth psychology system such as the theory of the individuation

process, not putting it into a new technique for dealing with mental patients. Rather, its revolutionary character was due to the new direction that was taken that the very creators of depth psychology had not even acknowledged as such, and to the fact that medical thinking was moving on the new road of psychotherapy towards a goal that was effective without even being recognized. This goal was the human being.

But how could this most familiar, most self-evident being that was known to everybody, how could the human being become a new goal of a discipline which never had to care about anything but man's weal and woe, how could it become the new meaning of medical practice? Obviously, there was no lack of formulas in which the recognition was expressed of this newness that was being approached. The new aspects of the crucial questions of life usually are as old as the hills. Man forfeits his knowledge in a thousand dubious ways, only to find it back again, totally surprised, as if such knowledge was never known and experienced. Nature is denied and with that man too has become a ghost. The spiritual is denied, and man ends up in nothingness and emptiness. The transcendental is denied, God is renounced, Christ is declared a mere genius, or otherwise a delusional patient, and the effect of all this is the distorted image of man, a caricature.

In the past decades of psychotherapeutic research ample formulas emerged intended to capture the newness. There was the slogan of the "whole human being," intended to mold a whole out of the body of scientific information about the human being. The theory of the mind–body unity emerged, undoubtedly a useful theory, but only a partial redress. Consequently, the theory of the whole human being was placed under the personality theories and the physician turned from a "doctor of the body" into a "doctor of the personality" (Speer); yet we know – one is reminded of the anthropological studies of Guardini and Ernst Michel – that the "personality" is only one aspect of the whole and integral human being and not the pinnacle of a philosophical or religious anthropology. The Swedish neurologist and sculptor Paul Bjerre, while comprehending the synthetically formative forces of creative life, placed the synthetic dream analysis in the center of his therapy; but the very point of convergence in which the digressing tendencies of human nature should be synthesized, in the end were left more or less to the blind aspirations of the liberated human nature. In Vienna, Viktor Frankl was the first to place the mind–body unity under the spiritual; psychotherapy became logotherapy. The will, the awareness of responsibility, and the decision, in his eyes – and correctly so – had again the task of integrating the human into the higher unity of freedom and truth, guided in its existence by the spiritual.

The fact that man in his pure egocentricity is a mere torso, that the self-realization of man requires the integration of the individual in the "us," that is, in a higher community, requires that the commitment of man to others is constitutive for personal life – this insight, in surpassing the so-called individual psychology of Adler, Künkel, and Kühnel, was finally infused into medical psychotherapy by Ernst Michel, the Catholic psychotherapist, and Martin Buber, the Jewish mystic.

The Christianization of medical anthropology had been prepared along the detour of a deepened theory of neuroses, slowly, and came as a total surprise. It clearly had become necessary to approach newly emerging therapeutic tasks with new conceptions of the human being, including the diseased human being, conceptions that differed considerably from those espoused in internal medicine, neurology, and psychiatry. What is highly astonishing, is that it became clear that these conceptions were nothing but the secularized basic principles of the old Christian personal theory of man and his destination. In one of those surprising turns of which the history of ideas is full, it became clear that even though there is a difference in the way questions are phrased when analyzing human existence from a metabiological and metapsychological perspective on the one hand, and a theological perspective on the other hand, there is no longer an incongruity. Both theories stand against one another in a relationship of mutual clarification and supplementation.

The Meaningful Stages of Medical Practice

At the base of medical practice, the soil on which it matures, is the encounter between physician and patient and the relationship which unfolds in this encounter. The meaningful stages of medical practice, therefore, are elaborations of a special situation with its particular meaning that appears in the threefold modulation of the relationship between doctor and patient. The three meaningful stages stand against one another in a dialectic relationship and are not deduced from the concept of disease, but in reference to the diseased human being. They are the following:

1. The elementary-sympathetic stage of being called by the need of an encountered human being: this is the immediate stage in the relationship.
2. The stage of true medical thinking, planning, acting, the diagnostic-therapeutic stage: this is the alienation stage in the relationship.
3. A stage which encompasses the former two modes of encounter, the stage of partnership between physician and patient: this is the personal stage of the relationship.

At each of these stages the physician and patient relate to one another differently; at each stage the physician is solicited differently. First as a fellow human being, called upon by the need of a fellow human being and thereby becoming a participant in that need; next as the technical executor of this call in the sense of combatant of need: the physician in the everyday use of the word; and finally as the personal partner of the patient, as "Thou" of a "Thou," in light of the solidarity of mankind in its relationship to the transcendental that encompasses guilt, suffering, death, and love. "Mastership" in the higher and true sense of the word develops when these three meaningful stages of medical practice are combined into a rank ordered comprehensive act.

The beginning, or original stage, is the sympathetic call stemming from the need of another being. In the acceptance of this call, acknowledging the need of a stranger, and through the elementary participation in this need, one becomes the fellow of the other (like the patient, inversely, turns from a stranger, the mere other, into a fellow as well). Strictly speaking, in this original state one is not really standing as a physician yet. It is only, upon being called by this need, when one feels instigated to help, that the undetermined, sympathetic solidarity takes the configuration of a physician. In and by itself the need has the character of a call, regardless of whether that call is audible or whether the need in painful muteness only cries out to the heavens. Even as a smothered call, the need searches for the listener, because the patient is smothered when he is caught in his own suffering; yet the patient recovers a breath through the sympathy of the other.

However, perceiving a stranger's need, the readiness to lend a favorable ear and a compassionate heart is not yet really a response to the call stemming from the need. The appealing presence of the need implies that it looks for a response, and this response is a named "help." The need of the fellow-human drives the one who does not suffer out of the pure *pathetic* communication between the one who suffers and the one who does not, into the *active* fight against the need, that is, into help. By its very nature, help is a responsive act. To be constituted as such, the possibility to master need must exist. Only the person who can swim can vigorously and effectively respond to the cry for help of a drowning person. The need of the human being that has the shape of disease has the character of a call as well. Without the call of such need, whether it stems from a pain, the threat of death, troubles or insufficiency, or, on a moral level, from the intrusion of nothingness into one's existence, nobody would ever seriously hit upon the idea that he is destined to consider as his life-work the observation of a physician's responsibilities. In the existential sense of the word, disease always is not-being-able-to-be somehow coming to power. And the call of this needful way of not-being-able-to-be provides the foundation of the medical profession. The physician has to call the patient back into uncurtailed being. Thus, at the elementary stage of the comprehensive medical act, an immediate needful encounter between doctor and patient takes place, which institutes an original, immediate vital unity between the two.

This bond and willingness, however, is again being lost in the medical management of the need at the second stage of the encounter between physician and patient, which I therefore named the "alienation stage." At first, this explanation will give rise to amazement, for in the art of diagnosis and therapy, the performance of the physician and his service to the patient is generally considered as being culminated. However, what this means shall be unfolded using the analogical example of pain.

If the need of the patient consists of physical or psychological pain, it is immediately evident that the physician's sympathetic rapport to the sufferer cannot undo the fact that the pain-free witness of the pain-stricken patient is separated in his existence from the existence of the other by an abyss which is called painlessness. Having suffered himself, he may be able to gain a more meaningful and realistic understanding of the pain of the stranger, but thereby the pain of the stranger will never become his own; sorrow for the suffering of the other does not become suffering with the other, if we leave aside the borderline case of an emotional affection which is pathological itself and ultimately deceitful. The fact irrefutably remains, that the pain-free person is assigned another place than the person overwhelmed by pain. The pain isolates the sufferer fully by chaining him to his situation, but likewise the pain separates the helper from the helpless.

Since the existential separation of the helper and helpless, which has now suddenly appeared, cannot be abrogated at the level of the pain or any other distress, as a thorn this separation urges the helper to remove the pain of the stranger. Thus, the pain appears to be a leap into the wellbeing of the sufferer as well as a leap into humane solidarity; and likewise, the call stemming from the need caused by disease urges one to fight the latter. This fight has the shape of a scientific and technically skilled act of help. The disease, instead of the diseased, becomes the enemy; and the act of help becomes a duel with the disease, like it is a duel for the patient; a duel with himself. The condition of the other person, the cause of his suffering, and the possibilities of removing them, all must be clarified in a process of objectification. In doing so, it can easily happen that the patient is no longer viewed as a person and has become the mere object of a technological contact.

Consequently, at this second stage of medical practice, though it represents the actual area of implementing medical rationality and the realm of its highest triumphs, the ethos of the physician is endangered. For the need which is calling for subjection is not a scientific construct, even if science understands all of its biological preconditions entirely; rather, it concerns a human being, and the fight against the need of the patient should be a service to him. However, when we look at the issue carefully, then in the sphere of diagnostic-therapeutical contact, the patient is actually not subjected as an individual to diagnostic-therapeutical procedures; he is only a case adapting to the general regularity and conformity laws, which make knowledge and technology possible in the scientific sense of the word. Careful as we may individualize and look for laws that apply in this case only, there remains the fact that physician and patient relate to one another as subject and object at the stage of separation. For it is not at this level that the higher meaningful unity can be found which is appropriate in overcoming the alienation stage. Thus, it can easily happen that this service to man, because at this stage there is no concern for man in his personal worth, is interpreted in an inhumane manner, as service to the state, the population, or the race; in which situation, the physician, being degraded to a functionary of society, is tempted to sacrifice the individual to the health of the population, the purity of the race, or the utility of the state.

Hence, the second stage of the act of help, in so far as it considers diagnosis and therapy the only important issues, prompts for a stronger grounding of medical practice. After all, it is not merely two individuals that are related to one another as physician and patient, but two persons, related at the level of personal existence, a style of communication is required other than the sympathetic rapport of the elementary stage, but also more than the mere diagnostic-therapeutic impact on the patient, skillful and exact as it may be. It is only in a practice which involves the person of the fellow man that the spiritual-pastoral and similarly the spiritual-medical comprehensive acts take place.

That man can be suffering terribly, despite unlimited disposition of his somatic and vital functions, that is, despite full physical health, from an agony which Kierkegaard (with staggering, nowadays still not fully understood, emphasis described as "Sickness unto Death") has opened our eyes to the third dimension of medical practice. Now the duel of the physician with the need of his fellow man enters a profundity formerly unknown to medicine, into the heart of personal existence – it enters its own meta-biological center. The notion then arose that it is God's call which called the person into existence.

The word of the Bible came alive: "I have called you by your name, you are mine." And it was furthermore recognized that it is up to man to anchor his life in this deepest existential foundation or to renounce it. Thus, a new form of need appeared; the need of an existential raggedness which divides the personality into a will to determine its final destination and an equally vehement counter-will.

The kind of need that characterizes the "existential neurosis" advances deeper into the interior of man than others and should be understood as the effect of a secret nihilism of personality. Since the appearance in the burning bush, the first time in history that the essence of the person has revealed itself in the expression: "I am that I am," there is for man, the image of God, a two-fold possibility: Either to realize the challenge of personal existence or to renounce this challenge and to maintain about oneself, "I do not want to be that I am." Of course such statements are usually not explicitly expressed. They exercise their power in the dark background of man: Their purpose is to dethrone God in man's own soul: Given man's actual stand, this dethronement is realized via the enthronement of one's own person. Thus, thoroughly hidden behind superficial disorders in man's psychological economy, deep lacerations are brought about in the dark will of the personality. This causes severe hindrance for the self-realization in love, community, and creative life-formation – the integrative process of the personality – that is, its completion. The nihilism of the central counter-will, which is hidden, yet present in every act of life, breaks through in the form of a multi-dimensional obstruction of man's development. That man heads towards nothingness, even desires it like an addict, and recklessly succumbs to it, is symptomatic of man's personality drifting away from its own center. Personal existence can prosper only in a Thou-relationship to the transcendental in its personal reality.

This is the only genuine, original psychological disease because the so-called psychological diseases are known to be primarily disorders with a somatic origin (Somatosen). The existential neurosis has revealed the third stage, which actually provides the very foundation of medical practice. We called it the stage of partnership, and this designation indicates that at this stage the physician is called to engage as a person in the communication with another person. Once this stage has been reached, it becomes clear that the technically oriented effort of the helper, to a large degree, is subordinated to the guidance of the existential effort. This is the only possible order that coincides with the very idea and essence of comprehensive medical practice. The effort required by neurosis must continue to determine in the background the essence of the doctor–patient relationship always and everywhere.

The neurosis illustrates the meaning of what has been said. For when the existential need of his partner calls for the responsibilities of the physician, the latter cannot abstain from first examining his own existential position. Unwillingly, the other in his need calls the physician into the same need. In this solidarity of need, which stems from the eternal dissatisfaction with our personal reference to the transcendental, the sufferer changes from being the object of skillful management to the personal partner of the physician, and then to a longing Thou who stands in the same reference to the transcendental as the I of the physician. The alliance between the helper and the helpless turns into the partnership between persons who are equal in regard to being, that is, in their attempts to find domicile in it. There thus emerges a community of partners between irreplaceable persons.

Although partnership is the genuine relationship between physician and patient, it cannot be initiated and achieved as diagnosis and therapy. The source of personal being is itself not the object of action. This source cannot be supplied by a moral institution or a new kind of therapy, such as the impetuous type of psychotherapist tired of psychoanalysis would favor. But Christianity can; for it is a reality beyond the applicability of practical-ethical norms, not an aggregate of moral guidelines and imperatives. Personal existence, from the perspective of man, is a venture of faith, and from the perspective of God, an act of love. This applies as well to the partnership between physician and patient. Whoever tries to establish it arbitrarily and violently is in danger of violating the law of freedom in the other, thereby calling into question the very partnership which he is trying to establish.

Merleau-Ponty, M. (1945), 'Cézanne's doubt'

From (1964) *Sense and Non-sense*. Translated by H. Dreyfus and P. A. Dreyfus. Evanston, IL: Northwestern University Press: 9–24. Originally published in book form as (1948) *Sens et non-sens*. Paris: Gallimard.

Editors' commentary

'Cézanne's doubt' was first published in 1945. In it Merleau-Ponty describes how Cézanne (and some of his friends and critics) had doubts about his talents. Merleau-Ponty suggests that the artist could well be described as schizoid in terms of his human relations and way of being in the world, but his art, although emerging from his character (he said that a face should be painted as an object), did not derive its meaning from it. Cézanne, he thinks, discovered what we perceive – the lived perspective – by recapturing and converting into visible objects what would remain walled up in the separate life of each consciousness. He felt that personality is seen in a glance. Therefore, Cézanne's doubt was not explained by his nervous

temperament, but by the purpose of his work: work that left him pondering 'for hours at a time before putting down a certain stroke'; Merleau-Ponty states that 'the work to be done called for this life'.

Here, the author says, we are beyond cause and effect in a realm of trying to understand the origins of creative freedom: 'A freedom which dawns in us without breaking our bonds with the world.' The latter part of the paper describes the bonds taken to have existed in Leonardo da Vinci's life. Following Freud's account he sees the artist as learning his detached powers of examination, solitude and curiosity, in 'assimilating the situation which his birth and childhood had made for him'. Merleau-Ponty finds himself in sympathy with psychoanalysis. He says that rather than giving us necessary relations of cause and effect, this approach has taught us to notice echoes, allusions, and repetitions from one moment to the next. He argues that it points to motivational relationships, and 'teaches us to think of freedom concretely, as a creative repetition of ourselves, always in retrospect, faithful to ourselves'.

He needed one hundred working sessions for a still life, five hundred sittings for a portrait. What we call his work was, for him, only an essay, an approach to painting. In September, 1906, at the age of 67 – one month before his death – he wrote: "I was in such a state of mental agitation, in such great confusion that for a time I feared my weak reason would not survive . . . Now it seems I am better and that I see more clearly the direction my studies are taking. Will I ever arrive at the goal, so intensely sought and so long pursued? I am still learning from nature, and it seems to me I am making slow progress." Painting was his world and his way of life. He worked alone, without students, without admiration from his family, without encouragement from the critics. He painted on the afternoon of the day his mother died. In 1870 he was painting at l'Estaque while the police were after him for dodging the draft. And still he had moments of doubt about this vocation. As he grew old, he wondered whether the novelty of his painting might not come from trouble with his eyes, whether his whole life had not been based upon an accident of his body. The uncertainty or stupidity of his contemporaries correspond to this effort and this doubt. "The painting of a drunken privy cleaner," said a critic in 1905. Even today, C. Mauclair finds Cézanne's admissions of powerlessness an argument against him.

Meanwhile, Cézanne's paintings have spread throughout the world. Why so much uncertainty, so much labor, so many failures, and, suddenly, the greatest success?

Zola, Cézanne's friend from childhood, was the first to find genius in him and the first to speak of him as a "genius gone wrong." An observer of Cézanne's life such as Zola, more concerned with his character than with the meaning of his painting, might well consider it a manifestation of ill-health.

For as far back as 1852, upon entering the Collège Bourbon at Aix, Cézanne worried his friends with his fits of temper and depression. Seven years later, having decided to become an artist, he doubted his talent and did not dare to ask his father – a hatter and later a banker – to send him to Paris. Zola's letters reproach him for his instability, his weakness, and his indecision. When finally he came to Paris, he wrote: "The only thing I have changed is my location: my ennui has followed me." He could not tolerate discussions, because they wore him out and because he could never give arguments. His nature was basically anxious. Thinking that he would die young, he made his will at the age of 42; at 46 he was for six months the victim of a violent, tormented, overwhelming passion of which no one knows the outcome and to which he would never refer. At 51 he withdrew to Aix, where he found landscape best suited to his genius but where also he returned to the world of his childhood, his mother and his sister. After the death of his mother, Cézanne turned to his son for support. "Life is terrifying," he would often say. Religion, which he then set about practicing for the first time, began for him in the fear of life and the fear of death. "It is fear," he explained to a friend; "I feel I will be on earth for another four days – what then? I believe in life after death, and I don't want to risk roasting in aeternum." Although his religion later deepened, its original motivation was the need to put his life in order and to be relieved of it. He became more and more timid, mistrustful, and sensitive: on his occasional visits to Paris he motioned his friends, when still far away, not to approach him. In 1903, after his pictures had begun to sell in Paris at twice the price of Monet's and when young men like Joachim Gasquet and Emile Bernard came to see him and ask him questions, he unbent a little. But his fits of anger continued. (In Aix a child once hit him as he passed by; after that he could not bear any contact.) One day when Cézanne was quite old, Emile Bernard supported him as he stumbled.

Cézanne flew into a rage. He could be heard striding around his studio and shouting that he wouldn't let anybody "get his hooks into me." Because of these "hooks" he pushed women who could have modeled for him out of his studio, priests, whom he called "sticky," out of his life, and Emile Bernard's theories out of his mind, when they became too insistent.

This loss of flexible human contact; this inability to master new situations; this flight into established habits, in an atmosphere which presented no problems; this rigid opposition in theory and practice of the "hook" versus the freedom of a recluse – all these symptoms permit one to speak of a morbid constitution and more precisely, as, for example, in the case of El Greco, of schizophrenia. The notion of painting "from nature" could be said to arise from the same weakness. His extremely close attention to nature and to color, the inhuman character of his paintings (he said that a face should be painted as an object), his devotion to the visible world: all of these would then only represent a flight from the human world, the alienation of his humanity.

These conjectures nevertheless do not give any idea of the positive side of his work; one cannot thereby conclude that his painting is a phenomenon of decadence and what Nietzsche called "impoverished" life or that it has nothing to say to the educated man. Zola's and Emile Bernard's belief in Cézanne's failure probably arises from their having put too much emphasis on psychology and their personal knowledge of Cézanne. It is quite possible that, on the basis of his nervous weaknesses, Cézanne conceived a form of art which is valid for everyone. Left to himself, he could look at nature as only a human being can. The meaning of his work cannot be determined from his life.

This meaning will not become any clearer in the light of art history – that is, by bringing in the influences on Cézanne's methods (the Italian school and Tintoretto, Delacroix, Courbet and the Impressionists) – or even by drawing on his own judgment of his work.

His first pictures – up to about 1870 – are painted fantasies: a rape, a murder. They are therefore almost always executed in broad strokes and present the moral physiognomy of the actions rather than their visible aspect. It is thanks to the Impressionists, and particularly to Pissarro, that Cézanne later conceived painting not as the incarnation of imagined scenes, the projection of dreams outward, but as the exact study of appearances: less a work of the studio than a working from nature. Thanks to the Impressionists, he abandoned the baroque technique, whose primary aim is to capture movement, for small dabs placed close together and for patient hatchings.

He quickly parted ways with the Impressionists, however. Impressionism tries to capture, in the painting, the very way in which objects strike our eyes and attack our senses. Objects are depicted as they appear to instantaneous perception, without fixed contours, bound together by light and air. To capture this envelope of light, one had to exclude siennas, ochres, and black and use only the seven colors of the spectrum. The color of objects could not be represented simply by putting on the canvas their local tone, that is, the color they take on isolated from their surroundings; one also had to pay attention to the phenomena of contrast which modify local colors in nature. Furthermore, by a sort of reversal, every color we perceive in nature elicits the appearance of its complement; and these complementaries heighten one another. To achieve sunlit colors in a picture which will be seen in the dim light of apartments, not only must there be a green – if you are painting grass – but also the complementary red which will make it vibrate. Finally, the Impressionists break down the local tone itself. One can generally obtain any color by juxtaposing rather than mixing the colors which make it up, thereby achieving a more vibrant hue. The result of these procedures is that the canvas – which no longer corresponds point by point to nature – affords a generally true impression through the action of the separate parts upon one another. But at the same time, depicting the atmosphere and breaking up the tones submerges the object and causes it to lose its proper weight. The composition of Cézanne's palette leads one to suppose that he had another aim. Instead of the seven colors of the spectrum, one finds eighteen colors – six reds, five yellows, three blues, three greens, and black. The use of warm colors and black shows that Cézanne wants to represent the object, to find it again behind the atmosphere. Likewise, he does not break up the tone; rather, he replaces this technique with graduated colors, a progression of chromatic nuances across the object, a modulation of colors which stays close to the object's form and to the light it receives. Doing away with exact contours in certain cases, giving color priority over the outline – these obviously mean different things for Cézanne and for the Impressionists.

The object is no longer covered by reflections and lost in its relationships to the atmosphere and to other objects: it seems subtly illuminated from within, light emanates from it, and the result is an impression of solidity and material substance. Moreover, Cézanne does not give up making the warm colors vibrate but achieves this chromatic sensation through the use of blue.

One must therefore say that Cézanne wished to return to the object without abandoning the Impressionist aesthetic which takes nature as its model. Emile Bernard reminded him that, for the classical artists, painting demanded outline, composition, and distribution of light. Cézanne replied: "They created pictures; we are attempting a piece of nature." He said of the old masters that they "replaced reality by imagination and by the abstraction which accompanies it." Of nature, he said that "the artist must conform to this perfect work of art. Everything comes to us from nature; we exist through it; nothing else is worth remembering." He stated that he wanted to make of Impressionism "something solid, like the art in the museums." His painting was paradoxical: he was pursuing reality without giving up the sensuous surface, with no other guide than the immediate impression of nature, without following the contours, with no outline to enclose the color, with no perspectival or pictorial arrangement. This is what Bernard called Cézanne's suicide: aiming for reality while denying himself the means to attain it. This is the reason for his difficulties and for the distortions one finds in his pictures between 1870 and 1890. Cups and saucers on a table seen from the side should be elliptical, but Cézanne paints the two ends of the ellipse swollen and expanded. The work table in his portrait of Gustave Geoffrey stretches, contrary to the laws of perspective, into the lower part of the picture. In giving up the outline Cézanne was abandoning himself to the chaos of sensations, which would upset the objects and constantly suggest illusions, as, for example, the illusion we have when we move our head that objects themselves are moving – if our judgment did not constantly set these appearances straight. According to Bernard, Cézanne "submerged his painting in ignorance and his mind in shadows." But one cannot really judge his painting in this way except by closing one's mind to half of what he said and one's eyes to what he painted.

It is clear from his conversations with Emile Bernard that Cézanne was always seeking to avoid the ready-made alternatives suggested to him: sensation versus judgment; the painter who sees against the painter who thinks; nature versus composition; primitivism as opposed to tradition. "We have to develop an optics," said Cézanne, "by which I mean a logical vision – that is, one with no element of the absurd." "Are you speaking of our nature?" asked Bernard. Cézanne: "It has to do with both." "But aren't nature and art different?" "I want to make them the same. Art is a personal apperception, which I embody in sensations and which I ask the understanding to organize into a painting." But even these formulas put too much emphasis on the ordinary notions of "sensitivity" or "sensations" and "understanding" – which is why Cézanne could not convince by his arguments and preferred to paint instead. Rather than apply to his work dichotomies more appropriate to those who sustain traditions than to those men, philosophers or painters, who initiate these traditions, he preferred to search for the true meaning of painting, which is continually to question tradition. Cézanne did not think he had to choose between feeling and thought, between order and chaos. He did not want to separate the stable things which we see and the shifting way in which they appear; he wanted to depict matter as it takes on form, the birth of order through spontaneous organization. He makes a basic distinction not between "the senses" and "the understanding" but rather between the spontaneous organization of the things we perceive and the human organization of ideas and sciences. We see things; we agree about them; we are anchored in them; and it is with "nature" as our base that we construct our sciences. Cézanne wanted to paint this primordial world, and his pictures therefore seem to show nature pure, while photographs of the same landscapes suggest man's works, conveniences, and imminent presence. Cézanne never wished to "paint like a savage." He wanted to put intelligence, ideas, sciences, perspective, and tradition back in touch with the world of nature which they must comprehend. He wished, as he said, to confront the sciences with the nature "from which they came."

By remaining faithful to the phenomena in his investigations of perspective, Cézanne discovered what recent psychologists have come to formulate: the lived perspective, that which we actually perceive, is not a geometric or photographic one. The objects we see close at hand appear smaller, those far away seem larger than they do in a photograph. (This can be seen in a movie, where a train approaches and gets bigger much faster than a real train would under the same circumstances.) To say that a circle seen obliquely is seen as an ellipse is to substitute for our actual perception what we would see if we were cameras: in reality we see a form which oscillates around the ellipse without being an ellipse. In a portrait of Mme Cézanne, the border of the wallpaper on one side of her body does not form a straight line with that on the other: and indeed it is known that if a line passes beneath a wide strip of paper, the two visible segments appear dislocated. Gustave Geoffrey's table stretches into the bottom of the picture, and indeed, when our eye runs over a large surface, the images it successively receives are taken from different points of view, and the whole surface is warped. It is true that I freeze these distortions in repainting them on the canvas; I stop the spontaneous movement in which they pile up in perception and in which they tend toward the geometric perspective. This is also what happens with colors. Pink upon gray paper colors the background green. Academic painting shows the background as gray, assuming that the picture will produce the same effect of contrast as the real object. Impressionist painting uses green in the background in order to achieve a contrast as brilliant as that of objects in nature. Doesn't this falsify the color relationship? It would if it stopped there, but the painter's task is to modify all the other colors in the picture so that they take away from the green background its characteristics of a real color. Similarly, it is Cézanne's genius that when the overall composition of the picture is seen globally, perspectival distortions are no longer visible in their own right but rather contribute, as they do in natural vision, to the impression of an emerging order, of an object in the act of appearing, organizing itself before our eyes. In the same way, the contour of an object conceived as a line encircling the object belongs not to the visible world but to geometry. If one outlines the shape of an apple with a continuous line, one makes an object of the shape, whereas the contour is rather the ideal limit toward which the sides of the apple recede in depth. Not to indicate any shape would be to deprive the objects of their identity. To trace just a single outline sacrifices depth – that is, the dimension in which the thing is presented not as spread out before us but as an inexhaustible reality full of reserves. That is why Cézanne follows the swelling of the object in modulated colors and indicates several outlines in blue. Rebounding among these, one's glance captures a shape that emerges from among them all, just as it does in perception. Nothing could be less arbitrary than these famous distortions which, moreover, Cézanne abandoned in his last period, after 1890, when he no longer filled his canvases with colors and when he gave up the closely-woven texture of his still lifes.

The outline should therefore be a result of the colors if the world is to be given in its true density. For the world is a mass without gaps, a system of colors across which the receding perspective, the outlines, angles, and curves are inscribed like lines of force; the spatial structure vibrates as it is formed. "The outline and the colors are no longer distinct from each other. To the extent that one paints, one outlines; the more the colors harmonize, the more the outline becomes precise . . . . When the color is at its richest, the form has reached plenitude." Cézanne does not try to use color to suggest the tactile sensations which would give shape and depth. These distinctions between touch and sight are unknown in primordial perception. It is only as a result of a science of the human body that we finally learn to distinguish between our senses. The lived object is not rediscovered or constructed on the basis of the contributions of the senses; rather, it presents itself to us from the start as the center from which these contributions radiate. We see the depth, the smoothness, the softness, the hardness of objects; Cézanne even claimed that we see their odor. If the painter is to express the world, the arrangement of his colors must carry with it this indivisible whole, or else his picture will only hint at things and will not give them in the imperious unity, the presence, the insurpassable plenitude which is for us the definition of the real. That is why each brushstroke must satisfy an infinite number of conditions. Cézanne sometimes pondered hours at a time before putting down a certain stroke, for, as Bernard said, each stroke must "contain the air, the light, the object, the composition, the character, the outline, and the style." Expressing what exists is an endless task.

Nor did Cézanne neglect the physiognomy of objects and faces: he simply wanted to capture it emerging from the color. Painting a face "as an object" is not to strip it of its "thought." "I realize that the painter interprets it," said Cézanne. "The painter is not an imbecile." But this interpretation should not be a reflection distinct from the act of seeing. "If I paint all the little blues and all the little maroons, I capture and convey his glance. Who gives a damn if they want to dispute how one can sadden a mouth or make a cheek smile by adding a shaded green to a red." One's personality is seen and grasped in one's glance, which is, however, no more than a combination of colors. Other minds are given to us only as incarnate, as belonging to faces and gestures. Countering with the distinctions of soul and body, thought and vision is of no use here, for Cézanne returns to just that primordial experience from which these notions are derived and in which they are inseparable. The painter who conceptualizes and seeks the expression first misses the mystery – renewed every time we look at someone – of a person's appearing in nature. In *La Peau de chagrin* Balzac describes a "tablecloth white as a layer of newly fallen snow, upon which the place-settings rise symmetrically, crowned with blond rolls." "All through youth," said Cézanne, "I wanted to paint that, that tablecloth of new snow . . . Now I know that one must will only to paint the place-settings rising symmetrically and the blond rolls. If I paint 'crowned' I've had it, you understand? But if I really balance and shade my place-settings and rolls as they are in nature, then you can be sure that the crowns, the snow, and all the excitement will be there too."

We live in the midst of man-made objects, among tools, in houses, streets, cities, and most of the time we see them only through the human actions which put them to use. We become used to thinking that all of this exists necessarily and unshakeably. Cézanne's painting suspends these habits of thought and reveals the base of inhuman nature upon which man has installed himself. This is why Cézanne's people are strange, as if viewed by a creature of another species. Nature itself is stripped of the attributes which make it ready for animistic communions: there is no wind in the landscape, no movement on the Lac d'Annecy; the frozen objects hesitate as at the beginning of the world. It is an unfamiliar world in which one is uncomfortable and which forbids all human effusiveness. If one looks at the work of other painters after seeing Cézanne's paintings, one feels somehow relaxed, just as conversations resumed after a period of mourning mask the absolute change and give back to the survivors their solidity. But indeed only a human being is capable of such a vision which penetrates right to the root of things beneath the imposed order of humanity. Everything indicates that animals cannot look at things, cannot penetrate them in expectation of nothing but the truth. Emile Bernard's statement that a realistic painter is only an ape is therefore precisely the opposite of the truth, and one sees how Cézanne was able to revive the classical definition of art: man added to nature.

Cézanne's painting denies neither science nor tradition. He went to the Louvre every day when he was in Paris. He believed that one must learn how to paint and that the geometric study of planes and forms is a necessary part of this learning process. He inquired about the geological structure of his landscapes, convinced that these abstract relationships, expressed, however, in terms of the visible world, should affect the act of painting. The rules of anatomy and design are present in each stroke of his brush just as the rules of the game underlie each stroke of a tennis match. But what motivates the painter's movement can never be simply perspective or geometry or the laws governing color, or, for that matter, particular knowledge. Motivating all the movements from which a picture gradually emerges there can be only one thing: the landscape in its totality and in its absolute fullness, precisely what Cézanne called a "motif." He would start by discovering the geological foundations of the landscape; then, according to Mme Cézanne, he would halt and look at everything with widened eyes, "germinating" with the countryside. The task before him was, first to forget all he had ever learned from science and, second through these sciences to recapture the structure of the landscape as an emerging organism. To do this, all the partial views one catches sight of must be welded together; all that the eye's versatility disperses must be reunited; one must, as Gasquet put it, "join the wandering hands of nature." "A minute of the world is going by which must be painted in its full reality." His meditation would suddenly be consummated: "I have my motif" Cézanne would say, and he would explain that the landscape had to be centered neither too high nor too low, caught alive in a net which would let nothing escape. Then he began to paint all parts of the painting at the same time, using patches of color to surround his original charcoal sketch of the geological skeleton. The picture took on fullness and density; it grew in structure and balance; it came to maturity all at once. "The landscape thinks itself in me," he said, "and I am its consciousness." Nothing could be farther from naturalism than this intuitive science. Art is not imitation, nor is it something manufactured according to the wishes of instinct or good taste. It

is a process of expressing. Just as the function of words is to name – that is, to grasp the nature of what appears to us in a confused way and to place it before us as a recognizable object – so it is up to the painter, said Gasquet, to "objectify," "project," and "arrest." Words do not look like the things they designate; and a picture is not a *trompe l'oeil*. Cézanne, in his own words, "wrote in painting what had never yet been painted, and turned it into painting once and for all." Forgetting the viscous, equivocal appearances, we go through them straight to the things they present. The painter recaptures and converts into visible objects what would, without him, remain walled up in the separate life of each consciousness: the vibration of appearances which is the cradle of things. Only one emotion is possible for this painter – the feeling of strangeness – and only one lyricism – that of the continual rebirth of existence.

Leonardo da Vinci's motto was persistent rigor, and all the classical works on the art of poetry tell us that the creation of art is no easy matter. Cézanne's difficulties – like those of Balzac or Mallarmé – are of a different nature. Balzac (probably taking Delacroix for his model) imagined a painter who wants to express life through the use of color alone and who keeps his masterpiece hidden. When Frenhofer dies, his friends find nothing but a chaos of colors and elusive lines, a wall of painting. Cézanne was moved to tears when he read *Le Chef-d'oeuvre inconnu* and declared that he himself was Frenhofer. The effort made by Balzac, himself obsessed with "realization," sheds light on Cézanne's. In *La Peau de chagrin* Balzac speaks of "a thought to be expressed," "a system to be built," "a science to be explained." He makes Louis Lambert, one of the abortive geniuses of the Comédie Humaine, say: "I am heading toward certain discoveries ..., but how shall I describe the power which binds my hands, stops my mouth, and drags me in the opposite direction from my vocation?" To say that Balzac set himself to understand the society of his time is not sufficient. It is no superhuman task to describe the typical traveling salesman, to "dissect the teaching profession," or even to lay the foundations of a sociology. Once he had named the visible forces such as money and passion, once he had described the way they evidently work, Balzac wondered where it all led, what was the impetus behind it, what was the meaning of, for example, a Europe "whose efforts tend toward some unknown mystery of civilization." In short, he wanted to understand what interior force holds the world together and causes the proliferation of visible forms. Frenhofer had the same idea about the meaning of painting: "A hand is not simply part of the body, but the expression and continuation of a thought which must be captured and conveyed ... That is the real struggle! Many painters triumph instinctively, unaware of this theme of art. You draw a woman, but you do not see her." The artist is the one who arrests the spectacle in which most men take part without really seeing it and who makes it visible to the most "human" among them.

There is thus no art for pleasure's sake alone. One can invent pleasurable objects by linking old ideas in a new way and by presenting forms that have been seen before. This way of painting or speaking at second hand is what is generally meant by culture. Cézanne's or Balzac's artist is not satisfied to be a cultured animal but assimilates the culture down to its very foundations and gives it a new structure: he speaks as the first man spoke and paints as if no one had ever painted before.

What he expresses cannot, therefore, be the translation of a clearly defined thought, since such clear thoughts are those which have already been uttered by ourselves or by others. "Conception" cannot precede "execution." There is nothing but a vague fever before the act of artistic expression, and only the work itself, completed and understood, is proof that there was something rather than nothing to be said. Because he returns to the source of silent and solitary experience on which culture and the exchange of ideas have been built in order to know it, the artist launches his work just as a man once launched the first word, not knowing whether it will be anything more than a shout, whether it can detach itself from the flow of individual life in which it originates and give the independent existence of an identifiable meaning either to the future of that same individual life or to the monads coexisting with it or to the open community of future monads. The meaning of what the artist is going to say does not exist anywhere – not in things, which as yet have no meaning, nor in the artist himself, in his unformulated life. It summons one away from the already constituted reason in which "cultured men" are content to shut themselves, toward a reason which contains its own origins.

To Bernard's attempt to bring him back to human intelligence, Cézanne replied: "I am oriented toward the intelligence of the *Pater Omnipotens*." He was, in any case, oriented toward the idea or the project of an infinite Logos. Cézanne's uncertainty and solitude are not essentially explained by his nervous temperament but by the purpose of his work. Heredity may well have given him rich sensations, strong emotions, and a vague feeling of anguish or mystery which upset the life he might have wished for himself and which cut him off from men; but these qualities cannot create a work of art without the expressive act, and they can no more account for the difficulties than for the virtues of that act. Cézanne's difficulties are those of the first word. He considered himself powerless because he was not omnipotent, because he was not God and wanted nevertheless to portray the world, to change it completely into a spectacle, to make visible how the world touches us. A new theory of physics can be proven because calculations connect the idea or meaning of it with standards of measurement already common to all men. It is not enough for a painter like Cézanne, an artist, or a philosopher, to create and express an idea; they must also awaken the experiences which will make their idea take root in the consciousness of others. A successful work has the strange power to teach its own lesson. The reader or spectator who follows the clues of the book or painting, by setting up stepping stones and rebounding from side to side guided by the obscure clarity of a particular style, will end by discovering what the artist wanted to communicate. The painter can do no more than construct an image; he must wait for this image to come to life for other people. When it does, the work of art will have united these separate lives; it will no longer exist in only one of them like a stubborn dream or a persistent delirium, nor will it exist only in space as a colored piece of canvas. It will dwell undivided in several minds, with a claim on every possible mind like a perennial acquisition.

Thus, the "hereditary traits," the "influences" – the accidents in Cézanne's life – are the text which nature and history gave him to decipher. They give only the literal meaning of his work. But an artist's creations, like a man's free decisions, impose on this given a figurative sense which did not pre-exist them. If Cézanne's life seems to us to carry the seeds of his work within it, it is because we get to know his work first and see the circumstances of his life through it, charging them with a meaning borrowed from that work. If the givens for Cézanne which we have been enumerating, and which we spoke of as pressing conditions, were to figure in the web of projects which he was, they could have done so only by presenting themselves to him as what he had to live, leaving how to live it undetermined. An imposed theme at the start, they become, when replaced in the existence of which they are part, the monogram and the symbol of a life which freely interpreted itself.

But let us make no mistake about this freedom. Let us not imagine an abstract force which could superimpose its effects on life's "givens" or which cause breaches in life's development. Although it is certain that a man's life does not explain his work, it is equally certain that the two are connected. The truth is that this work to be done called for this life. From the very start, the only equilibrium in Cézanne's life came from the support of his future work. His life was the projection of his future work. The work to come is hinted at, but it would be wrong to take these hints for causes, although they do make a single adventure of his life and work. Here we are beyond causes and effects; both come together in the simultaneity of an eternal Cézanne who is at the same time the formula of what he wanted to be and what he wanted to do. There is a rapport between Cézanne's schizoid temperament and his work because the work reveals a metaphysical sense of the disease: a way of seeing the world reduced to the totality of frozen appearances, with all expressive values suspended. Thus the illness ceases to be an absurd fact and a fate and becomes a general possibility of human existence. It becomes so when this existence bravely faces one of its paradoxes, the phenomenon of expression. In this sense to be schizoid and to be Cézanne comes to the same thing. It is therefore impossible to separate creative liberty from that behavior, as far as possible from deliberate, already evident in Cézanne's first gestures as a child and in the way he reacted to things. The meaning Cézanne gave to objects and faces in his paintings presented itself to him in the world as it appeared to him. Cézanne simply released this meaning: it was the objects and the faces themselves as he saw them which demanded to be painted, and Cézanne simply expressed what they wanted to say. How, then, can any freedom be involved? True, the conditions of existence can only affect consciousness by way of a detour through the *raisons d'être* and the justifications consciousness offers to itself. We can only see what we are by looking ahead of ourselves, through the lens of our aims, and so our life always has the form of a project or of a choice and therefore seems spontaneous. But to say that we are from the start our way of

aiming at a particular future would be to say that our project has already stopped with our first ways of being, that the choice has already been made for us with our first breath. If we experience no external constraints, it is because we are our whole exterior. That eternal Cézanne whom we first saw emerge and who then brought upon the human Cézanne the events and influences which seemed exterior to him, and who planned all that happened to him – that attitude toward men and toward the world which was not chosen through deliberation – free as it is from external causes, is it free in respect to itself? Is the choice not pushed back beyond life, and can a choice exist where there is as yet no clearly articulated field of possibilities, only one probability and, as it were, only one temptation? If I am a certain project from birth, the given and the created are indistinguishable in me, and it is therefore impossible to name a single gesture which is merely hereditary or innate, a single gesture which is not spontaneous – but also impossible to name a single gesture which is absolutely new in regard to that way of being in the world which, from the very beginning, is myself. There is no difference between saying that our life is completely constructed and that it is completely given. If there is a true liberty, it can only come about in the course of our life by our going beyond our original situation and yet not ceasing to be the same: this is the problem. Two things are certain about freedom: that we are never determined and yet that we never change, since, looking back on what we were, we can always find hints of what we have become. It is up to us to understand both these things simultaneously, as well as the way freedom dawns in us without breaking our bonds with the world.

Such bonds are always there, even and above all when we refuse to admit they exist. Inspired by the paintings of Da Vinci, Valéry described a monster of pure freedom, without mistresses, creditors, anecdotes, or adventures. No dream intervenes between himself and the things themselves; nothing taken for granted supports his certainties; and he does not read his fate in any favorite image, such as Pascal's abyss. Instead of struggling against the monsters he has understood what makes them tick, has disarmed them by his attention, and has reduced them to the state of known things. "Nothing could be more free, that is, less human, than his judgments on love and death. He hints at them in a few fragments from his notebooks: 'In the full force of its passion,' he says more or less explicitly, 'love is something so ugly that the human race would die out (la natura si perderebbe) if lovers could see what they were doing.' This contempt is brought out in various sketches, since the leisurely examination of certain things is, after all, the height of scorn. Thus, he now and again draws anatomical unions, frightful cross-sections of love's very act."[9] He has complete mastery of his means, he does what he wants, going at will from knowledge to life with a superior elegance. Everything he did was done knowingly, and the artistic process, like the act of breathing or living, does not go beyond his knowledge. He has discovered the "central attitude," on the basis of which it is equally possible to know, to act, and to create because action and life, when turned into exercises, are not contrary to detached knowledge. He is an "intellectual power"; he is a "man of the mind."

Let us look more closely. For Leonardo there was no revelation; as Valéry said, no abyss yawned at his right hand. Undoubtedly true. But in "Saint Anne, the Virgin, and Child," the Virgin's cloak suggests a vulture where it touches the face of the Child. There is that fragment on the flight of birds where Da Vinci suddenly interrupts himself to pursue a childhood memory: "I seem to have been destined to be especially concerned with the vulture, for one of the first things I remember about my childhood is how a vulture came to me when I was still in the cradle, forced open my mouth with its tail, and struck me several times between the lips with it."[10] So even this transparent consciousness has its enigma, whether truly a child's memory or a fantasy of the grown man. It does not come out of nowhere, nor does it sustain itself alone. We are caught in a secret history, in a forest of symbols. One would surely protest if Freud were to decipher the riddle from what we know about the meaning of the flight of birds and about fellatio fantasies and their relation to the period of nursing. But it is still a fact that to the ancient

Egyptians the vulture was the symbol of maternity because they believed all vultures were female and that they were impregnated by the wind. It is also a fact that the Church Fathers used this legend to refute, on the grounds of natural history, those who were unwilling to believe in a virgin birth, and it is probable that Leonardo came across the legend in the course of his endless reading. He found in it the symbol of his own fate: he was the illegitimate son of a rich notary who married the noble Donna Albiera the very year Leonardo was born. Having no children by her, he took Leonardo into his home when the boy was five. Thus Leonardo spent the first four years of his life with his mother, the deserted peasant girl; he was a child without a father, and he got to know the world in the sole company of that unhappy mother who seemed to have miraculously created him. If we now recall that he was never known to have a mistress or even to have felt anything like passion; that he was accused – but acquitted – of homosexuality; that his diary, which tells us nothing about many other, larger expenses, notes with meticulous detail the costs of his mother's burial, as well as the cost of linen and clothing for two of his students – then we are on the verge of saying that Leonardo loved only one woman, his mother, and that this love left no room for anything but the platonic tenderness he felt for the young boys surrounding him. In the four decisive years of his childhood he formed a basic attachment which he had to give up when he was recalled to his father's home and into which he had poured all his resources of love and all his power of abandon. His thirst for life could only be turned toward the investigation and knowledge of the world, and, since he himself had been "detached," he had to become that intellectual power, that man who was all mind, that stranger among men. Indifferent, incapable of any strong indignation, love or hate, he left his paintings unfinished to devote his time to bizarre experiments; he became a person in whom his contemporaries sensed a mystery. It was as if Leonardo had never quite grown up, as if all the places in his heart had already been spoken for, as if the spirit of investigation was a way for him to escape from life, as if he had invested all his power of assent in the first years of his life and had remained true to his childhood right to the end. His games were those of a child. Vasari tells how "he made up a wax paste and, during his walks, he would model from it very delicate animals, hollow and filled with air; when he breathed into them, they would

---

9 *Introduction à la méthode de Leonard de Vinci*, by Paul Valéry. Paris: Nouvelle revue française:, p. 185. (English translation by Thomas McGreevy: *Introduction to the Method of Leonardo da Vinci*, London, 1929.) [Original note]

10 *Un souvenir d'enfance de Leonard de Vinci*, by Sigmund Freud. Paris: Gallimard: p. 65. (English translation by A. A. Brill: *Leonardo da Vinci: A Study in Psychosexuality*, New York: Random House, 1947.) [Original note]

float; when the air had escaped, they would fall to the ground. When the wine-grower from Belvedere found a very unusual lizard, Leonardo made wings for it out of the skin of other lizards and filled these wings with mercury so that they waved and quivered whenever the lizard moved; he likewise made eyes, a beard, and horns for it in the same way, tamed it, put it in a box, and used this lizard to terrify his friends."[11] He left his work unfinished, just as his father had abandoned him. He paid no heed to authority and trusted only nature and his own judgment in matters of knowledge, as is often the case with people who have not been raised in the shadow of a father's intimidating and protective power. Thus even this pure power of examination, this solitude, this curiosity – which are the essence of mind – became Leonardo's only in reference to his history. At the height of his freedom he was, in that very freedom, the child he had been; he was detached in one way only because he was attached in another. Becoming a pure consciousness is just another way of taking a stand about the world and other people; Leonardo learned this attitude in assimilating the situation which his birth and childhood had made for him. There can be no consciousness that is not sustained by its primordial involvement in life and by the manner of this involvement.

Whatever is arbitrary in Freud's explanations cannot in this context discredit psychoanalytical intuition. True, the reader is stopped more than once by the lack of evidence. Why this and not something else? The question seems all the more pressing since Freud often offers several interpretations, each symptom being "over-determined" according to him. Finally, it is obvious that a doctrine which brings in sexuality everywhere cannot, by the rules of inductive logic, establish its effectiveness anywhere, since, excluding all differential cases beforehand, it deprives itself of any counter-evidence. This is how one triumphs over psychoanalysis, but only on paper. For if the suggestions of the analyst can never be proven, neither can they be eliminated: how would it be possible to credit chance with the complex correspondences which the psychoanalyst discovers between the child and the adult? How can we deny that psychoanalysis has taught us to notice echoes, allusions, repetitions from one moment of life to another – a concatenation we would

not dream of doubting if Freud had stated the theory behind it correctly? Unlike the natural sciences, psychoanalysis was not meant to give us necessary relations of cause and effect but to point to motivational relationships which are in principle simply possible. We should not take Leonardo's fantasy of the vulture, or the infantile past which it masks, for a force which determined his future. Rather, it is like the words of the oracle, an ambiguous symbol which applies in advance to several possible chains of events. To be more precise: in every life, one's birth and one's past define categories or basic dimensions which do not impose any particular act but which can be found in all. Whether Leonardo yielded to his childhood or whether he wished flee from it, he could never have been other than he was. The very decisions which transform us are always made in reference to a factual situation; such a situation can of course be accepted or refused, but it cannot fail to give us our impetus nor to be for us, as a situation "to be accepted" or "to be refused," the incarnation for us of the value we give to it. If it is the aim of psychoanalysis to describe this exchange between future and past and to show how each life muses over riddles whose final meaning is nowhere written down, then we have no right to demand inductive rigor from it. The psychoanalyst's hermeneutic musing, which multiplies the communications between us and ourselves, which takes sexuality as the symbol of existence and existence as symbol of sexuality, and which looks in the past for the meaning of the future and in the future for the meaning of the past, is better suited than rigorous induction to the circular movement of our lives, where the future rests on the past, the past on the future, and where everything symbolizes everything else. Psychoanalysis does not make freedom impossible; it teaches us to think of this freedom concretely, as a creative repetition of ourselves, always, in retrospect, faithful to ourselves.

Thus it is true both that the life of an author can teach us nothing and that – if we know how to interpret it – we can find everything in it, since it opens onto his work. Just as we may observe the movements of an unknown animal without understanding the law which inhabits and controls them, so Cézanne's observers did not guess the transmutations which he imposed on events and experiences; they were blind to his significance, to that glow from out of nowhere which surrounded him from time to time. But he himself was never at the center of himself:

---

[11] Freud, *Un souvenir d'enfance, op.cit.* p. 189. [Original note]

nine days out of ten all he saw around him was the wretchedness of his empirical life and of his unsuccessful attempts, the leftovers of an unknown party. Yet it was in the world that he had to realize his freedom, with colors upon a canvas. It was on the approval of others that he had to wait for the proof of his worth. That is the reason he questioned the picture emerging beneath his hand, why he hung on the glances other people directed toward his canvas. That is the reason he never finished working. We never get away from our life. We never see our ideas or our freedom face to face.

Epilogue

The questions motivating this *Reader* have been primarily clinical. Ten years ago, when we set out to prepare this book, we were concerned about how to organize our clinical experiences. Like many other psychiatric trainees, we were astonished by what seemed like a vast variety of human experience and expressions of suffering in our patients. Searching for tools to navigate this multitude of clinical phenomena revealed a limited number of options.

The biological approach to psychiatry was one and it was undoubtedly fascinating. Advances such as the mapping of basic mental functions to brain regions or networks and the application of technology to identify genetic polymorphisms offered promises for psychiatry. However, most of these developments were and remain far away from clinical application. Clinically, knowledge of brain pathology or genetics mainly helped to identify and exclude rare neuropsychiatric cases. The reality of the emergency clinic and the psychiatric ward were largely untouched by such progress.

The psychoanalytic approach was another alternative that offered a solid clinical focus. Its particular emphasis on the patient–doctor relationship, the here and now of the consultation room, was a strength that biological approaches lacked. However, it came with a series of theoretical commitments that seemed at the time remote from clinical reality and had yet to develop an organized evidence base, in order to compete on equal terms with other branches of psychology and therapeutics.

Phenomenology was presented as an enigmatic third approach. We were taught the basics of Jasperian phenomenology and learnt about empathy and the distinction between 'form' and 'content'. It offered the immediate way we were looking for, to organize complex clinical phenomena; it was close to what we were actually encountering. Furthermore, it did not seem to require theoretical commitments. We were taught that phenomenology aspired to being a-theoretical (which fitted well with our overall sceptical outlook at the time) and could be learnt relatively quickly.

This feeling of things falling into place by studying phenomenology was short-lived and with increasing clinical exposure came new questions. The standard phenomenology syllabus had little to say about mood or anxiety disorders and seemed to be moving within the narrow boundaries of the current classification systems. Moreover, there was a feeling that the philosophical foundations of phenomenology were underplayed. References to philosophy were fleeting and confined to Husserl.

It therefore seemed plausible to ask whether there was more to phenomenology than we were being presented with in our training. Indeed, there were indications that made us expect something of a hidden treasure from the phenomenological tradition. In the readings organized by the Maudsley Philosophy Group there was a chance to read primary texts of, among others, Husserl, Heidegger and Scheler with other clinicians and philosophers. At the same time, mainly through the writings of Spiegelberg (1972) and Cutting (1997) we were pointed to previous attempts to incorporate such philosophical knowledge into clinical psychiatry.

We also wanted to access the primary clinical phenomenology texts that were being cited by contemporary phenomenological psychopathologists, such as Sass, Parnas, Stanghellini and Fuchs, and philosophers such as Gallagher, Ratcliffe and Zahavi. However, these texts seemed largely inaccessible. Most were untranslated from the German and of the few that were available in English, most were out of print. Making these texts available to ourselves was the first step. We found them in a variety of places including private collections held at the Institute of Psychiatry library. The idea of a *Reader* emerged that would allow psychiatrists (particularly trainees) and philosophers ready access to this material.

Five years on and with the *Reader* in hand, it is probably reassuring to know that we don't believe we have recovered a lost ark. However, we have a sense that important discoveries have been made. In part it involved discovering that, in spite of our expectations, these texts from the past left several of our initial questions unanswered. Conversely, we found that taken together they contained profound insights that point at a new range of opportunities for psychiatry.

Perhaps the most important discovery for us lies in the plurality that exists within the phenomenological tradition. This range has long been underacknowledged. Below, we outline how the texts in this *Reader* contribute to a novel understanding of these varied phenomenological themes and how they could be of relevance to clinicians, philosophers and researchers.

Variation in origin

Trainees are taught that phenomenological theory was developed by Husserl and applied to psychiatry by Jaspers, an account exemplified by the following textbook excerpt:

> Descriptive psychopathology ... owes a great deal to the philosophical discipline called 'phenomenology' – a method (developed by Husserl) of scrupulously inspecting one's own conscious processes, without assuming anything about external causes or consequences of those 'phenomena' and without altering the phenomena by observational methods. This school of thought has influenced psychiatry through the philosopher/psychiatrist Karl Jaspers. The development of sympathy and intuitive understanding allows for the objective observation of phenomena in others, by relating them to phenomena in ourselves
>
> (Buckley 2005).

The focus on the Husserl–Jaspers nexus is partly understandable. There is hardly a text in phenomenological psychiatry that cannot be ultimately traced back to them. However, this *Reader* also shows that most of these routes to Husserl and Jaspers are not direct. Instead, the links occur via other authors – Binswanger can be traced back to Husserl via Heidegger (please refer to pp. 48–84 and pp. 155–158 and 197–203) and some of Schneider's (please refer to pp. 36–47 and 203–207) links to Jaspers and Husserl are less obvious than his debt to the philosopher Scheler. But there are other reasons why phenomenological psychiatry is a more complex story than the Husserl–Jaspers nexus would suggest. The philosophical texts in this *Reader* serve as a reminder that Jaspers' own approach to psychiatry was informed by a range of thinkers (Husserl alongside others such as Kant, Dilthey and Weber – please refer

to Section 1, pp. 3–12).[1] Moreover, such an account of phenomenology fails to notice the tradition of what may be called an existential or structural phenomenology (please refer to Section 2, pp. 13–84). This is crucially distinct from what Jaspers and Schneider aspired to – a relatively theory-neutral approach to the description of the subjective experience of patients. Instead, authors such as Minkowski (please refer to Chapter 12, pp. 102–116), Binswanger (please refer to pp. 155–158 and 197–203) or von Gebsattel (please refer to pp. 232–240 and 250–256) seemed to want to make sense of patients' experience in metaphysical and "whole-person" terms. Whereas Jaspers and Schneider aspired to the value neutrality advocated by Weber in his methodology of social science (please refer to Chapter 4, pp. 8–9), Minkowski took up Bergson's metaphysics of the human being and Binswanger Heidegger's notions of the thrownness and facticity of Dasein.

This variation in origins may be of particular interest to philosophers and historians of philosophy: what accounts for this branching out from Husserl and Jaspers? Similarly, what explains the fact that the Jaspers–Schneider approach remains more influential than the (more recent) existential or structural approaches?

Variation in methodology

Closely linked to the point above is the fact that the phenomenological method is varied. Clinicians will tend to doubt the relevance that complex philosophical texts and methodology might have for their thinking and practice, but the texts presented here show how previous generations of clinicians have integrated knowledge from such texts into their own clinical approaches. It is interesting to see that the Husserlian approach (please refer to Chapter 6, pp. 13–35) of the reduction, of bracketing out causal theories and the 'natural attitude' is rarely used and whenever it is, it is not used consistently. Empathy, the paradigmatic approach since Dilthey, Weber and Jaspers (please refer to Chapter 10, pp. 91–100), is explored further in texts, such as Rumke's (please refer to Chapter 16,

---

[1] Indeed, there is a wide-ranging academic debate as to whether the method of Jaspers' *General Psychopathology* is more indebted to these philosophers and social scientists than to Husserl and phenomenology. See Rickman (1987), Walker (1988, 1993) and Wiggins and Schwartz (1997).

pp. 193–196), on the value of the 'praecox feeling' as a diagnostic approach. Other approaches that take the human being as a whole (please refer to passages from Bergson, Scheler, Heidegger from Sections 1 and 2) are more commonly adopted – see, for example, Minkowski's (please refer to Chapter 12, pp. 102–116), von Gebsattel's (please refer to pp. 214–218, 232–240, 250–271) and Binwanger's (please refer to pp. 155–158 and 197–203). It seems that phenomenology provided a sufficiently elastic frame within which clinicians could generate various mappings of their patients' pathological experiences. The texts presented here also show how such methodology could be a fruitful area for empirical research. For example, remarkably little has been done to determine the predictive value that empathy might have in diagnosis or to explore empathy from the perspective of social psychology or biology. Do 'whole-person' approaches, such as those of Minkowsi or Binswanger, provide a more valid account of patients' experience – including their suffering? Do they bias observation or keep observation attuned and checked against the biases that may be introduced by the (often unacknowledged) models of mental disorder extant in clinical psychiatry? How do they relate to clinical decision-making where the person as a moral agent is at stake – for example in mental health law?

Variation in diagnostic topics

The diagnosis that is traditionally approached in phenomenological terms is schizophrenia. In this reader we have shown how the phenomenological approach can encompass a wide range of diagnoses and offer a comprehensive approach. The texts presented show how clinicians working with patients suffering from mood disorders (e.g. Schneider; please refer to Chapter 17, pp. 203–207) or anxiety disorders (please refer to Part 3, Chapter 18, pp. 224–240) where symptoms such as delusions or hallucinations are not present can draw on phenomenology. Yet there are also gaps; learning disability and childhood disorders have received little phenomenological attention. Interestingly, many of the texts concern phenomenological accounts within established diagnoses. Hence, we have descriptions of the experiences of patients with schizophrenia (Blankenburg; please refer to pp. 158–176), or reports about time perception in melancholia (Straus; please refer to pp. 207–214), and the phenomenology of brain injury (Goldstein; please refer to pp. 132–141). The implication is that many texts have treated diagnoses as if they were examples of nature carved at its joints. Indeed, many of these texts seem to have been less concerned about the boundaries and robustness of these diagnoses. It was also surprising to see that given Husserl's calls for the phenomenological method to step outside the natural attitude, clinical phenomenologists based a lot of their theory on existing taxonomies. However, it seems reasonable to suggest that phenomenological psychiatry should make a point of approaching phenomena unconstrained by existing diagnostic systems, and perhaps by putting to one side causal accounts of disorders, whether cognitive, psychoanalytic, neuroscientific or genetic. Yet phenomenological psychiatry may also have a role in discovering phenomenological structure in diagnostic categories that have, for pragmatic reasons, endured. In any case, phenomenological psychiatry will need freedom to move outside, and inside, of existing diagnostic concepts.

Variation in ways of carving up psychopathology

Phenomenological analysis may also identify patterns in psychopathology that are missed by existing diagnostic categories. Examples can be found, at least in partial form, in some of the texts provided in the *Reader*. A fascinating and only little-studied notion is that of temporality: of how time and its perception may provide an alternative grouping of psychopathological phenomena, for example in the area of depressed mood (Straus; please refer to p. 207), The same could apply to the pathology of 'common sense' (Blankenburg; please refer to p. 158). It seems pertinent to ask about the developmental phenomenology of 'common sense': how is it shaped, how does it relate to other notions of understanding others and their thoughts, and are there other forms of pathology of 'common sense', beyond what is posited here about schizophrenia? Clinicians will be particularly interested to know how much what they perceive as a disturbed 'common sense' may just be a difference in cultural or other expectations. Similarly, could a phenomenology of time provide an opportunity for a shared patient–doctor temporality with therapeutic implications?

Can phenomenology be longitudinal?

The traditional view of phenomenology (descriptive psychopathology) is that it is cross-sectional – it is the delusions and hallucinatory experiences that the patient describes in the consultation room that are usually the focus. However, the accounts provided here show longitudinal approaches, as the text by Conrad (please refer to p. 176) on stages of illness exemplifies. Perhaps a more general question concerns how one could develop longitudinal or developmental phenomenology and integrate it into clinical practice. Clinicians see patients in the here and now – often in an emergency room, ward or clinic – and are asked to provide a diagnosis. Retrospective accounts, while telling about a patient's current perspective on his/her life, don't offer a solid basis for a phenomenology of the life course. However, clinicians often also follow up patients over time – creating a common past and present with them. Phenomenology would seem particularly suited to study the way future and past experiences are perceived and constructed and of how contextual effects can influence the perception of reality. This could be fruitfully applied to better understand environmental influences throughout life and offer a dynamic view of the patient–doctor relationship over time.

Variations and complexities in the relationship of phenomenology with the natural sciences

The texts presented in this *Reader* demonstrate the emphasis that is placed on the patient's experience. The weight given to clinical descriptions and the patient's perspectives in the clinical texts is in stark contrast to the often reductive approach that is typical of contemporary psychiatric research papers. Indeed, it seems hard to imagine how the rich and often tortuous clinical descriptions of some of these texts could be contained in a modern scientific discourse. One of the questions, therefore, is whether the two are somehow incompatible. Kurt Schneider (1926) writing an overview of the relationship between phenomenology and biological psychiatry in the 1920s thought of them as complementary for the following reasons:

> There is only one side for the psychiatrist to take, and, for the purposes of clinical psychiatry, it is the side of biological psychiatry. Only in biological psychiatry flourish the possibilities of treating psychoses.

> *****

> It would, at the same time, be very wrong, it would in fact be impossible, to try to erase phenomenological psychiatry from what psychiatrists do. Not only

because, by doing so, phenomenological psychiatry would be left to philosophers, paedagogians and theologians, but, more importantly, because the psychiatrist needs phenomenological psychiatry. Not only because of the feeble neurological grasp we have today; phenomenological psychiatry will always be necessary, because all the medicalising in the world will not gain us access to our patients' experiences, their soul.

In Schneider's sense, then, phenomenology is a critical tool enabling the psychiatrist to value and perhaps understand their patients' experiences. He contrasts this to the biological approach, from which, to his mind, innovation in diagnosis and treatment can emerge. The texts in this *Reader* provide several reasons to be critical of Schneider's polarizing of natural science and phenomenology. From a research perspective, phenomenology seems to provide a range of opportunities for building new scientific hypotheses. Indeed, it is difficult to imagine how certain research areas in psychiatry or psychology could do without at least some phenomenology. It is not just the phenotypic refinement that remains central to genetic research, but also the building of testable alternative models in areas such as experimental psychology. Also, as mentioned above, phenomenology goes well beyond descriptive psychopathology, offering a guide for reconsidering nosological boundaries in their own right. It is often argued that advances in laboratory methods, such as in neuroimaging, might reduce the need for phenomenology in clinical psychiatry. This may well be true and biomarkers could become more useful for clinical psychiatry and help reshape nosology. However, even in those areas of medicine where laboratory medicine has become highly useful (for example haematology or oncology), the equivalents of phenomenology, that is, clinical observation and examination remain central to a doctor's daily activity. The texts by Minkowski (please refer to pp. 102–116, 143–155), von Gebsattel (please refer to pp. 232–240, 250–257) and Binswanger (please refer to pp. 197–203) in this *Reader* also reveal another aspect of the relationship between psychiatry and the natural sciences that may be the most complex so far. These authors posit that understanding alien worlds (such as the world of someone with mental disorder) requires, from the outset, a whole-person approach, that of a philosophical anthropology. It is the philosophical level of understanding the human being, which, to these authors, opens up a new space of possibilities for psychiatry and other areas of medicine. These writings are rooted in some of the scepticism about the scientific approach that is also prevalent in Heidegger's work (Heidegger 1994). For these writers, the usual 'simplifying and condensing' (please refer to p. 250) approach of medicine does not do justice to the phenomena. Instead, Binswanger for example, calls for a stance that seems different from today's medical approaches: 'devote yourself to the sick fellow human confronting you with your entire *being* and complete *love*' (please refer to p. 198). This insistence on the irreducibility of the human and the approach to the 'whole being' seems fairly radical. Here, phenomenology is not resorted to because biology has not advanced enough, it is rather seen as essential in its own right if justice is to be done to the patient as a human being. Authors like Binswanger and von Gebsattel emphasize meaning in psychopathology; they see attempts at making sense of patients' experiences as a psychiatrist's central endeavour. However, this priority on meaning may be at odds with the scope of the natural sciences. It has recently been argued that search for meaning may have very little to do with causal explanations (Kendler *et al.* 2011) and, perhaps even worse, it may hinder rational interventions (Lyketsos and Chisolm 2009). Indeed, many would argue – along with the philosopher Nicolai Hartmann (1965, pp. 152–3) – that

phenomenology's major flaw is that it cannot account for causality or more generally non-experiential connections. It is unclear whether this apparent gap between phenomenology and the natural sciences is unbridgeable. It did not seem so in the 1910s/20s when Scheler (1933), who was himself broadly embracing of scientific discovery, proposed that the natural sciences could themselves be a topic of phenomenological enquiry along with, say, mathematics or politics. Neither did it seem so to Jaspers, who produced a majestic overview of psychiatry that continues to speak to us after almost a century (Jaspers 1963). One could argue that phenomenology brings forth a kind of meta-psychiatry that stands beyond the clinical discipline of psychiatry and the different empirical sciences at work in psychiatry. However, neither Jaspers nor Scheler delivered an entirely clear demonstration of how this could work and whether phenomenology could, or should, play such a role in psychiatry. Nonetheless, much of their impetus and their spirit has been imprinted upon psychiatry and getting close to that history has left a marked impression upon us. The relationship between phenomenology and psychiatry remains a matter of debate and further enquiry. We hope that the texts of this *Reader* will provide a useful basis for such important discussions.

References

Aschoff, J. (1954). Zeitgeber der tierischen Tagesperiodik. *Naturwissenschaften* **41**: 49–56.

Aschoff, J. (1970). Circadiane Periodik als Grundlage des Schlafwach Rhythmus. In *Ermüdung, Schlaf und Traum*, ed. W. Baust. Stuttgart: Wissenschaftliche Buchgesellschaft: 59–98.

Baeyer-Katte, W. von. (1966). Immanuel Kant über das Problem der abnormen Persönlichkeit. In *Conditio humana: Erwin W. Straus on his 75th birthday*, eds. W. von. Baeyer and R. M. Griffith. Berlin: Springer: 35–54.

Bergson, H. *Ecrits et paroles*, vol. 1, ed. R. M. Mosse-Bastide. Paris: Presses Universitaires de France: 84ff.

Beringer, K. (1924). Beitrag zur Analyse schizophrener Denkstörungen. *Zeitschrift fur die gesamte Neurologie und Psychiatre* **93**: 55–61.

Beringer, K. (1926). Denkstörungen und Sprache bei Schizophrenen. *Zeitschrift fur die gesamte Neurologie und Psychiatre* **103**: 185–97.

Berrios, G. E. (1993). Phenomenology and psychopathology: was there ever a relationship? *Comprehensive Psychiatry* **34**(4): 213–0.

Binder, H. (1936). *Zur Psychologie der Zwangsvorgänge*. Berlin: Karger.

Binswanger, L. (1933). *Über Ideenflucht*. Zurich: Orell Füssli.

Binswanger, L. (1956). *Drei Formen missglückten Daseins: Verstiegenheit, Verschrobenheit, Manieriertheit*. Tübingen: Niemeyer.

Binswanger, L. (1963). Über das Wahnproblem in rein phänomenologischer Sicht. *Schweizer Archiv für Neurologie, Neurochirurgie und Psychiatrie* **91**: 85–8.

Binswanger, L. (1965). *Wahn*. Pfullingen: Neske.

Binswanger, W. (1960). *Melancholie und Manie*. Pfullingen: Neske.

Blattner, W. (2006). *Heidegger's Being and Time*. London: Continuum.

Bleuler, E. (1911). Dementia praecox oder die Gruppe der Schizophrenien. In *Handbuch der Psychiatrie*, vol. 4, ed. G. Aschaffenburg. Leipzig: Deuticke.

Bolton, D., Hill, J. (2004). *Mind, Meaning, and Mental Disorder: The Nature of Causal Explanation in Psychology and Psychiatry*. Oxford: Oxford University Press.

Bräutigam, W. (1965). *Erlebnisvorfeld und Anlässe schizophrener Psychosen*, vol. 7. Psychiatertagung des Landschaftverbandes Rheinland: Suchteln.

Broome, M. R. (2006). Taxonomy and ontology in psychiatry: a survey of recent literature. *Philosophy, Psychiatry and Psychology* **13**(4): 303–19.

Broome, M. R. (2008). Philosophy as the science of values: Neo-Kantianism as a guide to psychiatric interviewing. *Philosophy, Psychiatry and Psychology* **15**(2): 107–16.

Buckley, P. (2005). Descriptive psychopathology. In *Examination Notes in Psychiatry*, 4th edn, eds. P. Buckley, D. Prewette, J. Bird and G. Harrison. Oxford, UK: Oxford University Press: 10–21.

Burger, T. (1976). *Weber's Theory of Concept Formation: History, Laws, and Ideal Types*. Durham, NC: Duke University Press.

Cassirer, E. (1957). Toward a pathology of the symbolic consciousness. In *The Philosophy of Symbolic Forms*, vol. 3, *The Phenomenology of Knowledge*, trans. R. Manheim. New Haven, CT: Yale University Press: Chapter 6.

Cerbone, D. R. (2003). Phenomenology: straight and hetero. In *A House Divided: Comparing Analytic and Continental Philosophy*, ed. C. G. Prado. Amherst, NY: Humanity Books: 105–38.

Cohen, M. B., Baker, G., Cohen, R. A., *et al.* (1954). An intensive study of twelve cases of manic-depressive psychosis. *Psychiatry* **17**: 103–37.

Conrad, K. (1958). *Die beginnende Schizophrenie*. Stuttgart: Thieme.

Crowell, S. (2009). Husserlian phenomenology. In *A Companion to Phenomenology and Existentialism*, eds. H. L. Dreyfus and M. A. Wrathall. Oxford: Wiley-Blackwell: 9–30.

Cutting, J. (1997). *Principles of Psychopathology: Two Worlds – Two Minds – Two Hemispheres*. Oxford, UK: Oxford University Press.

Dennett, D. (1991). *Consciousness Explained*. Boston, MA: Back Bay Books.

Descartes, R. (1931). *Philosophical Works*, 2 vols. New York: Dover.

Descartes, R. (1953). *Oeuvres et letters*. Paris: Gallimard.

Dreyfus, H. L. (1991). *Being-in-the-world: A Commentary on Heidegger's Being and Time, Division I*. Cambridge, MA: MIT Press.

Engel, G. E. (1977). The need for a new medical model: a challenge for biomedicine. *Science* **196**: 129–36.

Figal, G. (2010). Phenomenology: Heidegger after Husserl and the Greeks. In *Martin Heidegger: Key Concepts*, ed. B. W. Davis. Durham: Acumen: 33–43.

Fish, F. (1966). Experimentelle Untersuchung der formalen Denkstörung bei der Schizophrenie. *Fortschritte Neurologie Psychiatrie* **34**: 427–45.

Fring, M. (1995) *Max Scheler: A Concise Introduction into the World of a Great Thinker*, 2nd edn. Milwaukee, WI: Marquette University Press.

Funk and Wagnall (1964). *Standard Dictionary*. New York.

Gadamer, H. G. (1965). *Wahrheit und Methode: Grundzüge einer philosophischen Hermeneutik*, 2nd edn. Tübingen: Mohr.

Gadamer, H.G. *Philosophical Apprenticeships*, trans. R. Sullivan. Cambridge, MA: MIT Press.

Gebsattel, V. von (1954). *Prolegmena zu einer medisinischen Anthropologie*. Berlin: Springer.

Ghaemi, S. N. (2009). Nosologomania: DSM and Karl Jaspers' critique of Kraepelin. *Philosophy, Ethics, and Humanities in Medicine* **4**(10).

Glendinning, S. (2007). *In the Name of Phenomenology*. Oxford: Routledge.

Goeppert, H. (1960). *Zwangskrankheit und Depersonalisation*. Basel: Karger.

Guerlac, S. (2006). *Thinking In Time: An Introduction to Henri Bergson*. Ithaca, NY: Cornell University Press.

Gutting, G. (2001). *French Philosophy in the Twentieth Century*. Cambridge: Cambridge University Press.

Harland, R., Antonova, E., Owen, G. S., *et al.* (2009). A study of psychiatrists' concepts of mental illness. *Psychological Medicine* **39**: 967–76.

Hartmann, N. (1965). *Zur Grundlegung der Ontologie*, 4th edn. Berlin: De Gruyter.

Heidegger, M. (1927). *Sein und Zeit*. Halle: Niemeyer.

Heidegger, M. (1972). *Being and Time*. New York: Harper and Row.

Heidegger, M. (1977). *Sein und Zeit*, 14th edn. Tübingen: Niemeyer.

Heidegger, M. (1984). *The Metaphysical Foundations of Logic: In Memoriam Max Scheler*, trans. M. Heim. Bloomington, IN: Indiana University Press.

Heidegger, M. (1994). *Zollikoner Seminary: Protokolle-Zwiegespräche-Briefe*. Frankfurt am Main: Klostermann.

Held, K. (2003). Husserl's phenomenological method. In *The New Husserl: A Critical Reader*, ed. D. Welton. Bloomington, IN: Indiana University Press: 1–31.

Hofer, G. (1954). Phänomen und Symptom. *Nervenarzt* **25**: 342–4.

Hofer, G. (1968a). *Der Mensch im Wahn*. Basel: Karger.

Hofer, G. (1968b). Der Wahnende als Mitmensch. *Psychiat. Clin.* **1**: 253–62.

Husserl, E. (1929). Formale und transzendentale Logik. In *Jahrbuch für Philosophie und phänomenologische Forschung* 10, 222; (1969) *Formal and Transcendental Logic*, trans. D. Cairns. The Hague: Nijhoff.

Husserl, E. (1954). *Die Krisis der europäischen Wissenchaften und die transzendentale Phänomenologie*. The Hague: Nijhoff.

Husserl, E. (1973/1999). Eidetic variation and the acquisition of pure universals. In *The Essential Husserl*, ed. D. Welton. Bloomington, IN: Indiana University Press: 292–300.

Jacquette, D. (2004). Brentano's concept of intentionality. In *The Cambridge Companion to Brentano*, ed. D. Jacquette. Cambridge: Cambridge University Press: 98–130.

Jaide, W. (1937). *Das Wesen des Zaubers in den primitiven Kulturen und in der Islandssaga*. Leipzig: Borna.

Janzarik, W. (1959). *Dynamische Grundkonstellationen in endogenen Psychosen*. Berlin: Springer.

Jaspers, K. (1963a). *General Psychopathology*, 7th edn, trans. J. Hoenig and M. W. Hamilton. Manchester: Manchester University Press.

Jaspers, K. (1963b). Philosophical memoir. In *Philosophy and the World: Selected Essays and Lectures*, trans. E. B. Ashton. Chicago, IL: Henry Regnery.

Jaspers, K. (1981). Philosophical autobiography. In *The Philosophy of Karl Jaspers, Augmented Edition*, ed. P. A. Schilpp. La Salle, IL: Open Court: 55–8.

Kafka, G. (1929). Zur Psychologie des Ekels. *Zeitschrift für angewandte Psychologie* **34**.

Kant, I. (1799). *Kritik der Urteilskraft*, 3rd edn. (C). Königsberg.

Kant, I. (1800). *Anthropologie in pragmatischer Hinsicht*, 2nd edn. (B). Königsberg.

Kendler, K. S., Myers, J., and Halberstadt, L. J. (2011). Do reasons for major depression act as causes? *Molecular Psychiatry* **16**: 626–33.

Kisiel, T. (2010). Hermeneutics of facticity. In *Martin Heidegger: Key Concepts*, ed. B. W. Davis. Durham: Acumen: 17–32.

Kisker, K. P. (1957). Kants psychiatrische Systematik. *Psychiat. Neurol. Basel* 133: 17–28.

Kisker, K. P. (1960). *Der Erlebniswandel des Schizophrenen.* Berlin: Springer.

Klages, L. (1960). *Der Geist als Widersacher der Seele,* 4th edn. Bonn: Bouvier.

Klein, M. (1960). Zur Psychogenese der manisch-depressiven Zustande. *Psyche* 14: 156.

Kosik, K. (1967). *Die Dialektik des Konkreten.* Frankfurt am Main: Suhrkamp.

Kraepelin, E. (1906). Katatonic excitement. In *Lectures on Clinical Psychiatry,* 2nd edn, ed. T. Johnstone. London: Ballière, Tindall & Cox.

Kraepelin, E. (1913). *Lectures on Clinical Psychiatry.* Bristol: Thoemmes Press.

Kühn, H. (1943). Über Störungen des sympathiefuhlens bei Schizophrenen: Ein Beitrag zur Psychologie des schizophrenen Autismus und der Defektsymptome. *Zeitschrift für die gesamte Neurologie und Psychiatre* 174: 418–59.

Kunz, H. (1966). Über vitale und intentionale Bedeutungsgehalte. In *Conditio humana: Erwin W. Straus on his 75th Birthday,* eds. W. von Baeyer and R. M. Griffith. Berlin: Springer.

Laing, R. D. (1990). *The Divided Self.* London: Penguin.

Litt, T. (1926). *Individuum und Gemeinschaft,* 3rd edn. Leipzig: Teubner.

Lukacs, G. (1964). *Die Eigenart des Ästhetischen.* Berlin: Luchterhand.

Lyketsos, C. G., and Chisolm, M. S. (2009). The trap of meaning: a public health tragedy. *Journal of the American Medical Association* 302: 432–3.

Makkreel, R. A. (1998). Dilthey. In *A Companion to Continental Philosophy,* eds. S. Critchley and W. R. Schroeder. Oxford: Blackwell: 425–32.

Matthews, E. (1996). *Twentieth-Century French Philosophy.* Oxford: Oxford University Press.

Merleau-Ponty, M. (2002). *Phenomenology of Perception,* 2nd edn. London: Routledge.

Michaelis, R. (1965). Zur Typologie der Hypersommen. *Fortschritte Neurologie-Psychiatrie* 33: 587.

Minkowski, E. (1970). *Lived Time: Phenomenological and Psychopathological Studies,* trans. N. Metzel. Evanston, IL: Northwestern University Press.

Moore, G. E. (1969). *Die Verteidigung des Common Sense.* Frankfurt am Main: Suhrkamp.

Moran, D. (2000). *Introduction to Phenomenology.* London: Routledge.

Mullarkey, J. (2010). Henri Bergson. In *The History of Continental Philosophy,* vol. 3, *The New Century: Bergsonism, Phenomenology and Responses to Modern Science,* eds. K. Ansell-Pearson and A. D. Schrift. Durham: Acumen: 19–46.

Mulligan, K. (2004). Brentano on the Mind. In *The Cambridge Companion to Brentano,* ed. D. Jacquette. Cambridge: Cambridge University Press: 66–97.

Natanson, M. (1963). Philosophische Grundfragen der Psychiatrie. I. Philosophie und Psychiatrie. In *Psychiatrie der Gegenwart,* vol. 1/2. Berlin: Springer: 903–25.

Oesterreigh, K. and Tellenbach, H. (1967). Die Behandlung hirnatrophisch begründeter Versagenszustände mit Infusionen von Beta-Pyridyl Carbinol (Ronicol). *Nervenarzt* 38: 34.

Outhwaite, W. (1986). *Understanding Social Life: The Method called Verstehen,* 2nd edn. Lewes: Jean Stroud.

Owen, G. (2008). Karl Jaspers' methodological pluralism and its exclusion of philosophy. *Philosophy, Psychiatry and Psychology* 14(1): 67–70.

Parkin, F. (2002). *Max Weber,* revised edn. London: Routledge.

Parnas, J., Zahavi, D. (2002). The role of phenomenology in psychiatric classification and diagnosis. In *Psychiatric Diagnosis and Classification,* eds. M. Maj, W. Graebel and J. J. Lopez-Ibor. Chichester: John Wiley: 137–62.

Payne, R. W. (1966). The measurement and significance of over inclusive thinking and retardation in schizophrenic patients. In *Psychopathology of Schizophrenia,* ed. P. H. Hoch and J. Zubin. New York: Grune and Stratton: 77–97.

Polt, R. (1999). *Heidegger: An Introduction.* London: UCL Press.

Ratcliffe, M. (2009). Understanding existential changes in Psychiatric illness: the indespensability of phenomenology. In *Psychiatry as Cognitive Neuroscience: Philosophical Perspectives,* eds. M. R. Broome and L. Bortolotti. Oxford: Oxford University Press: 223–44.

Reid, T. H. (1846). *The Philosophical Works,* vol. 2. Edinburgh.

Rickman, H. P. (1987). The philosophic basis of psychiatry: Jaspers and Dilthey. *Philosophy of the Social Sciences* 17: 173–96.

Russell, M. (2006). *Husserl: A Guide for the Perplexed.* London: Continuum.

Scheler, M. (1933). Phänomenologie und Erkenntnistheorie. In *Schriften aus dem Nachlass, Gesammelte Werke,* vol. 10, ed. Maria Scheler. Bonn: Bouvier: 263–312.

Scheler, M. (1958) *Philosophical Perpectives*, trans. O. Haac, Boston, MA: Beacon Press.

Scheler, M. (1973a). Phenomenology and the theory of cognition. In *Selected Philosophical Essays*, trans. D. Lacterman, Evanston, IL: Northwestern University Press: 136–201.

Scheler, M. (1973b). *Formalism in Ethics and Non-Formal Ethics of Values*, trans. M. Frings and R. L. Funk, Evanston, IL: Northwestern University Press.

Scheler, M. (1973c). The idols of self-knowledge. In *Selected Philosophical Essays*, trans. D. Lacterman, Evanston, IL: Northwestern University Press.

Scheler, M. (1973d). On the ideas of man, trans. C. Nabe. *Journal of the British Society for Phenomenology* 9(3): 184–98.

Scheler, M. (1973e). Idealism and realism. In *Selected Philosophical Essays*, trans. D. Lacterman, Evanston, IL: Northwestern University Press.

Scheler, M. (1980). *Die Wissenformen und die Gesellschaft.* London: Routledge.

Scheler, M. (2007). *Ressentiment*, trans. W. H. Holdheim, Milwaukee, WI: Marquette University Press.

Scheler, M. (2009a). *The Human Place in the Cosmos*, trans. M. Frings. Evanston, IL: Northwestern University Press.

Scheler, M. (2009b). *The Constitution of the Human Being*, trans. J. Cutting, Milwaukee, WI: Marquette University Press.

Schneider, K. (1926). Die phänomenologische Richtung in der Psychiatrie. *Philosophischer Anzeiger* 4: 382–404.

Schneider, K. (1959). *Clinical Psychopathology*, trans. M. W. Hamilton. New York: Grune and Stratton.

Schwartz, M. A., Wiggins, O. P. (1987). Diagnosis and ideal types: a contribution to psychiatric classification. *Comprehensive Psychiatry* 28(4): 277–91.

Scott, C. E. (2010). Care and authenticity. In *Martin Heidegger: Key Concepts*, ed. B. W. Davis. Durham: Acumen: 57–68.

Shaftesbury, A, Earl of (1711). *Characteristics of Men, Manners, Opinions, Times*, vols 1–3. London.

Simmel, E. (1909). *Die Mode: Philosophische Kultur*, 2nd edn. Leipzig.

Smith, B. (1994). *Austrian Philosophy: The Legacy of Franz Brentano.* La Salle, IL: Open Court.

Smith, D. W. (2007). *Husserl.* Oxford: Routledge.

Spiegelberg, H. (1964). Phenomenology through vicarious experience. In *Phenomenology: Pure and Applied*, ed. E. Straus. Pittsburgh, PA: Duquesne University Press.

Spiegelberg, H. (1965). *The Phenomenological Movement*, 2nd edn. The Hague: Martinus Nijhoff.

Spiegelberg, H. (1972). *Phenomenology in Psychology and Psychiatry.* Evanston, IL: Northwesteren University Press.

Stapleton, T. (2010). Dasein as being-in-the-world. In *Martin Heidegger: Key Concepts*, ed. B. W. Davis. Durham: Acumen: 44–56.

Stein, E. (1989) *On the Problem of Empathy*, trans. W. Stein. Washington, DC: ICS Publications.

Stekel, W. (1930). Die Psychologie der Zwangskrankheiten. *Zeitschrift für die gesamte Neurologie und Psychiatric* 57.

Stoning, G. E. (1933). Ein Beitrag zum Problem der Zwangspsychopathie. *Zeitschrift für die gesamte Neurologie und Psychiatric* 139.

Straus, E. (1960). *Psychologie der menschlichen Welt.* Berlin: Springer.

Tatossian, A. (1979) *La phénoménologie des psychoses.* Paris: L'art du comprendre, 1997. An English translation has been provided by John Cutting and is available at: http://maudsleyphilosophygroup.org/resources/texts.html.

Tellenbach, H. (1956). Die Räumlichkeit der Melancholischen. *Nervenarzt* 27: 12 and 289.

Tellenbach, H. (1967). Zur Phänomenologie der Eifersucht. *Nervenarzt* 28: 133.

Tellenbach, H. (1968). *Geschmack und Atmosphäre: Medien menschlichen Elementarkontakts.* Salzburg: Muller.

Tellenbach, H. (1969). Zur Freilegung des melancholischen Typus im Rahmen einer kinetischen Typologie. In *Das depressive Syndrom*, eds. H. Hippius and H. Selbach. Munich: Urban and Schwarzenburg: 173–81.

Tellenbach, H. (1974). On the nature of jealousy. *Journal of Phenomenological Psychology* 4: 461–8.

Tellenbach, H. (1976). *Melancholie.* Berlin: Springer.

Tellenbach, R. (1975). Untersuchungen zur prämorbiden Persönlichkeit von Psychotikern, unter besonderer Berücksichtigung Manisch Depressiver. *Confinia Psychiatrica* 18: 1–15.

Vico, G. (1963). *De nostri temporis studiorum ratione, 1708.* Darmstadt: Wissenschaftliche Buchgesellsch.

Vico, G. (1966) [1924]. *La Scienza Nuova (1725/1744).* Berlin: de Gruyter.

Walker, C. (1988). Philosophical concepts and practice: the legacy of Karl Jaspers' psychopathology. *Current Opinion in Psychiatry* 1: 624–9.

Walker, C. (1993). Karl Jaspers as a Kantian psychopathologist. I. The philosophical origin of the concept of form and content. *History of Psychiatry* 4: 209–38.

Weber, M. (1904/2004). *The Methodology of the Social Sciences.* Jaipur, India: ABD Publishers.

Wiggins, O. P., Schwartz, M. A. (1997). Edmund Husserl's influence on Karl Jaspers's phenomenology. *Philosophy, Psychiatry, and Psychology* 4(1): 15–36.

Wittgenstein, L. (1969). *On Certainty*. Oxford: Blackwell.

Wittkoiver, E. D. and Hugel, R. (1969). Transkulturelle Aspekte des depressiven Syndroms. In *Das depressive Syndrom*, eds. H. Hippius and H. Selbach. Munich: Urban and Schwarzenberg.

World Health Organization (1992). *The ICD-10 Classification of Mental and Behavioural Disorders: Clinical Descriptions and Diagnostic Guidelines*. Geneva: World Health Organization Divion of Mental Health.

Wyrsch, J. (1940). Über die Psychopathologie einfacher Schizophrenien. *Monatsschrift für Psychiatrie und Neurologie* 102: 75–106.

Wyrsch, J. (1949). *Die Person des Schizophrenen*. Bern: Haupt.

Zahavi, D. (2003). *Husserl's Phenomenology*. Stanford, CA: Stanford University Press.

Zerssen, D. von, Koeller, D. M. and Rey, E. R. (1969). Objektivierende Untersuchungen zur prämorbiden Personlichkeit endogen Depressiver. In *Das depressive Syndrom*, eds. H. Hippius and H. Selbach. Munich: Urban and Schwarzenberg

Zerssen, D. von, Koeller, D. M. and Rey, E. R. (1970). Die prämorbide Personlichkeit von endogen Depressiven. *Confinia Psychiatrica* 13: 156.

Index

Printed in the United States
By Bookmasters